VICTORY OVER VESTIBULAR MIGRAINE

The ACTION Plan for Healing & Getting Your Life Back

Third Edition

Shin C. Beh, MD

ISBN-13: 9798661210616

Cover design by: Shin C. Beh, MD

Library of Congress Control Number: 2018675309

Printed in the United States of America

내 소중한 사랑 Yessie

Table of Contents

PREFACE

Vestibular migraine is the most common neurological cause of vertigo in adults, affecting almost 10 million Americans and causing significant economic impact and disability. Unfortunately, it is under-recognized and under-diagnosed. It has been estimated that only about 20% of sufferers are correctly diagnosed with vestibular migraine, leading to long delays in treatment.

I cannot begin to count how many patients have told me about losing years of their lives to vertigo, dizziness, brain fog, and migraine without being given any clear diagnosis or treatment. They are universally shocked and surprised when the diagnosis of vestibular migraine is made. How can it be migraine? How can migraine cause dizziness and vertigo? How come they don't have headaches? When I explain that it is a very treatable condition, shock turns to relief and hope; once we formulate a customized treatment plan, the healing journey begins and the vast majority of my patients return to normal lives. There is so much I have learned from helping them on their journeys toward healing. Because of the limited time I had with my patients in a clinical setting, I wished for a resource that could provide them with the knowledge they need.

I wanted a resource that would help my patients understand the disorder. I wanted a single, comprehensive reference that answered all their questions. I wanted a book that distilled the research on vestibular migraine into an easily understood, user-friendly format. I wanted a book that not only described the symptoms, but covered the treatments, supplements, and lifestyle changes needed. I wanted a book that discussed the potential impact of vestibular migraine on someone's job, school, family, and future. I wanted a comprehensive go-to reference for the holistic treatment of vestibular migraine.

I could not find anything that fulfilled these goals. Because the book I sought did not exist, I wrote *Victory Over Vestibular Migraine*. With it, I endeavor to share my knowledge, experience, and observations, as well as the lessons I have learned from my many, wonderful patients. I want to help you not only understand vestibular migraine, but also have an actionable, concise, and lucid plan on how to deal with it.

The **ACTION** plan comprehensively covers all aspects of vestibular migraine, and provides an all-encompassing treatment strategy:

A: *Alternative* drug-free therapies that can heal your vestibular migraine, including supplements, and exercises.

C: Life *Changes*. Identify your triggers and what life changes you need to make to fortify your brain against vestibular migraine. You will also learn about foods and vestibular migraine and how to design a diet to heal your brain.

T: *Therapeutic* options (preventive and rescue therapies) you can choose from. Learn about available preventive treatments as well as rescue treatments.

I: *Interictal* & Co-morbid Disorders. Understand what symptoms can occur during the attack-free and how to treat them. Learn about the relationship between hormones and vestibular migraine.

ON: *ONward!* Harness the power of your mind to heal your body, build a network of support, and plan for the future.

The information provided in this book is to educate and not provide any specific medical advice or to diagnose. Before starting any treatment or exercise, always consult your physician. The characters and names used in the stories and case studies are fictionalized but their stories are based on my patients' experiences and struggles. I have not been paid to endorse any of the products discussed in this book.

There is so much that we have learned about vestibular migraine and there is so much more to learn. To ensure this book remains an information-packed resource for people with vestibular migraine, the third edition was needed to keep abreast with new developments. Besides updates to available treatments, this edition delves further into the neuroscience of vestibular migraine, acupressure, the gut-brain axis, neuroplasticity, how thinking patterns affect those with this disorder, and the impact of COVID-19. For people living with vestibular migraine and their loved ones, I hope this book will be a guide to understanding this disorder and help you prepare for your journey to healing.

Shin C. Beh, MD, FAAN, FAHS

Chapter 1: The Invisible Illness

Nancy was at the pinnacle of her career as a corporate lawyer. She loved her job and her colleagues loved her. There was nothing more satisfying than sinking her teeth into a complex legal case, slowly dissecting it, and finally synthesizing a winning strategy for grateful clients.

One beautiful spring morning, it hit her like a bolt of lightning. A stomach-turning sensation that her world had flipped upside down, and like she was about to spin off the face of the earth. It felt like she was being sucked into a vortex, further and further down a bottomless pit. She lost her bearings, and fell off her rolling armchair onto the floor, grabbing onto the rug for dear life. Nauseous, sweating bullets, with a jackhammer pounding her skull, she finally managed to weakly call out. Her secretary screamed for help and called 911.

As Nancy waited for what seemed an eternity for emergency services, she thought she was going to die. Do I have a brain tumor? Did I burst an aneurysm? Did I have a stroke? What will happen to my kids? My husband?

When she finally arrived at the emergency department of a nearby hospital, she was whisked from test to test... EKG, blood tests, CT scans, MRIs... it was all a blur. Her head was still pounding. She still felt as though she were on the edge of Earth, about to be flung into the void of space.

An emergency physician appeared. "All your tests are negative. You're not having a heart attack, there is no stroke, there is nothing wrong with the blood vessels in your neck and head, ma'am."

"Then what's wrong with me? Why am I so dizzy?" she asked.

A shrug. "Sounds like vertigo. We're going to admit you to the hospital to keep an eye on you," came the reply.

She spent the night in the hospital. By morning, the awful spinning and falling sensations subsided and her head was no longer pounding. She felt queasy, discombobulated, just "not right". Another doctor popped in to see her, a neurologist. He basically repeated what the emergency physician had told her.

"Vertigo". Everything was normal. There was nothing wrong with her. She was going home. A prescription for meclizine, and a referral to a few doctors.

Following that fateful day, nothing was the same. Using a computer, reading, walking past the wide glass windows of her office, walking across the shiny floors in her building, getting in an elevator, driving over bridges, and even going to the grocery store made her dizzy and nauseous. It was constant and made her life hell. Every errand she took for granted was now a monumental task.

The worst thing was that her colleagues, friends, and some family members didn't, couldn't, or wouldn't understand.

"It can't be that bad. You look completely healthy!"

"But you LOOK pretty okay!"

"All the tests are normal. It's all in your head"

"I've been dizzy before. It can't be that bad."

"You look fine to me!"

While no one said it, their comments and expressions told Nancy that they thought she was making this all up. She could *hear* them think "hypochondriac".

Nancy sought help from many physicians to figure out why she was dizzy. She started with the obvious, her internist, who referred her to an otolaryngologist. The otolaryngologist ran a battery of tests and told her it was not her inner ear and told her to see a neurologist. The neurologist checked another MRI, performed an EEG to see if it were seizures, and did a nerve conduction test to see if it was neuropathy. Nothing. She began exploring other specialties.

Could it be hormonal? An endocrinologist said no.

Could it be her heart? A cardiologist said no.

Maybe an autoimmune disease? Not according to a rheumatologist.

How about a blood vessel problem or (God forbid) a brain tumor? A neurosurgeon reassured her it was not.

Perhaps some mysterious infection like Lyme disease? An infectious disease specialist told her the tests did not reveal any infection.

TMJ problems, maybe? An oral and maxillofacial surgeon took scans of her jaw and felt it was highly unlikely that her symptoms were due to TMJ dysfunction.

So, what in the world was going on? How could she be fine one day, suffer from the most awful vertigo ever, and now be constantly dizzy with attacks of vertigo practically every week? She lost faith in mainstream medicine and began seeking out alternative medicine.

These practitioners were different. They always told her they knew exactly what was wrong and promised cures. One said her cerebellum had escaped and gave her a cocktail of expensive intravenous vitamins. Another said it was a chronic black mold allergy and told her to consume a mixture of herbs, whilst brushing her body every night with what appeared to be a kabuki make-up brush. One blamed chronic Lyme disease, and she had to receive intravenous antibiotics (not covered by insurance, of course), and bounce on a trampoline to "release the toxins". Yet another said her sacrum was misaligned and promised massages would restore it to its rightful place. The final straw came when one literally threw ice at her body with the assurance of 100% relief.

Nothing worked. She had quit her job and her husband cared for her. Gnawing guilt grew inside her. She felt like a burden, an inconvenience, a bad wife, a failed mother.

Her long journey led to me, but she was clearly exhausted and almost defeated. I went through all her symptoms, her history, and all the tests that were performed. I finally diagnosed her with vestibular migraine. She was shocked. Migraine? But isn't migraine a headache?

Unfortunately, Nancy's experience is not uncommon in vestibular migraine sufferers. Vestibular migraine is an *invisible illness*. On the surface, everything looks calm and "normal", but beneath, vestibular migraine stirs like a serpent, ready to strike at any time with the violence of a tornado.

It does not care about your job.

It does not care about your friends.

It does not care about your family.

It does not care about your life.

A pervasive dizziness hangs like a dark cloud between attacks of ferocious vertigo constantly reminding you of that lurking serpent. The fear of that serpent is paralyzing – what if it strikes while you are driving? Or when you are in public? Or when there is no one around to help you?

It shames you for missing your child's recital.

It haunts you with the guilt that you have failed as a spouse.

It condemns you for being an inconvenience, or worse, a burden to others.

Obvious illnesses like cough, rash, or a broken leg are observable to onlookers. On the other hand, conditions that cause pain, vertigo, dizziness, and fatigue are invisible illnesses – they rob you of your well-being, but you appear "fine" to outsiders. Those suffering from vertigo and dizziness cannot perform tasks that others take for granted but look "fine". Many are unable to perform their jobs, but look "healthy". Many cannot engage in family functions, and withdraw from social engagements, but look "normal".

Unfortunately, human nature compels outsiders to judge by what they can see, demeaning those who appear "disabled" but who are completely capable, and frustrating those who appear "able" but are not. For example, they automatically assume a person in a wheelchair is pitifully incapable, even though the person may be independent and able to manage quite well. Likewise, they fail to understand how someone with vestibular migraine who "looks fine" can suffer from debilitating dizziness when performing seemingly simple tasks like scrolling through multiple Excel spreadsheets, flipping back and forth from three computer screens, playing with children, or driving in heavy traffic.

Complicating matters, the impact of such invisible disabilities varies from person to person. A headache to a person without chronic migraine is often mild and more of a nuisance, but a headache to a chronic migraine sufferer (who has central pain sensitization) can be terribly debilitating. Similarly, almost everyone has experienced brief and often mild dizziness (like getting up too fast or after spinning around as a child), but disorders like vestibular migraine can cause horrible vertigo and dizziness that wreak havoc on a person's job and family life. Even within vestibular migraine itself, different people may be afflicted by its symptoms to different degrees. To one, it may cause a bothersome attack or two per year. To another, vestibular migraine may result in almost daily vertigo attacks, turning their lives upside down and bringing misery in its wake. Some may have constant light and sound sensitivity, some describe interminable nausea and brain fog, while some are perfectly well between attacks.

I admit that the medical profession has failed those with chronic invisible illnesses, especially vestibular migraine. The vague, subjective symptoms of dizziness and vertigo, brain fog, blurry vision, light intolerance, sound sensitivity, and motion sickness, are difficult to communicate and express. In busy practices, such subjective symptoms are often dismissed or ignored, as long as life-threatening diseases like stroke, epilepsy, and heart disease are ruled out.

Invisible illnesses often do not have any clear diagnostic tests, not because there is nothing wrong with the sufferer, but because medical science has not yet come up with an appropriate test for the condition, and thus, the diagnosis relies on recognizing a particular pattern of symptoms. Before the 1970s, multiple sclerosis (MS) could only be definitively diagnosed at autopsy; MS is now easily diagnosed with MRIs. Early in the COVID-19 pandemic, vast numbers of people fell sick but reliable tests for SARS-CoV-2 were severely lacking and healthcare professionals had to rely on clinical symptoms and signs (e.g., loss of smell, shortness of breath, fever, cough, or pneumonia) to diagnose COVID-19.

Vestibular migraine is a condition that is diagnosed clinically (i.e., based on a patient's symptoms and history) and not with any particular test. In fact, traditional tests for vestibular disorders are performed to rule out other conditions as part of the evaluation, and as such, are often normal or only show non-specific abnormalities. This unfortunately results in a misguided idea: "If all the tests are normal, you must be normal". The lack of a specific test that can prove a person has vestibular migraine is frustrating for patients, confusing for healthcare providers and employers, and allows rapacious insurance companies to deny disability claims. The misguided idea that vestibular migraine is a "diagnosis of exclusion" creates the false belief that vestibular migraine is a trashcan diagnosis that one is put in once every other diagnosis is excluded. Vestibular migraine is *not* a diagnosis of exclusion; it has a unique set of symptoms and clinical history.

As an invisible illness becomes chronic, initial goodwill and sympathy ferment into nagging doubt and impatience, and soon, accusations of being a hypochondriac grow louder. Furthermore, because mood disorders like anxiety and depression often co-exist with almost all vestibular disorders, physicians are quick to ascribe all your symptoms to purely psychiatric problems.

Medical trauma is defined as the psychological response to a negative or traumatic experience, involving illness, pain, injury, procedures, and/or distressing or dismissive medical care. For example, medical trauma can emerge after intensive care unit (ICU) stays, medical emergencies (e.g., heart attacks, strokes), cancer treatment, birth, childhood health complications, or surgery. In fact, such traumatic experiences can, and often, trigger vestibular migraine. For many with vestibular migraine, there is a more insidious form of medical trauma arising from dealing with chronic, medically unexplained symptoms and dismissive medical professionals. It is driven by the sense of powerlessness from unpredictable, unexplained symptoms, and the feeling of being abandoned by the healthcare system. "Doctors look at me as if I'm crazy!" is a common (and unfortunate) refrain. I can often tell who has been exposed to these experiences when they use prefaces like "Now, please don't think I'm crazy", or "I know this sounds crazy, but..." before describing their symptoms. Because it is often insidious and ongoing, this form of medical trauma is often missed by the sufferer, just like the proverbial frog slowly boiling to death.

Women are at much higher risk of this form of medical trauma because suspicions about women's health have pervaded human culture for millennia. Ancient Egyptians blamed many symptoms in women to a "wandering uterus" that ventured out of the pelvis to cause mischief. To return the uterus to its rightful abode, Egyptian physicians placed pleasant-smelling herbs in patients' vulvas to entice it or gave them disgusting-smelling substances to chase the uterus back. The Greeks adopted this view, and the word *hysteria* originates from the Greek word for uterus, *hystera*. They believed that the uterus was afflicted by bad humors and became sad (uterine melancholy) due to a lack of orgasms and children. Similar views spread to the Romans, and later to the Byzantines, the Middle East, and Andalusia. It made its way back to Europe in the Middle Ages, and with the backdrop of religious superstition, hysterical women were considered witches, interrogated, tortured, and executed.

Things began to change in the 16th century when French physician Charles Le Pois hypothesized that hysteria was neurological, not gynecological. The father of neurology, Jean-Martin Charcot (1825-1893) ardently supported this idea and used hypnosis to treat hysteria. While we have come a long way, and the term hysteria is no longer used in medicine, the hardwired tendency to attribute any unexplained symptom, particularly in women, to a psychiatric disorder continues. Early in my training, I too was subject to this close-mindedness – anything medically unexplained must be psychiatric, according to my simplistic reasoning. When I opened my mind to the diverse complexity of symptoms that affected patients with neurological disorders, I realized that I had so much to learn from my patients.

In the 1983 movie *Yentl*, Barbra Streisand plays a young Jewish woman who is compelled to masquerade as a man to receive an education. Yentl syndrome (coined by Dr. Bernadine Healy in 1991) describes how women are misdiagnosed and dismissed by healthcare providers because their symptoms or disease do not conform with those of men. The failure to appreciate the differences in how diseases affect women has real-world consequences. Life-threatening conditions like heart attacks are often missed in women because the symptoms are dissimilar from men. Men tend to experience chest pain and left arm pain (which we always associate with heart attacks) but women may experience difficulty breathing, nausea, fatigue, and abdominal pain. Such gender differences also impact the immune system; for example, men have a higher risk of mortality in acute COVID-19 infection but women are at higher risk of long COVID.

Additionally, diseases like vestibular migraine and fibromyalgia, which affect women much more than men often receive much less attention and research dollars. Yentl syndrome is a huge problem in vestibular disorders because they predominantly affect women. Not only does the medical establishment lack a clear understanding of the symptoms and impact of vestibular disorders, Yentl syndrome undermines the veracity of women's symptoms. Instead of being believed, their symptoms are labeled as "psychosomatic" or "emotional". Many women with vestibular migraine are told, "There's nothing wrong with you" or "It's all in your head'. I'm not saying the same situation does not affect men with vestibular disorders; it definitely does, and many men with dizziness and vertigo are often told they are just "anxious". However, the burden disproportionately affects women because of the female preponderance of these disorders and this cultural bias.

People with a history of PTSD, anxiety, and depression are more vulnerable to medical trauma. In addition, higher levels of stress from other sources augment the risk for medical trauma. In vestibular migraine, the stress of having to cope with the impact on one's job and personal life can increase the chances of medical trauma from dismissive care. Many studies confirm that anxiety and depression are common in vestibular migraine and very often amplify the impact of the disease. Anxiety commonly afflicts people with vestibular disorders. It causes hypervigilance, heightening one's awareness of dizziness and elevating one's perception of the severity of the dizziness, which in turn exacerbates the anxiety. This results in a vicious feed-forward cycle of ever-increasing dizziness and anxiety. Depression is also very common in vestibular migraine. The longer the disease lasts, the more severe its symptoms, and the greater the depression.

Chapter 2: What's in a Name?

Diagnosis is not the end, but the beginning of practice
Dr. Martin H. Fischer

The first step in conquering vestibular migraine is getting the right diagnosis. Vestibular migraine is a great mimicker, often appearing like and co-existing with many other illnesses. One study [Rocha, 2023] showed that only 3.8% of patients with acute vertigo who see non-neurotologists are correctly diagnosed with vestibular migraine. The diagnoses my patients receive before they are finally diagnosed with vestibular migraine include Meniere's disease, perilymph fistula, vestibular neuritis, benign paroxysmal positional vertigo, ear infections, allergies, sinus problems, deviated septum, endolymphatic hydrops, Eustachian tube dysfunction, multiple sclerosis, mini-stroke, heart problems, epilepsy, anxiety, depression, Chiari malformation, pseudotumor cerebri, and, of course, the dreaded diagnosis - cancer.

Getting the right diagnosis is essential. Firstly, it eliminates doubt and the fear of the unknown. The lack of any clear diagnosis is extremely stressful – the mind is left to wonder about catastrophic scenarios: Will I be in a wheelchair? Will I have a stroke? Will I lose my job? Who will take care of my family? Will I end up in a nursing home? Will my family be able to care of me? Will I die from this? Getting the correct diagnosis removes all these doubts and distractions, allowing the mind to focus on the next steps in conquering vestibular migraine.

Secondly, the right diagnosis ends the incessant search for answers and a cure. Many vestibular migraine patients end up seeing multiple specialists like cardiologists, otolaryngologists, ophthalmologists, optometrists, endocrinologists, neurologists, rheumatologists, neurosurgeons, and orthodontists. Getting the right diagnosis will save precious time and resources. The correct diagnosis will also save you from unnecessary and potentially dangerous tests or treatments. I have seen vestibular migraine patients who went deaf after undergoing inner ear surgery for Meniere's disease. It also protects you from the unscrupulous vultures waiting to prey on your desperation and suffering by peddling nonsensical, *wu wu* cures like wands that shoot red laser lights, magnetic hats, and magical apps that make your heart beat in sync with the universe (yes, these exist!).

Thirdly, it validates your experience. Not only have you suffered from symptoms of vestibular migraine, but you have also endured the barbs of doubt and suspicions of many, including physicians, bosses, colleagues, and even family members. Some may have even accused you, directly or indirectly, of being a hypochondriac, making it all up, or being crazy. Getting the correct diagnosis validates your suffering, your pain, and your journey – and proves the doubters wrong. It confirms that you are not a crazy hypochondriac. It will also help you realize that you are not alone in this; there are many people with vestibular migraine!

Tis but thy name is mine enemy;
What's Montague? It is not hand nor foot,
Nor arm, nor face, nor any other part.
What's in a name? That which we call a rose,
By any other name would smell as sweet
William Shakespeare, Romeo & Juliet, Act II Scene II

Unlike Juliet, names and jargon are important in medicine. To guide me to the correct diagnosis, I need to understand what vestibular symptoms you experience. Terms like "vertigo", "dizziness" and "giddiness" are common, but mean different things to different people. To me, giddiness and dizziness can be used interchangeably, and according to the International Classification of Diseases (the source of disease codes used by insurance companies), "Dizziness and Giddiness" is coded as a diagnosis. One of my patients was upset at that diagnosis since to her, "giddy" referred to silly giggling girls. Thankfully, she calmed down after I explained that it was the diagnostic code that I had no control over.

Another problem is that the term "vertigo" has been misused by many, including healthcare professionals. Any vestibular symptom is labeled as "vertigo". Furthermore, almost all healthcare professionals are trained to ask "Is the room spinning?" when a patient complains of dizziness or any vestibular symptom. Most answer "yes" and from then on, they receive a diagnosis of "vertigo" and every physician they see assumes the person experiences spinning sensations.

I always ask my patients to describe what they feel. There is a multitude of vestibular symptoms, and many people experience more than one. To make the right diagnosis, I need to understand what someone's vestibular symptoms feel like.

Incomprehensible jargon is the hallmark of a profession.
Kingman Brewster, Jr.

To help you understand how to describe your vestibular symptoms, I will define them based on the definitions set by the International Barany Society, an organization of scientists, neurologists, and otolaryngologists dedicated to advancing collaborative research in vestibular disorders.

Vertigo

Vertigo is defined as the illusion of motion, either of self, or the environment. For example, if you feel that you are spinning, or if your world is spinning around you, you have vertigo. However, vertigo does not only mean "spinning". It encompasses a variety of sensations including tumbling, falling through space, rocking, swaying, bobbing, swimming, shimmering, floating, ground-shifting, and jolting. The most evocative description I've heard is 'it feels like the devil has grabbed me by the arms and is throwing me around".

Vertigo can be spontaneous or triggered. Spontaneous vertigo occurs without any clear precipitating factor (not to be confused with a migraine trigger). Triggered vertigo occurs in relation to a specific precipitating event. For example, head motion-induced vertigo is vertigo that occurs during head movement. Positional vertigo is vertigo that occurs once the head assumes the offending head position (not during head movement). Visually-induced vertigo is vertigo that is provoked by complex, busy, distorted, or moving visual stimuli.

Dizziness

Dizziness is defined as non-specific disorientation without the illusion of motion. It is a very broad term that encompasses sensations like disorientation, discombobulation, lightheadedness, or feeling "tipsy". It can be rather vague e.g., feeling like one is not wearing the right pair of glasses, feeling "off" or feeling as if "things are not right". Some describe feeling like their brains are vibrating, wobbling, or jiggling like jelly.

Similar to vertigo, dizziness can be spontaneous or triggered. Spontaneous dizziness occurs without a clear provoking factor, while triggered dizziness occurs in relation to a specific precipitating event.

Pre-Syncope/Syncope

Pre-syncope is the medical term for feeling faintness (as if one may blackout), and syncope refers to fainting. Although pre-syncope and syncope may occur if vertigo is severe enough, these symptoms do not typically indicate a vestibular disorder. Many people with vestibular migraine describe feeling as though they may pass out, but never actually faint.

Instead, presyncope/syncope usually suggests a cardiovascular cause, especially if associated with chest discomfort, chest pain, chest pressure, difficulty breathing (or shortness of breath), or palpitations.

Presyncope or syncope can also be due to low blood pressure, especially if an antihypertensive medication was just started or increased in dose. These can be signs of a serious, potentially life-threatening, cardiovascular disorder, and should be addressed with an internist or cardiologist.

Postural Symptoms

Postural symptoms are defined as balance symptoms related to maintaining an upright posture. These are symptoms that usually occur when a patient stands, walks, or sometimes tries to sit upright.

Unsteadiness is a term that encompasses symptoms like instability, "can't walk a straight line, "walking like a drunk", and disequilibrium. It is essentially a feeling of imbalance when standing or walking.

Directional pulsion refers to a tendency to fall or veer in a particular direction, or sometimes a feeling that a force is pushing or pulling oneself. For example, a person may experience feeling like he/she is being pulled backward, forward, rightward, or leftward. It may be one specific direction (e.g., always feeling like one is veering to the right) or non-specific (i.e., experiencing a pulling sensation when walking that can vary in direction).

Balance-related fall or *near fall* refers to a fall or an imminent fall related to particularly severe vestibular symptoms. Near falls are not always reported since patients and physicians focus on actual falls. It is important to pay attention to near falls because they increase the risk of an actual fall. Intervening before actual falls occur can prevent severe injury.

Visual-Vestibular Symptoms

This refers to visual symptoms that are caused by vestibular disease, or from a disturbance in the interaction between the visual and vestibular systems. Symptoms that fall under this category include:

Oscillopsia is a Greek-Latin combination word that means "swinging vision". This is a perception of a jerky back-and-forth movement of the visual environment. This symptom is usually a manifestation of nystagmus.

Nystagmus is a condition where the eyes make rhythmic, repetitive, involuntary movements; it is a sign of a vestibular disorder, and its pattern can often provide crucial clues about which part of the vestibular system is affected. Nystagmus is the movements of the eyes observed by others; oscillopsia is the bouncing vision experienced by the patient.

Visual lag is the sensation that the eyes don't precisely follow the movements of the head. It can be understood as a sensation that the visual environment takes a tad longer to catch up with a head movement. This is an odd sensation that patients often hesitate before describing it to me, worried that I would think them crazy, but once I indicate that I understand it, they heave a sigh of relief.

Movement-induced blur is a momentary disturbance in visual acuity during or just after head movement. The vestibular system is responsible for ensuring crisp, sharp vision by stabilizing the eyes and keeping the image of a visual target right on a tiny area of the eye called the fovea, which has the densest collection of cones (an eye cell that detects color). If the image slips from the fovea, it becomes blurry. Disorders of the vestibular system impair this ability and cause transient blurring of vision with head movements.

Diagnosis: "Vertigo"

Patients are often told that they have "vertigo" when they seek medical attention, and everything stops there as if vertigo were a diagnosis. Vertigo is *not* a diagnosis. Vertigo is a symptom, just like a swollen arm. If your arm was swollen, you wouldn't be satisfied if a physician diagnosed "arm swelling" – you will want to know why it was swollen so it can be fixed! Similarly, figuring out why a person has vertigo or dizziness is important – the right diagnosis leads to the right treatment, which in turn, leads to proper control of vertigo.

Details make perfection, and perfection is not a detail.

Leonardo da Vinci

Specialists like myself rely on a detailed history to make the right diagnosis. We need as much information as possible. It is not enough to just tell me you are dizzy, or that you have vertigo. Understanding the temporal evolution, accompanying symptoms, triggers, previous tests, and your medical and family history can provide crucial clues to the diagnosis. What details should you pay attention to? Here is a list of questions, and symptoms that you should take note of:

1. What vestibular symptoms do you experience? Describe them in detail based on the points outlined in this chapter.

2. Do you have more than one vestibular symptom? If so, describe them.

3. When did the vestibular symptom(s) start?

4. The temporal profile of the vestibular symptom(s):

a. Acute (within days): if this is the first time you suffered the vestibular symptom(s), how long has the symptom(s) been going on?

b. Chronic, episodic: "spells" or "attacks" that occur repeatedly over a course of time. What is the average duration of each episode (minutes, hours, days)? It can feel like an eternity when you're spinning but try to estimate the duration as accurately as possible. This will ensure an accurate diagnosis.

c. Chronic, constant (weeks to months or years): the vestibular symptoms have not abated since they began.

5. Accompanying symptoms: take note of symptoms that accompany the vestibular symptoms. Examples include ear pressure (fullness), tinnitus, muffled or loss of hearing, headache (describe the quality, location, aggravating factors, relieving factors), light sensitivity, sound sensitivity, difficulty thinking, vision changes, nausea, vomiting, sensory changes (numbness, tingling), motor changes (muscle weakness), and difficulty speaking.

6. Triggers: Are the vestibular symptoms triggered or do they occur without warning? Is there a specific head position or

movement? Is it triggered by pressure maneuvers, like coughing, sneezing, bearing down, and lifting heavy objects? How about migraine triggers?

7. Tests performed: if you have had any tests (e.g., CT, MRI, labs, hearing tests), have the reports ready. For CTs and MRIs, keep a copy of the CD (radiology centers often provide these but be sure to ask). Routine blood tests (e.g., complete blood count, metabolic panel) are usually not very useful.

8. Medications tried: It is essential to have a list of medications that have been tried, including responses (side effects, any improvement or lack thereof). It will save a lot of time. I won't start a medication you've failed or could not tolerate.

9. Medical History: a list of your medical problems (e.g., hypertension, asthma).

10. Family History: are there diseases that run in your family? A family history of neurological problems, or diseases that cause vertigo, dizziness, and imbalance is of particular interest to me.

Chapter 3: What Is Vestibular Migraine?

Who in the world am I?
Ah. That's the great puzzle.
Lewis Carroll, Alice's Adventures in Wonderland

What is Migraine?

Migraine affects about 15% of the population and is the second most common cause of disability among working-age adults in the world, after back pain. Migraine affects women about 3 times more frequently than men. Unfortunately, the prevalence of migraine is likely higher because it is often undiagnosed. Many people go on with life believing that they have "sinus headaches" when they actually suffer from migraine.

According to the International Classification of Headache Disorders, a person can be diagnosed with migraine after experiencing at least 5 attacks of unprovoked headache lasting 4 to 72 hours, severe enough to impair or restrict routine daily activity, accompanied by nausea or light/sound sensitivity. Now, this is the formal way of *diagnosing* migraine, but it doesn't really tell us *what* migraine is. We will get into this more later.

The term migraine is derived from the Greek word *hemicrania* which means "disease affecting half the skull". Humans have suffered from migraine since the beginning of our species, and the earliest description of migraine is contained in the oldest medical manuscript in the world, the Ebers Papyrus of Egypt. It blames the disorder on demons and recalls a remedy from even older sources dating back to about 3000 years B.C. that prescribes binding a clay crocodile figurine to the head of a patient. While we have come a long way since the days of blaming migraine on demons, we still have so much to learn about migraine. The biggest misconception that lingers is that migraine is only a headache or just a type of headache.

A migraine attack can be divided into four phases: premonitory, aura, attack, and postdrome. The premonitory phase can begin up to 3 days prior to the headache. The aura is characterized by transient neurological changes that last from 5 to 60 minutes, commonly manifesting as visual phenomena. The attack or headache phase usually lasts 4 to 72 hours, and is typically characterized by a one-sided throbbing headache that is aggravated by routine activity and can be accompanied by nausea, vomiting, light sensitivity, sound sensitivity, and smell sensitivity. The headache phase is usually debilitating enough that a person will need to lie down to rest. The postdrome of a migraine involves the "after-shocks" of the migraine attack; people usually experience lethargy, trouble concentrating, depressed mood, and in rare cases, euphoria.

Migraine is not *just* a headache.

The most common misconception is that migraine equals headache. Migraine is much more than a headache. While headaches are a common symptom of migraine, migraine can affect a person in many other ways. The best definition of migraine is "a complex neurologic disorder arising from metabolic and biochemical derangements that affects multiple brain regions that control sensory, autonomic, emotional, cognitive, and even motor, function". As such, people with migraine can experience symptoms that span across divergent neurological domains.

Childhood Migraine Syndromes

These conditions are migraine variants that usually occur in children. Children who suffer from these conditions are at higher risk of developing migraine later in life. Childhood migraine syndromes support the concept of migraine being a genetic disorder that manifests differently across a person's life; its permutations depend on the brain's maturity, and hormonal influences. Most children with these conditions have a close family member with migraine.

Infantile Colic

Colic is now believed to be a migraine variant that manifests in infants. A study showed that over 70% of children (6 to 18 years old) with migraine had a history of colic [Romanello, 2013]. In fact, infantile colic is associated with a threefold increase in the risk of developing migraine later in life [Sillanpaa, 2015]. Genetic predisposition underlies infantile colic. Mothers (not fathers) with migraine are twice as likely to have a baby with colic [Gelfand, 2012; Gelfand, 2019]. However, fathers with depression or anxiety are about twice as likely to have a child with colic [Gelfand, 2019]. These fascinating observations underscore the complex role genes play in migraine.

Benign paroxysmal torticollis

Benign paroxysmal torticollis is an uncommon neurological disorder that affects infants (usually between 2 to 8 months old). It can occur in early childhood, but not beyond 5 years of age. It causes episodes of head and sometimes trunk tilting and may be accompanied by vomiting, unsteadiness (in those who can walk), pallor, upward eye deviation, irritability, and nystagmus. The episodes can last from a few minutes to a few days and may occur every few weeks or months.

Benign paroxysmal vertigo of childhood

In this condition, a child (usually between 2 to 7 years of age) experiences episodes of vertigo lasting minutes. These episodes occur suddenly and resolve on their own. The child is often terrified during the episode. Thankfully, benign paroxysmal vertigo of childhood usually stops about 18 months after the onset.

Abdominal Migraine

This condition is characterized by repeated attacks of abdominal pain accompanied by symptoms like pallor, light sensitivity, sound sensitivity, headache, nausea, or vomiting. A poorly localized dull pain or soreness is usually described in the central abdominal region. The episodes last between 1 to 72 hours, and sufferers are asymptomatic between attacks.

Abdominal migraine usually occurs in children between 3 to 10 years of age, with a peak age of 7. However, adults also may be affected. Triggers are similar to those for migraine, including bright lights, sleep deprivation, and stress. Interestingly, eating high-fiber cereal before bed ("breakfast at bedtime") prevents attacks that occur upon awakening, suggesting a possible role of diminished blood glucose levels as a trigger. Before making the diagnosis of abdominal migraine, a gastrointestinal evaluation is important to exclude other causes of abdominal pain, like appendicitis or gastroenteritis.

Cyclic vomiting syndrome

This is commonly seen in children between the ages of 3 and 7, but may also occur in adults. It is characterized by episodes of vomiting lasting hours to several days. The frequency of vomiting can range from once every 2 hours to 10-20 times per hour. Vomiting and retching can be severe enough that bile and stomach acid are regurgitated, and some people become dehydrated to the point of requiring intravenous fluids.

Some people experience a prodrome, or warning, which may consist of fatigue, nausea, pallor, sweating, diarrhea, flushing, anxiety, appetite loss, irritability, thirst, insomnia, shivering, abdominal pain, or muscle pain. During attacks, migraine symptoms like light and sound sensitivity may occur. Some experience intense thirst and drink so much water it makes them vomit. Interestingly, hot baths or showers temporarily relieve the vomiting. The episodes are stereotypical (the symptoms follow a set pattern) and can be provoked by typical migraine triggers.

The episodes can be separated by a week to a month in children, or several months in adults. Most children are asymptomatic between attacks, but adults may suffer from nausea and abdominal discomfort. The episodes are, of course, extremely unpleasant and distressful; many sufferers live in fear of the next attack. In severe cases, the episodes become so frequent that nausea and vomiting are almost constant. Sufferers can often go undiagnosed for a long time because awareness of this condition is lacking.

Many patients undergo repeated gastrointestinal evaluations, which are almost always unremarkable. Cyclic vomiting syndrome can have a significant impact on school and work, and unsurprisingly, is associated with a high prevalence of anxiety and depression.

What is Vestibular Migraine?

The most basic definition of vestibular migraine is a type of migraine that predominantly manifests with vertigo and dizziness. While headaches may occur with vestibular migraine, headaches are not the most significant feature. Instead, vertigo and dizziness are the main, and most disabling, symptoms of the disorder.

Vestibular migraine is not just migraine headache plus vertigo/dizziness. It is a distinct entity from migraine with several unique characteristics. It is less common than migraine (by the most conservative estimates), affecting about 3% of the adult population, making it the most common neurologic cause of vertigo among adults. The female predominance of vestibular migraine is also much higher than migraine headache, with studies reporting almost six times more female than male sufferers. Furthermore, vestibular migraine tends to affect an older age group. While migraine afflicts those in their late teens to the early 30s, vestibular migraine usually occurs in the late 30s to mid-40s. The reason for this difference is unknown but is likely hormonal and/or epigenetic. Most vestibular migraine sufferers tend to suffer from migraine headaches early in life, but as they go through menopause, the headaches improve (or even disappear) but vertigo and dizziness begin to manifest. We will discuss how the diagnosis of vestibular migraine is made in Chapter 4.

What Causes Vestibular Migraine?

Why me, Lord? Don't answer that!

Charles M. Schulz

I am often asked "Why did I get vestibular migraine?" and "What did I do that caused me to have vestibular migraine?". It is not your fault that you have vestibular migraine. There was nothing you could have done to avoid getting it. The precise causes of migraine and vestibular migraine remain elusive but it is believed that a confluence of several different factors. The word *pathophysiology* refers to the dysfunctional physiological processes that underlie a specific illness. In this section, we will discuss the pathophysiological underpinnings of vestibular migraine to help you understand what causes this condition.

Migraine brains are different from non-migraine brains. There are two systems in the brain – the excitatory system (that increases the activity of nerve cells), and the inhibitory system (which calms and reduces the activity of nerve cells). Migraine brains are wired to favor the excitatory system. It is like the dial for migraine brains is turned on "high" by default. They inherently have a heightened sensitivity to many sensory stimuli. For example, many people with migraine describe a history of childhood motion sickness, long before they develop any symptoms of either disorder. Furthermore, many people with either disorder also note that they have been more sensitive to sound, light, and/or strong odors from an early age. The migraine brain is essentially a "hot brain" – one that is more excitable and as such, more sensitive to various sensory stimuli, and more prone to migraine attacks.

Genetic predisposition is partly responsible for migraine and vestibular migraine. That is why there is typically a family history of migraine in sufferers. Highlighting the relationship between migraine and vertigo, as well as the complexity of the role of genetics, is the gene responsible for the voltage-gated calcium channel (CACNA1A) on chromosome 19. A specific mutation of this gene causes familial hemiplegic migraine (a form of migraine that causes temporary stroke-like paralysis). Another mutation can cause episodic ataxia type 2 (a rare condition characterized by attacks of vertigo, nystagmus, and imbalance), and fascinatingly, a different mutation results in a neurodegenerative condition called spinocerebellar ataxia type 6 (resulting in slowly progressive loss of balance). However, single-gene mutations causing migraine and vertigo are rare. There are many genes (over 30 at the time of this writing) suspected to cause migraine, and vestibular migraine, but the exact role and interactions between these genes remain a mystery at this time.

The genetic makeup of an individual determines his or her vulnerability to migraine attacks. The British naval vessel, HMS Bounty, left England in 1787 to set sail for Tahiti. During a long layover in Tahiti, the British crew developed relationships with local Polynesian women. On the journey from Tahiti to the West Indies, some of the crew finally had enough of Captain William Bligh's harsh command, mutinied, and sent the captain and his loyalists adrift. The saga, including how Captain Bligh survived and how HMS Pandora pursued the mutineers has been portrayed in two major films, Mutiny on the Bounty (1962), and The Bounty (1984).

Of more interest to migraine research was a group of 11 British mutineers and six Polynesian women who settled on Pitcairn Island in the South Pacific, and built a small community that moved to Norfolk Island when Pitcairn Island became too small for the population. The current population of Norfolk Island is descended from that original group of settlers. The incidence of migraine among people on Norfolk Island is twice as high as that of the usual prevalence among Caucasians. Genetic studies have revealed several genetic traits that predispose the population to migraine, including genes involved in serotonin metabolism [Cox, 2013].

However, genes are not the whole story. Many other factors conspire to cause migraine. Stress and trauma play a huge role in migraine. Generational stress is a new, fascinating area of study that explores how the effects of trauma can be transmitted through the generations. The children of people who survived the

Holocaust display high levels of behavioral disturbances like anxiety, guilt nightmares, and trouble with interpersonal functioning. Children of parents with PTSD have a higher chance of developing PTSD. While it is tempting to attribute this to growing up with traumatized parents, the roots of intergenerational trauma go beyond that. The babies of stressed mother rats have brains with fewer corticosteroid receptors; they are less able to inhibit the body's stress reaction, leading to higher and longer responses to stressors. This may explain why children of pregnant women who lived through the Dutch famine of World War II had a higher risk of obesity and diabetes [Yehuda, 2018]. Blunted corticosteroid responses are also found in the children of women with PTSD and women who were abused as children [Yehuda, 2018].

Childhood trauma also plays an important role in migraine. Lab rats are more sensitive to pain if they are traumatized at a very young age by removing them from their mothers. Childhood trauma (including physical, sexual, and emotional abuse) increases the risk of developing migraine and other pain disorders. In fact, many with a history of childhood abuse have a much higher risk of frequent and disabling headaches, as well as chronic migraine. Childhood stress alters gene expression in the hypothalamic-pituitary-adrenal (HPA) axis, serotonin production, estrogen receptors, and neuroplastic pathways, resulting in long-term dysfunction in these systems. In other words, early traumatic experiences set the physiological stage for how the brain and body respond to stress for the remainder of the lifespan, making it more vulnerable to the effects of stress, and increasing the risk of depression, anxiety, and migraine. A new frontier in medicine, the gut-brain axis, gives us another intriguing window into how generational, maternal or childhood trauma causes disease states by altering the gut microbiome (see Chapter 13).

Acute stress often precedes the onset of vestibular migraine. Many of my patients experience their first vestibular migraine attack during periods of unusually high stress. Stress changes the brain's activity, putting it in a hyper-excitable state (the flight or fight response) by ramping up the levels of excitatory neurotransmitters, and diminishing the levels of inhibitory neurotransmitters. The already hyperexcitable hot migraine brain is more prone to the effects of stress. Chronic stress leads to permanent structural changes in the brain, particularly in regions responsible for the perception of pain and vertigo, lowering the threshold for attacks even further.

Depression also plays an important role in migraine genesis. There is an interesting chicken-egg relationship between depression, and migraine. People with depression are at higher risk of migraine, and people with migraine have an increased incidence of depression. Both disorders are associated with changes in similar regions of the brain, and similar biochemical derangements (e.g., low serotonin, low vitamin D). This association also likely explains why antidepressants can be an effective migraine preventive.

Suboptimal vitamin and nutrient levels play an important part in migraine development. A lesson about the importance of nutrition in neurologic disease is found in the story of vitamin D and multiple sclerosis (MS), an autoimmune condition that causes immune cells to strip the brain and spinal cord of myelin (the substance that insulates nerves). People who live farther away from the Equator, where the levels of sunlight are lower (our skin uses sunlight to synthesize vitamin D) suffer from a higher incidence of MS. A Veterans' Affairs system study found a clear relationship between low vitamin D levels and the risk of developing MS later in life. A fascinating study of Ashkenazi Jewish children who migrated from Europe to Israel showed that those who moved to Israel (with its sunny Mediterranean weather) before puberty have a risk for MS similar to people who grew up in Israel. However, children who moved to Israel after puberty have a higher risk of developing MS, closely approximating the risk in Europeans. This study proved that a vitamin deficiency at a crucial point in life can elevate the risk of developing certain diseases. We know that people with migraine have lower vitamin D, riboflavin, coenzyme-Q10, and magnesium levels. Could low vitamin levels at a crucial age in life (perhaps before puberty) predict who will go on to develop migraine? Could suboptimal vitamin or nutrient levels during periods of stress predict who will go on to migraine? This is an exciting area for migraine research.

Hormonal changes play a very important role in migraine and most likely play an important role in its genesis. Migraine headaches are uncommon in children; instead, they may have conditions called childhood migraine variants, which are precursors of migraine. After puberty, the incidence of migraine headaches increases in girls but decreases in boys. Around the time of menopause, migraine headaches often improve or disappear, but vertigo and dizziness become the dominant migraine manifestations in some.

The hormonal changes during the menstrual cycle are a well-known migraine trigger. Many women experience more migraine attacks, increased motion sickness, and vertigo episodes around the time of menses. Pregnancy provides another window into the role of hormones in migraine. The majority of migraine patients experience a welcome reduction in migraine frequency during pregnancy (particularly after the first trimester) but suffer more attacks in the post-partum period. I have seen patients whose vestibular migraines were well-controlled for a long time suddenly experience a surge in vestibular migraine attacks after delivering a baby.

Various other factors also need to be considered. Concussions or traumatic brain injury can cause migraines in vulnerable brains. I have seen many college and high school athletes who developed migraine after suffering concussions, as well as adults who began suffering from migraine after car wrecks or hitting their heads. With all the publicity surrounding concussions, we should pay attention to children and teens with vulnerable migraine brains. Several questions need to be studied: Do children of a parent with migraine have a higher risk of developing migraine if they suffer concussions? Do children with migraine equivalents have a higher risk of developing migraine or more severe migraine if they suffer concussions?

Neck injuries can sometimes contribute to the development of migraine. The nerves of the upper cervical spine control sensation over the scalp and are intimately connected with the trigeminal system. Pain from the neck can often aggravate the trigeminal system which then provokes migraine.

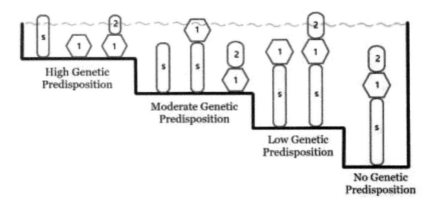

The swimming pool diagram illustrates why some people develop migraine and others don't. The depths of the pool indicate inherent genetic predispositions (i.e., the vulnerability); in the shallowest end are people with high genetic propensity and as such, most vulnerable to migraine, and in the deepest end are those with no genetic inclination whatsoever. The surface of the water is the threshold – as long as causative agents remain below the surface, one does not develop migraine but if these agents breach the surface, migraine emerges. After genetic predisposition, traumatic events and stress (S) appear to be a huge contributing factor. Other factors involved in starting migraine are denoted by (1) and (2) in the diagram. In those most vulnerable (high genetic predisposition) to migraine, a high level of stress may be enough to cause migraines to manifest. In the absence of this high stress, a combination of two factors (e.g., depression and hormones, or a lack of essential vitamins combined with hormonal changes) may be needed to provoke migraines; a single agent is unlikely to result in migraine. Those with a moderate genetic predisposition may require a high level of stress combined with another agent (e.g., hormonal changes, or low vitamin levels) to set migraines off. People with a low genetic predisposition may require high stress levels combined with multiple causative agents to push them into migraines. In the deepest end of the pool, those with no genetic predisposition will not develop migraine even when exposed to high stress, and all known causative agents.

The Neuroscience of Vestibular Migraine

To understand the symptoms and treatments of vestibular migraine, it helps to understand the basic neuroscience of the disease. A detailed, complex discussion is not necessary, but a broad overview of the nature of the beast will help you understand many points discussed in this book. This section may be a bit heavy and is fine to skip. As you read other chapters, you can always refer back to this section to get a better understanding.

Neuroanatomy

The trigeminal system plays a central role in migraine. The second largest cranial nerve (after the vagus nerve), it is predominantly responsible for sensation of the face, head, meninges (covering of the brain), and the surface of the blood vessels inside the skull. The branches of the trigeminal collect sensory information from these regions and convey them to the brainstem, where they are processed and sent to other parts of the brain to be interpreted. The trigeminal system contains many neurotransmitters and neuropeptides implicated in migraine, including calcitonin gene-related peptide (CGRP), glutamate, serotonin, amylin, and pituitary adenylate cyclase-activating polypeptide (PACAP). The CGRP pathway is central to migraine.

A migraine attack begins with neuronal dysfunction called cortical spreading depression. This is a phenomenon where a wave of electrical hyperactivity begins in one brain region, and then propagates across the brain, leaving areas of abnormally depressed activity in its wake. The effects of cortical spreading depression can be observed in certain forms of visual aura; a bright colorful jagged wave begins in a corner of one's visual field and marches across the visual field leaving darkened or blurry areas in behind it. Cortical spreading depression triggers activation of the trigeminal system, leading to changes in the dura (part of the meninges), and upper cervical cord.

An important concept in migraine pathophysiology is neurogenic inflammation, which is triggered by cortical spreading depression. Neurogenic inflammation in the meninges leads to the release and leakage of pro-inflammatory chemicals, which irritate sensitive nerves, dilate blood vessels, and stimulate immune cells (e.g., mast cells). Blood vessel dilation and the release of even more pro-inflammatory compounds from triggered immune cells further exacerbate the inflammatory cascade, worsening the headache, and leading to a feed-forward loop that drives and sustains neurogenic inflammation and migraine.

Migraine-related changes also take place within the upper cervical cord (upper neck). The nerves from this region are intimately linked to the trigeminal system and are often referred to together as the trigeminocervical complex. Migraine-associated dysfunction then spreads to other parts of the brain, including the thalamus, hypothalamus, locus coeruleus, and various brainstem regions (especially the vestibular system).

The thalamus receives and processes all sensory information (except for smell) before conveying it to the part of the cortex responsible for interpreting that information. The thalamus plays an important role in light sensitivity and cutaneous allodynia (the misperception of normal touch as being painful) in migraine. Furthermore, the thalamus plays an important role in relaying vestibular information from the brainstem to the higher centers of the brain. It is obvious how disrupted signaling in the thalamus can affect a multitude of sensory information, including balance and pain.

The hypothalamus is of particular interest since it controls many essential functions including our sleep-wake cycle, hunger, thirst, body temperature, digestion, heart rate, and blood pressure. Migraine-induced changes in the hypothalamus can explain why migraines can be accompanied by food cravings, loss of appetite, fatigue, and depression.

The autonomic nervous system can be divided into the sympathetic and the parasympathetic systems. The sympathetic system drives the flight-or-fight response. In stressful or threatening situations, the limbic system triggers the sympathetic response, resulting in a flood of epinephrine (adrenaline), norepinephrine, and cortisol to prepare the body for flight or fight. The parasympathetic system is activated when the organism feels safe and controls the "rest-and-digest" or "feed-and-breed" responses; essentially, it controls digestion, defecation, urination, salivation, and reproduction. The sympathetic and parasympathetic systems function in a yin-and-yang relationship. A balance between these systems ensures the organism survives and thrives in an ever-changing environment.

The hypothalamic-pituitary-adrenal (HPA) axis is the body's main stress response mechanism. Stress refers to a state in which homeostasis (the balance in the body's environment) is disturbed due to an actual or perceived threat. When a stressor is encountered, the amygdala activates the hypothalamus to stimulate the pituitary gland to secrete adrenocorticotropic hormone (ACTH), which signals the adrenal glands to produce glucocorticoids (the most important of which is cortisol). Glucocorticoids prepare the body for stress by mobilizing energy supplies. They increase blood pressure, heart rate, and blood sugar levels (inducing a craving for sweets and carbs) to ensure the muscles are well-prepared for fight or flight. Bodily functions not essential to immediate survival (e.g., digestion, bone formation, reproductive function, and muscle building) are suppressed. Once the threat has abated, the brain turns off the sympathetic response and HPA axis and returns the reins to the parasympathetic system. Heart rate, blood pressure, and blood sugar return to normal, and the organism can focus on digesting food, eliminating waste, and reproducing.

This ancient stress response mechanism is found in fish, reptiles, amphibians, birds, and mammals. To these creatures, stressors are simple: find food, avoid predators, and reproduce. To the human brain, the pinnacle of evolution, stressors are anything that *could* disrupt homeostasis. Stressors are no longer limited to surviving predators, reproducing, and finding sustenance, but now include paying one's bills, working a job (and the maddening challenges it entails), raising kids, and keeping up with the Joneses. The stress response was designed to be quick. Turning on the stress response for three minutes to escape a hungry tiger does not cause long-term harm. Unfortunately, if the brain constantly and mistakenly believes it is encountering stressors, a chronic state of sustained psychological stress ensues, an all-too-common feature of modern life. Having the same response perpetually turned on to deal with the demands of your job, family, and financial commitments will lead to serious health problems, like diabetes, hypertension, obesity, infertility, and increased vulnerability to infections.

The locus coeruleus is located in the brainstem. Its involvement in migraine is also notable since it produces norepinephrine, a neurotransmitter that plays a crucial role in controlling arousal (wakefulness), attention, memory, stress responses, emotions, and balance. Many of the symptoms of vestibular migraine affect these domains.

Other brainstem centers involved in pain regulation include the nucleus raphe magnus and periaqueductal gray. These areas help suppress pain perception in normal states but are impaired in migraine, explaining why headache and pain are such prominent features of the disorder.

The vestibular system is a complex network of nerves that helps us maintain balance by controlling how we perceive motion and our spatial relationship to the surrounding environment. The vestibular system starts in the inner ear with two tiny, but highly important organs – the semicircular canals and the otolithic organs. The semicircular canals detect angular acceleration (i.e., head motion), while the otolithic organs detect linear acceleration (e.g., gravity). Information from these organs travels via the vestibular nerve to the brainstem, where the vestibular nuclei and cerebellum integrate this subconscious information with visual and proprioceptive (joints and muscles) data. This information is then sent to the thalamus before being relayed to the higher centers of the brain, where it is processed and interpreted to help us make sense of our relationship to the environment. For example, when you ride a bicycle, information about your head movements and relationship to gravity is integrated with what you see and information from the joints and muscles on a subconscious level to keep you from falling. This information is also conveyed to the higher centers of the brain that help you consciously decide how fast to pedal, where to go, and what to pay attention to.

The trigeminocervical system is intimately connected to many structures in the vestibular system. The abnormal electrical activity responsible for triggering migraine spread between the vestibular and trigeminocervical systems causes the vestibular symptoms that characterize vestibular migraine.

Biochemistry

The biochemistry of migraine is fascinating, and a brief explanation is needed to understand why certain medications are effective. When you read about migraine treatments later in the book, you can refer back to this section to better understand why certain treatments help migraine.

The hot migraine brain is an essentially "hyper-excitable" brain due to the factors outlined earlier. The "hyper-excitable" state means that the usual balance between excitatory and inhibitory pathways is tilted in favor of the former. Different neurotransmitters (the chemicals used by nerves to "talk" to each other) control the excitatory and inhibitory pathways. The hot migraine brain thus has an excess of excitatory neurotransmitters (like glutamate and aspartate), and a deficiency of inhibitory neurotransmitters (like GABA and glycine).

A central player in the chemistry of a migraine attack is CGRP. The discovery of CGRP's role in migraine has been nothing short of revolutionary. CGRP levels spike with migraine attacks, and infusion of CGRP in vulnerable individuals triggers migraines. In fact, the levels of CGRP change with different migraine attack phases. CGRP is released from the trigeminal ganglion and along the nerves that run along blood vessels in the dura. It is found in many brainstem locations related to migraine. Intriguingly, the vestibular system, including the cerebellum and inner ear, has numerous CGRP receptors suggesting a central role for CGRP in vestibular migraine.

Serotonin is also an important neurotransmitter in migraine. It is produced predominantly in the gut and carried in the circulation by platelets; a small amount is produced by the brainstem. Low serotonin levels increase the likelihood of cortical spreading depression, abnormal trigeminal activation, and blood vessel dilation. It is interesting to note that low serotonin levels are linked to migraine, motion sickness, irritable bowel syndrome, and depression. Sudden changes in estrogen levels can lower serotonin levels and trigger migraine attacks.

Norepinephrine (also called noradrenaline) is the neurotransmitter that controls wakefulness and attention. Its levels are lowest when we sleep and rise when we are awake. Norepinephrine peaks in response to fight-or-flight stimuli. Migraine patients generally have lower norepinephrine levels than the general population. Furthermore, decreased norepinephrine be the cause of fatigue and brain fog in people with migraine.

Dopamine is the reward system neurotransmitter. It makes you "feel good" when you buy the latest Gucci bag, or devour a cheesecake. Dopamine is the neurotransmitter that makes us want to do things that we know make us feel good. It is also involved in cognition, sleep, mood, motivation, and pain perception. There is a link between migraine and the dopamine system, but the exact relationship between dopamine levels and migraine remains unclear. Dopamine levels drop during the migraine attack but interestingly, rise and intensify pain perception if heat is applied to the forehead. Furthermore, dopamine-blocking medications like prochlorperazine and metoclopramide relieve migraine attacks. This suggests that perhaps low dopamine levels increase the likelihood of a migraine attack but high levels may sustain an attack once it has occurred.

If you know the enemy and know yourself, you need not fear the result of a hundred battles.
Sun Tzu, The Art of War

Chapter 4: Diagnosing Vestibular Migraine - What Happens During Attacks?

If darkness possesses the eyes, and if the head be whirled round with dizziness, and the ears ring as from the sound of rivers rolling along with a great noise, or like the wind when it roars among the sails, we call the affection Vertigo, a bad complaint indeed... the mode of vertigo is heaviness of the head, sparkles of light in the eyes along with much darkness, ignorance of themselves and of those around; and, if the disease go on increasing, the limbs sink below them, and they crawl on the ground; there is nausea and vomitings...
Aretaeus the Cappadocian, *De Causis et Signis Diuturnorum Morborum* (Book II)

The ancient Greek physician Aretaeus, wrote about vertigo and migraine in his renowned medical work "De Causis et Signis" and may have provided the first written account of a vestibular migraine attack. He presciently observed attacks of vertigo that were associated with headache ("heterocrania"), photophobia ("avoid light and feel relief when in the dark"), possible visual aura ("flying threads float before their eyes"), nausea, vomiting, and even nystagmus ("the eyes... move to and fro forcedly").

Even though the relationship between vertigo and migraine has been recognized for centuries, the entity we now call vestibular migraine did not receive much attention until very recently. Many names were used to describe it, including migraine-related vertigo, migraine-associated dizziness, vertiginous migraine, migrainous vertigo, benign recurrent vertigo, and migraine-related vestibulopathy. As you may imagine, the absence of a uniform name and diagnostic criteria led to a lot of confusion. Could we diagnose any patient with dizziness and migraine as having this condition? And which name should be used?

In 1999, the term vestibular migraine was used for the first time in a seminal study by Drs. Dieterich and Brandt [Dieterich, 1999] and the first set of diagnostic criteria were published by Dr. Neuhauser and colleagues in 2001 [Neuhauser, 2001]. Finally, with a name and a formal set of diagnostic criteria, vestibular migraine was studied in greater detail, leading to a remarkable expansion in our knowledge of the disorder. Finally, in 2012, the International Barany Society and International Headache Society collaborated to produce the diagnostic criteria set that we use today [Lempert, 2012].

The Diagnostic Criteria for Vestibular Migraine

A. At least 5 episodes of vestibular symptoms of moderate or severe intensity, lasting 5 minutes to 72 hours.

B. Current or previous history of migraine with or without aura.

C. One of more migraine features with at least 50% of the vestibular episodes:

• Headache with at least two of the following characteristics: unilateral, pulsating or throbbing, moderate or severe intensity, aggravated by routine physical activity

• Photophobia and phonophobia

• Visual aura

D. Not better accounted for by another diagnosis

Important points and caveats:

• Vestibular symptoms that can qualify for the diagnosis of vestibular migraine include all forms of vertigo and head motion-induced dizziness resulting in nausea.

• The vestibular symptoms must be severe enough to impair (moderate intensity) or completely restrict (severe intensity) one's ability to perform activities

• Nausea, while considered a diagnostic criterion for migraine headache, is not considered for vestibular migraines since dizziness and vertigo trigger nausea, regardless of their cause.

Vestibular migraine in children may seem obvious and intuitive but the lack of formal diagnostic criteria complicates efforts to study the disorder. Since the second edition of this book, the International Headache Society and Barany Society again collaborated to formulate criteria to diagnose vestibular migraine in children [van de Berg, 2021]. The diagnosis of "vestibular migraine of childhood" can be used in all children under 18 years of age who meet the same criteria for vestibular migraine in the adult population (see above). Note that most children with migraine tend to experience bilateral headache. The term "probable vestibular migraine of childhood" is used when an individual below 18 years of age experiences at least 3 episodes of vestibular symptoms of moderate or severe intensity lasting between 5 minutes and 72 hours, who meets either criterion B or C. A diagnosis of "recurrent vertigo of childhood" is used for children who have experienced at least 3 episodes of vestibular symptoms of moderate or severe intensity, lasting between 1 minute to 72 hours) without the other criteria.

The challenge of diagnosing vestibular migraine in the pediatric population is the patient's difficulty in describing their symptoms (a tough task for most adults). In very young children, observing the loss of balance, nystagmus, vomiting, and pallor can be useful. In older children, I find it useful to have them mimic the vestibular symptom for me (e.g., imitating a motion with their hands) if they are unable to put it in words.

We will first discuss what symptoms occur during vestibular migraine attacks since these pertain to the diagnostic criteria and diagnosis. In the following chapter, we will discuss what symptoms may occur in between these attacks.

Please note that many of these symptoms can also occur in serious, life-threatening conditions like strokes; if you suddenly experience them for the first time, you must always seek medical attention - do not automatically assume these are due to vestibular migraine until you have discussed them with your neurologist.

The Phases of a Migraine Attack

Recall that we alluded to the four phases of a migraine attack: premonitory (or prodrome), aura, attack (or headache), and postdrome. Not everyone experiences all these phases, and symptoms may overlap between the phases. Don't be too dogmatic and try to classify every symptom in these phases. This is a useful framework to help us understand how vestibular migraine attacks evolve.

The Premonitory (Prodrome) Phase

The premonitory phase affects about two-thirds of people with migraine. It can begin anywhere between two hours up to 3 days prior to the aura or attack phase and may include fatigue, food cravings or aversion, loss of appetite, excessive yawning, cognitive symptoms, mood alterations, changes in bowel habits, increased urinary frequency, insomnia, or excessive sleep.

Abnormal activity in the limbic system and the hypothalamus occurs during the prodrome. The limbic system is the part of the brain responsible for emotions, behavior, motivation, smell, and memory. The hypothalamus is a tiny part of the brain that plays a huge role in controlling numerous physiological and hormonal functions vital to our survival. Limbic system dysfunction can lead to mood changes, memory difficulties, and feeling demotivated. Hypothalamic abnormalities can cause a variety of manifestations, including changes in energy levels, sleep, appetite, urination, and bowel function, as well as food cravings or aversion and yawning.

It is interesting to consider if some of the foods blamed as migraine triggers, may not be true migraine triggers after all, but foods that we crave in the lead-up to a migraine attack. One patient described how she would crave blue cheese and red wine a day before a migraine attack. She realized that these were food cravings and not migraine triggers because she would experience the migraine attack regardless if she gave in to the cravings or not. Recognizing your prodrome can be very valuable. You can use your migraine rescue treatments to nip the attack in the bud.

The Aura Phase

My migraine aura was now so severe that the world on the left had ceased to exist, except as an intermittent yellow flash.

Hilary Mantel

The word "aura" is ancient Greek for "breeze", which is a very apt description of this phenomenon. The aura is the metaphoric "breeze" that warns of the impending storm of a migraine attack. However, in some, the aura occurs with the headache, i.e., during the attack phase. The aura is characterized by transient neurological changes that last from 5 to 60 minutes. About 20% of people with migraine experience aura.

The most common aura is visual and affects about 98% of people with migraine with aura. It can manifest as seeing sparkles, shimmers (like looking at heat waves), mosaic patterns, tunnel vision, stars, zig-zag lines, squiggly lines, flashing lights, dark or blind spots, floaters, flickering, deformed edges and lines, and fortification spectra (a jagged C- or bean-shaped pattern that begins in one corner of the vision and slowly spreads across the field of vision). Sometimes, Alice in Wonderland-type visual symptoms may occur (see later).

The visual aura begins in one part of the visual field and gradually expands. Interestingly, this gradual expansion follows the velocity of cortical spreading depression, which is the wave of abnormal electrical activity that cascades across the brain regions affected by migraine. The visual aura involves both eyes, although it may be mistaken as occurring in one eye because it begins in a part of the visual field and spreads.

The term "retinal migraine" should not be used for visual aura; it refers to a specific condition where the visual aura symptoms occur only in ONE eye (i.e., monocular). As a rule of thumb, monocular visual symptoms are usually caused by an ocular problem and should prompt evaluation by an ophthalmologist. When you have an aura, close each eye to determine if the aura is in one or both eyes.

Sensory aura is less common. Tingling or numbness may occur on part of the body and spread. Typically, it occurs on one arm and then spreads to the face or the body (usually on the same side as the affected arm). The numbness can be perceived as weakness due to the impaired sensory feedback from the affected limb.

Language auras are uncommon and manifest as trouble thinking, finding the right words, or difficulty speaking (sometimes talking gibberish). Other auras are rare and include ringing in the ears, ear pressure, dizziness, vertigo, or olfactory hallucinations (perceiving odors that are not actually present). The bizarre symptoms of Alice in Wonderland syndrome (discussed later) can also occur during the aura phase of an acute migraine episode.

Remember, although symptoms like dizziness, vertigo, trouble thinking, sensory changes, and ear pressure are rare as auras, these symptoms are not uncommon as part of the attack (headache) phase.

The Attack (Headache) Phase

And then a throb hits you on the left side of the head so hard that your head bobs to the right... There's no way that came from inside your head, you think. That's no metaphysical crisis. God just punched you in the face.

Andrew Levy

The attack or headache phase usually lasts between 4 to 72 hours, and is characterized by the typical headache of a migraine attack, accompanied by symptoms like nausea, vomiting, light sensitivity, sound sensitivity, and smell sensitivity. Even though the diagnostic criteria state that the headache should last between 4 to 72 hours, in real life, it varies, and headaches may last for days.

The headache of a migraine attack is often described as a pounding, throbbing, or pulsating pain. Some of my patients have described it as sharp, pressure-like, or squeezing as well. Most commonly, it affects one side of the head. It is not typically "side-locked" which means that although it is one-sided, it can affect either side of the head and usually does not constantly affect the same side. Headaches that exclusively occur on one side of the head raise the possibility of other diagnoses.

In some, the headache affects the whole head, the front of the head, both temples, or the back of the head (occipital). People with vestibular migraine who experience headache with their attacks tend to experience occipital headaches. Occasionally, the pain can radiate to the neck or face. I have patients who actually see their scalp or neck swell up during migraine attacks.

The key characteristic of migraine headaches is that the headache worsens with routine physical activity. This means that if you try to go about your day or move around the house as you usually do if you are having a migraine attack, the headache will get worse. Migraine headaches compel a person to stop what they are doing and rest. Some headaches are not aggravated by physical activity (e.g., tension-type headaches) and a person is able to push through what they need to do. Other headaches compel the sufferer to pace about restlessly (e.g., cluster headache) to distract themselves from the horrible pain.

Light sensitivity (photophobia – Greek for "dread of light") is an abnormal sensitivity to light, often causing significant discomfort or even pain (in the eye or head) in sufferers. Light sensitivity is very problematic and is usually rated as the most bothersome migraine symptom in clinical trials. Glare, fluorescent lighting, and LED lights are particularly uncomfortable, and are often triggers for migraine.

Sound sensitivity (phonophobia – Greek for "dread of noise") refers to aversion to noise or even noise levels that others would perceive as "normal". Light and sound sensitivity compel many to seek quiet, dark rooms to rest during migraine attacks.

Nausea is another common symptom during migraine attacks, affecting over 90% of people. Vomiting is less common and occurs in about one-third of people during migraine attacks. Interestingly, vomiting can often relieve a migraine attack in some. There are many theories as to why vomiting can ameliorate a migraine attack. One suggests that vomiting does not actually terminate an attack but rather, marks the end of a migraine attack as the digestive tract (which slows down significantly during the attack) begins moving again.

Another theory suggests that vomiting stimulates the vagus system which then terminates the migraine attack, or stimulates the release of a hormone called arginine-vasopressin (AVP) that constricts the dilated blood vessels responsible for driving the inflammatory changes underlying a migraine attack. As a migraine sufferer myself, I do not believe that vomiting merely marks the ending of a migraine attack. I intentionally vomit when I have an acute migraine episode and always feel much better after, and therefore suspect that the act of vomiting may induce certain neurological or hormonal changes that serve to halt a migraine attack.

Note that headaches may not occur, or may not be severe during the attack phase of vestibular migraine. Vestibular symptoms (discussed later) usually predominate and are accompanied by other migraine features. Studies of vestibular migraine report that anywhere from one- to three-quarters of patients consistently experience a headache with their attacks [Beh, 2019]. Migraine headaches tend to improve and lessen with age, and may even disappear altogether after menopause. As such, vestibular migraine attacks may be accompanied by a mild or moderate headache that is far less severe than vertigo or may not be associated with a headache at all. Some people describe head pressure but not actual pain.

Many patients and physicians are confused by the lack of headache and are perplexed at how migraine can manifest without a headache. Often, physicians (even neurologists) tell patients that they could not possibly have vestibular migraine because of the absence of significant headache. Remember, the diagnostic criteria for vestibular migraine require *one* migraine feature only – it can be a headache, visual aura, or light and sound sensitivity. A headache is *not* required to make the diagnosis of vestibular migraine. Don't forget: migraine is more than just a headache.

Barbara is a 64-year-old woman, with no medical problems other than infrequent migraine headaches when she was in her 20s but these stopped when she was 40. In her late 40s, she experienced episodes where she felt she was spinning violently, and falling through space. These sensations were aggravated by moving her head in any direction, and by looking at her blinds, ceiling fan, or dog running around. During these episodes, she found that lights hurt her eyes, and she could not bear to have the TV volume on or listen to her husband speaking. She did not have any headaches during such spells. For relief, she had to lie down in a dark, quiet room during these attacks, which lasted for between 1 hour to half a day. She has had an attack every 2-3 months.

Diagnosis

Barbara meets the diagnostic criteria for vestibular migraine. The attacks are characterized by both spontaneous (spinning and falling through space) and triggered (head motion- and visually-induced) vertigo, accompanied by light and sound sensitivity. The absence of headache does NOT rule out vestibular migraine; recall that according to the diagnostic criteria, only one migraine feature is required and in Barbara's case, she has photophobia and phonophobia.

The Postdrome Phase

The postdrome of a migraine consists of the "after-shocks" of the migraine attack and affects the majority of people with migraine. These are the symptoms that occur once the attack phase has subsided and can last from a few hours to 1-2 days. It can be likened to, and often feels like, a hangover. The most common postdrome symptoms are fatigue, feeling withdrawn, feeling down, and wiped out. People also may experience brain fog, trouble concentrating, irritability, and depressed mood. Some experience neck soreness or stiffness, while others report scalp tenderness and pain. Food cravings, thirst, constipation, pallor, dizziness, frequent urination, yawning, diminished appetite, nausea, and even euphoria have been described in the postdrome phase of a migraine attack. In other words, the symptoms can be similar to those in the premonitory phase.

It is important to recognize postdrome phase symptoms to not incorrectly attribute them to the side effects of rescue medications. For example, while triptans can cause drowsiness in rare instances, postdrome fatigue and sleepiness may be incorrectly blamed on triptans.

Right there is the usefulness of migraine, there in that imposed yoga, the concentration on the pain. For when the pain recedes, ten or twelve hours later, everything goes with it, all the hidden resentments, all the vain anxieties. The migraine has acted as circuit breaker, and the fuses have emerged intact. There is a pleasant convalescent euphoria.

Joan Didion

Symptoms of Vestibular Migraine Attacks

Now that we have a framework for understanding the phases of a migraine attack, let us discuss the many other symptoms that occur during vestibular migraine attacks.

Vestibular Symptoms

A myriad of vestibular symptoms may occur during vestibular migraine attacks. This can often cause confusion among both patients and physicians. A wide range of vertigo sensations occur [Beh, 2019], including spinning, tumbling, falling, floating, shimmering, floating, sliding, tilting, swimming, and multi-directional motion. These vertigo sensations may be spontaneous or triggered (usually by head movement or visual stimuli).

Positional vertigo may also occur; patients may describe triggering or worsening vertigo if they lie on their back, or sides, and often have to sit in a recliner for relief. Other vestibular symptoms include dizziness, postural unsteadiness, oscillopsia, and directional pulsion. Making matters more confusing, my study found that vestibular migraine sufferers often experience more than one vestibular symptom during an attack [Beh, 2019]. For example, a person may suffer from spinning vertigo, oscillopsia, lightheadedness, and a rightward pulling sensation during the attack.

Pop Quiz:

When do vestibular symptoms occur in relation to a vestibular migraine attack?

A. The premonitory phase

B. The aura phase

C. The attack phase

D. The postdrome phase

Answer: All the above. The vestibular symptoms are not limited to a specific part of a migraine attack. They can occur at any time, or last throughout the whole attack.

Ear Symptoms

Besides phonophobia, a variety of other ear or hearing symptoms may accompany vestibular migraine attacks. Tinnitus (ringing in the ears), muffled hearing, and a sensation of fullness or pressure in the ears are frequently reported in vestibular migraine [Beh, 2019]. These ear symptoms are usually associated with Menière's disease, a condition related to swelling of the inner ear (endolymphatic hydrops), and as such, their presence in vestibular migraine often leads to misdiagnosis as Meniere's disease.

Ear pressure or fullness is being recognized more as a symptom of migraine [Mostaghi, 2018; Risbud, 2021]. Up to half of patients with vestibular migraine experience ear pressure/fullness during attacks. In some, it may occur in the interictal period. In migraine patients, this is usually experienced bilaterally (both ears) whereas Menière's disease tends to cause more unilateral (one-sided) ear pressure.

There is also emerging evidence of tinnitus in migraine patients. Studies have shown that between 10-22.5% of people with migraine have tinnitus. The incidence of tinnitus in people with vestibular migraine is even higher, with an estimated 40-50% of patients experiencing it. Some studies report that most patients experience bilateral tinnitus, while others found that it was unilateral in the majority.

Hearing loss is not uncommon in people with vestibular migraine. In vestibular migraine, this tends to be a milder high-frequency hearing loss [Radtke, 2012]. One possible explanation is that vestibular migraine tends to affect an older cohort, compared to migraine. Another possible explanation is that vestibular migraine may be associated with mild inner ear injury. While not proven in humans, trigeminal stimulation in lab animal studies results in inflammatory changes in the inner ear.

The relationship between migraine and Menière's disease is complicated and fascinating. Half of Menière's disease patients suffer from migraine, and a subset of patients suffer from both vestibular migraine and Menière's disease. A person diagnosed with migraine is twice as likely to develop Menière's disease in the future compared to a non-migraine sufferer. A person with diagnosed Menière's disease is also twice as likely to have migraine in the future compared to someone without Menière's disease. Some have even postulated that Meniere's disease is a form of migraine! I tend to disagree with that but it highlights the close, confusing, and complicated relationship between Menière's disease and vestibular migraine. Distinguishing these two disorders is crucial since the treatments are quite different.

Ear pain (otalgia) is another underappreciated symptom in those with migraine. Patients with unexplained ear pain have a high prevalence of migraine symptoms and often respond to migraine treatments [Teixido, 2011; Sussman, 2022]. Ear pain in migraine is usually one-sided and can also be found in some people with vestibular migraine. In my experience, other unusual ear symptoms may also be described by vestibular migraine patients, including strange sensations (bubbling, pulsations, itching, tingling) inside the ears, and popping noises.

<u>Case Study</u>

Lisa is a 46-year-old woman with episodic migraine with visual aura, who describes a 6-year history of episodes of tumbling vertigo lasting hours and occurring about once a week. These episodes are accompanied by head pressure, light, and sound sensitivity, as well as pressure inside both ears (as if she were on a plane and could not pop her ears), and a loud ringing noise. She was diagnosed with Menière's disease by multiple ENT specialists but never improved with diuretics. She has had multiple normal hearing tests over this duration.

Diagnosis

Lisa has vestibular migraine and meets the diagnostic criteria discussed previously. How about her ear pressure and ringing? How do we distinguish vestibular migraine from Menière's disease? Firstly, the ear symptoms in Menière's disease tend to be one-sided (unilateral); typically, someone with Menière's disease experiences a pressure building up within one ear, accompanied by difficulty hearing and a roaring noise in that ear leading up to a vertigo attack. The ear symptoms in vestibular migraine tend to be bilateral, i.e., affecting both ears. Secondly, Menière's disease usually results in low-frequency hearing loss in one ear; the absence of any hearing loss with repeated audiograms over the years makes Menière's disease highly unlikely in Lisa. Thirdly, the presence of photophobia and phonophobia during vertigo attacks suggests vestibular migraine, not Menière's disease.

Visual Symptoms

Aside from visual aura and photophobia, a variety of visual symptoms can occur in vestibular migraine.

Blurry vision. A vague sensation of a lack of visual clarity, that makes it difficult for people to read, or appreciate small details. This is a fairly common symptom in most of my patients.

Impaired depth perception. A feeling of being unable to visually judge distances. Sufferers often describe difficulty when trying to step on uneven surfaces or reach for objects accurately. This symptom is less common in my patients.

Eye strain. This is another commonly reported visual symptom in my patient population. It is a sensation of eye discomfort, fatigue, and tiredness, similar to what you may experience from intense use at a close distance (e.g., reading, using a computer) for a prolonged time.

Visual snow. Recently accepted as a migraine phenomenon, visual snow is also known as visual static or aeropsia. It is characterized by persistent tiny flickering white and black dots in the whole visual field, similar to the appearance of static on old television sets.

Double vision. When a person sees a double image when there should be only one. Double vision may be horizontal (the false image lies to the side of the real image), vertical (the false image lies above or below the real image), or oblique (images overlap diagonally). It is not very common in vestibular migraine.

Polyopia. This rare symptom refers to a visual phenomenon where multiple (more than two) images arranged in rows, columns, or diagonals are seen when looking at an object.

Palinopsia. Derived from the Greek words that mean "seeing again", it refers to persistent visual images after the stimulus has been removed. For example, someone with palinopsia who looks at an object will report that the object still appears in his or her vision for a period of time, even with the eyes closed, or after looking away. It is not uncommon in people with visual snow syndrome. Light streaking and visual trailing may also occur in palinopsia. *Light streaking* is characterized by streaks of light when looking at a bright object against a dark background and in *visual trailing*, multiple after-images are seen behind a moving object.

Neuropsychiatric Symptoms

Neuropsychiatric symptoms refer to symptoms that affect mood and cognitive abilities. These commonly occur during migraine attacks (either during the prodrome or attack phases) and are often very disruptive.

Brain fog is a general term that describes difficulty thinking. It encompasses a variety of cognitive problems. These include confusion, an inability to clearly articulate thoughts (things seem to be at the tip of the tongue), trouble multitasking, impaired attention, slowed processing speed (taking longer and more effort to mentally process anything), and dysfluency ("can't find the right words"). One of my patients beautifully described brain fog as "thinking through pea soup".

Word-finding difficulties (dysfluency) refer to trouble speaking during a migraine attack. This is not difficulty with enunciation or pronunciation – difficulty articulating words is called slurred speech or dysarthria. Dysfluency refers to the phenomenon where a person uses the wrong words, garbles a sentence structure, speaks gibberish, and/or finds it extremely hard to think of and use the appropriate words.

Fatigue can occur during migraine attacks but usually hits during the postdrome. My patients often describe feeling utterly drained and exhausted after an attack. Cognitive fatigue refers to mental exhaustion after performing cognitively challenging tasks.

Mood disturbances are not uncommon during migraine attacks. Depression, irritability, anxiety, or panic are common. In my experience, depression and irritability are frequently described in the premonitory or postdrome phase. It is not hard to find migraine sufferers who describe feeling depressed, anxious, or just "blah" leading up to or after a migraine attack.

Autonomic Symptoms

The autonomic nervous system controls and regulates bodily functions that are crucial to life, like temperature regulation, sweating, digestion, breathing, heart rate, urination, sexual function, and pupillary changes. The vestibular system shares numerous connections with the autonomic nervous system – that is why vertigo is commonly accompanied by nausea, vomiting, sweatiness, clamminess, and pallor. It is thus unsurprising that vestibular migraine attacks are associated with autonomic symptoms like sweating, diarrhea, feeling hot or cold, and pallor. Other autonomic symptoms like hunger, loss of appetite, excessive yawning, and dry mouth tend to occur in the premonitory phase and can be useful as warnings of an impending attack. Excessive tear production, runny nose, eye redness, and eyelid droopiness may occur during the attack phase of vestibular migraine; unlike cluster headache, these are usually bilateral in migraine.

Sensory Symptoms

A variety of non-specific sensory symptoms can occur during migraine attacks and may affect any part of the body, limbs, or head. Altered sensations can either be positive (feeling too much), or negative (not feeling enough). On their own, these sensory symptoms are not specific to any particular disorder but may be part of vestibular migraine attacks.

Positive sensory symptoms may include tingling, pins and needles, burning, electrical sensations, vibrations, itchiness, weird non-specific feelings, burning, pain, or allodynia (a phenomenon where normal touch is perceived as pain). These may occur on part of the body or face, or all over. Some of my patients experience brain zaps, a shock-like electrical sensation that shoots through the inside of the head; this may occur during migraine attacks but is also described as a side effect or withdrawal symptom of antidepressants.

Negative sensory symptoms are usually described as numbness or a loss (or diminishment) of sensation. Similar to positive sensory symptoms, this can occur on part of the face or body, or all over.

Alice in Wonderland Syndrome

Mad Hatter: Have I gone mad?

Alice: I'm afraid so. You're entirely bonkers.

But I'll tell you a secret: all the best people are.

Lewis Carroll, Alice's Adventures in Wonderland

Alice in Wonderland syndrome refers to a set of bizarre misperceptions (distortions of sensory input). It is commonly caused by migraine and occurs in vestibular migraine [Beh, 2018]. Many children who experience Alice in Wonderland phenomena later go on to develop migraine. Alice in Wonderland syndrome can be categorized based on the types of misperceptions that occur.

Extrapersonal misperceptions include out-of-body experiences (where a person feels like they are outside their actual bodies, and sometimes even "see" the body they left behind), depersonalization (a feeling that one becomes detached and is no longer part of reality), and derealization (feeling like the world and one's surroundings become unreal). One patient described depersonalization as feeling as though she were separated from the world and looking at it through a two-way mirror. Another described derealization as feeling like she was on a movie set and everyone but she had the movie script. Depersonalization and derealization may be difficult to distinguish and are sometimes referred to as depersonalization-derealization disorder.

Visual misperceptions are the most common manifestation of Alice in Wonderland syndrome. More commonly, people may describe objects as appearing larger, smaller, closer, or farther than they actually are. Other possible visual misperceptions include illusory splitting (objects appear split down the middle), misperceptions of color (where everything becomes a single color, or everything loses color), mosaic vision (as though everything is fragmented into crystalline mosaics), underwater vision (as if looking at things underwater), zoopsia (seeing animals that are not there), enhanced stereoscopic vision (everything appearing in much greater detail – described as "super 3D" or "4K" vision by some of my patients), and closed eye visual hallucinations (seeing objects that are not there when the eyes are closed).

Somesthetic misperceptions are misperceptions of body image and are common Alice in Wonderland symptoms in vestibular migraine. In Lewis Carroll's classic novel, Alice drinks a bottle on a table that says "Drink Me" and shrinks to tiny proportions, and later eats a cake labeled "Eat Me" and grows so big her head hits the ceiling. In another chapter, eating part of a mushroom made her smaller than ever, but eating the other side of the mushroom caused her neck to grow so high above the trees she looked like a serpent. While attending the trial of the Knave of Hearts, she grows larger and larger until she is "a mile high".

Macro- or micro-somatognosia refers to illusions of one's entire body appearing bigger or smaller than it actually is (respectively). One patient with micro-somatognosia described feeling like he shrinks into "molecular size". Partial body macro- or micro-somatognosia affects specific body parts. I have patients who feel like their heads swell up like balloons, feel like their hands are too small, or their feet are too big. One described feeling like she had "Munchkin legs" and was a foot tall. Aschematia is feeling like a body part is missing; a patient I saw reported feeling like he had no eyes during his vestibular migraine attack, while another described feeling like half her body was missing. Quite a few describe feeling like their hands did not belong to them; it remains a mystery to me as to why the hands are more affected than other body parts. Body image splitting refers to the illusion of one's body being split in half.

Misperceptions of time refer to alterations in one's perception of time. Some of my patients experience decelerations, where time appears to move at a much slower pace or everything seems to move in slow motion. One patient described it as suddenly feeling like she was driving at 20 mph even though she was driving at 80 mph on a highway. Accelerations of time feel like time is moving much faster than it actually is, almost like moving at warp speed.

It is very interesting that Lewis Carroll himself suffered from migraine and his own migraine-related misperceptions may have inspired Alice's adventures [Blom, 2016].

Diagnosis: My Approach

I will detail here how I typically approach people with vertigo and dizziness. Diagnosing vestibular disorders takes time. I need enough time to ensure I obtain enough historical data, review tests that have been performed, explain the diagnosis to my patients and discuss treatment options. I'll admit that I am not smart enough to do all of that in the 15-20 minutes typically allocated for a clinic visit.

Today's medical profession is beset by the need to see more patients because greedy insurance companies keep reducing reimbursements for patient visits. As a consequence, doctors have to see more patients in a day to maintain revenue. Even universities and academic medical centers have fallen victim. Institutions that should take pride and effort in investigating complex medical problems have degenerated into businesses driven solely by a desire to generate revenue through increased patient volume. Managers and administrators who have zero clinical experience get to dictate how physicians should see their patients. Patients and physicians are caught between the small-minded bureaucrats in healthcare organizations focused on maximizing revenue, and the mindless automatons of greedy insurance companies aiming to pay as little as possible. Gluttonous insurance companies churn out an endless stream of soul-sucking paperwork for physicians – prior authorizations, denials, appeals, etc. This robs physicians of the time and resources they need to focus on diagnosing and helping their patients.

I like to hear your story from you. You may have told it to many other healthcare professionals, and expect that it is all in your records. I have news for you: it is not. Most physicians cannot write everything single you say. We extract what we feel is relevant and write down what they believe your symptoms are. As you can see, vital information and historical data needed for an accurate diagnosis are often lost in translation. Even if you have seen other physicians, I have to go over your story to find the important clues that others may have missed just like how a detective investigates a cold case. After I get your history, I more or less have a good idea of what the diagnosis is, most of the time.

The bedside neuro-otologic examination can help me refine my diagnosis and confirm that I did not miss anything else. Tests are not diagnostic for vestibular migraine but can help rule out other problems.

If migraine patients have a common and legitimate second complaint besides their migraines, it is that they have not been listened to by physicians. Looked at, investigated, drugged, charged, but not listened to.

Dr. Oliver Sacks (1933-2015)

Chapter 5: Interictal Symptoms & Comorbid Disorders – What Happens Between Attacks?

Really? You think migraine is just a headache?
And I suppose Godzilla is just a lizard?
Anonymous

In a previous chapter, we discussed what happens during migraine attacks. In this chapter, we will discuss what symptoms occur in the periods between migraine attacks, or the attack-free periods. These are referred to as interictal symptoms. We will also discuss disorders that are often comorbid (i.e., coexisting) with migraine.

There is so much overlap between some of these symptoms and comorbid disorders that I will discuss both in this chapter. While it may seem that you have a migraine all the time, what is more likely is a combination of interictal symptoms with superimposed attacks of vestibular migraine.

Learning to differentiate interictal symptoms from vestibular migraine attacks is important. Firstly, you will be able to assess the efficacy of a migraine preventive treatment; if a particular treatment stops all your migraine attacks (but not your interictal symptoms), that means it is successful and should not be abandoned. Secondly, by distinguishing interictal symptoms from attacks, you will know when to use your migraine rescue treatment; these are medications that you only use for migraine attacks, not interictal symptoms. Thirdly, there are treatments specifically targeted at interictal symptoms (e.g., vestibular rehabilitation therapy) that can be considered if they are severe enough.

It is also vital to recognize conditions that can be comorbid with migraine. This allows you to recognize them and seek appropriate care for them, and not just attribute them to migraine or confuse them with migraine symptoms. A holistic, comprehensive treatment plan for migraine not only addresses symptoms directly arising from migraine, but also all comorbid conditions.

Additionally, identifying comorbid disorders can help guide treatment choices; for example, a person with depression and migraine may choose a medication that can address both conditions. On the other hand, if you have bipolar disorder, consider migraine preventives that can also help control it and avoid those that could worsen it.

Aura

While a migraine aura is usually accompanied by a full-blown migraine attack, it is not uncommon for an aura to occur in isolation. Other aura symptoms that can be experienced include sensory phenomena, or language problems. An aura usually lasts between 5 and 60 minutes. In rare cases, it can last longer than an hour, and is referred to as "prolonged aura". It is important to contact your neurologist if this occurs, to ensure that no other neurological disorders may be causing it. Migraine aura status is a very rare condition characterized by aura lasting for days and is a medical emergency.

Visual Symptoms

Light sensitivity

Visual information is processed in the part of the brain known as the occipital cortices (also called the visual cortices). The neurons in the visual cortices respond to various features of visual input, including brightness, color, contrast, edges, the orientation of the edges, and motion. Just as each person's brain is unique, the visual cortex of each person is unique, and has different thresholds and sensitivities to these stimuli. The visual cortices of people with migraine are structurally and functionally different from people who do not.

Even during attack-free periods, the visual cortices in people with migraine remain hyperexcitable and more sensitive. The visual system and pain processing systems in migraine brains also appear to be more interconnected; this may be why bright lights can often be perceived as actual pain and not just discomfort.

Not all light is created equal when it comes to migraine. Light comes in a variety of wavelengths; different wavelengths are perceived as different colors. The spectrum of light that causes the most discomfort is blue light, which is about 480 nanometers in wavelength. Blue light is found in sunlight, fluorescent lights, energy-saving bulbs, and electronic screens. Blue light is detected by a specialized group of retinal cells called the intrinsically-photosensitive retinal ganglion cells that travel from the retina to the suprachiasmatic nucleus (our biological clock) in the hypothalamus and to the thalamus. This pathway is responsible for producing melatonin, the hormone that causes sleepiness when it gets dark. These retinal ganglion cells are also connected to the nerves that process pain information in the thalamus, which can explain the link between migraine and sensitivity to blue light. Abnormalities in this pathway may also explain why sleep disturbances are more common in migraine and why melatonin can improve migraines. Green light is the spectrum of light that is least bothersome to people with migraine.

It is common for people with vestibular migraine to be sensitive to light even when they are not experiencing a migraine attack. In addition, sudden changes in ambient lighting (e.g., going from a dark to a bright environment, or vice versa) can be very unpleasant. In over half of people with migraine, bright light triggers migraine attacks.

Visual snow

Visual snow may occur during migraine attacks or be a constant interictal symptom. As discussed in the prior chapter, it appears as small TV static dots in the entire visual field. People with visual snow syndrome experience other visual symptoms like light sensitivity, floaters, difficulty with night vision, visual trailing, and palinopsia. It can start in childhood, but most tend to start in the 20s.

Blurry vision

Some people report visual blurriness or feeling as if things look "off", or as if looking through a mist. They consult with optometrists and ophthalmologists, and are often told that they have "normal vision". Many spend a large amount on changing their prescription glasses, without any improvement. I often find that controlling migraine leads to improvement in visual blurriness.

Palinopsia

There is evidence that migraine patients have a higher incidence of palinopsia compared to the general population. As discussed in the previous chapter, palinopsia can occur during a migraine attack. It can also occur intermittently in the interictal period, but some suffer from almost constant palinopsia.

Ear Symptoms

Noise Sensitivity

Noise sensitivity refers to an increased sensitivity to sound with intolerance or discomfort for noise at levels that typically do not bother a normal person. Noise sensitivity is a well-recognized symptom of migraine attacks. What may be less well-known is that many people with migraine have interictal noise sensitivity.

The severity of interictal noise sensitivity appears to correlate with the frequency of migraine attacks. With frequent attacks, the brainstem and cortical regions that control sound perception become more and more sensitive; this process is called central sensitization (see later). Connections between the thalamus (the relay station for all sensory information except smell) and the amygdala (the threat detection area) grow stronger. Studies show that people with migraine have a much lower threshold for sound-induced discomfort and pain, compared to those without migraine. In addition, loud sounds or noisy environments can often trigger migraine attacks.

Hyperacusis refers to the intolerance for certain everyday sounds that causes distress and adversely affects a person's job, family, social, and everyday activities. People with hyperacusis experience ear pain, annoyance, and sound distortions for many sounds that do not affect normal people. At times, this intolerance may trigger crying spells or panic attacks.

There is a close relationship between hyperacusis and tinnitus: almost all patients with hyperacusis have tinnitus, and half of patients with tinnitus have hyperacusis. Both conditions tend to occur in hearing loss because it leads to increased activity in the central auditory pathways (the brain networks responsible for sound perception), resulting in the maladaptive neuroplasticity that causes tinnitus and hyperacusis. In vestibular migraine, those with hyperacusis and tinnitus tend to be those who have some degree of hearing loss. Furthermore, mild high-frequency hearing loss is known to occur in vestibular migraine, although the reasons for that remain unclear.

Misophonia (literally "hatred of sound") is a psychiatric disorder where a person experiences an emotional aversion to specific sounds (e.g., chewing, breathing). People with misophonia are not just sensitive to noises, they have a visceral emotional reaction to certain sounds.

Tinnitus

Tinnitus and migraine have a lot in common. Like migraine, tinnitus appears to be caused by a hyperexcitable brain. Central sensitization is a feature of migraine, a condition where pain processes in the brain become established, leading to headache persistence and allodynia (a condition where even the lightest touch is perceived as pain).

Similarly, tinnitus can start from a specific disorder, but maladaptive re-organization of the brain, causes it to be entrenched in the brain circuitry. Also, like migraine, stress can both cause and exacerbate tinnitus. Just like migraine, vestibular migraine, and dizziness, people suffering from tinnitus are at higher risk of anxiety, depression, and insomnia.

In addition. people with migraine and vestibular migraine are at higher risk of developing tinnitus. One reason for this may be the connections between the sensory system and auditory centers. This link can explain why the loudness and pitch of tinnitus can be temporarily changed by muscle contractions of the head, neck, and limbs, by facial movements, eye movements, pressure on certain muscle trigger points, and sensory stimulation of the face, or hands. This link also most likely explains why migraine, neck pain, and TMJ disorders can often cause or aggravate tinnitus.

Red Ear Syndrome

Red ear syndrome is a rare condition linked to migraine. It causes one or both ears to turn bright red accompanied by a burning sensation. The burning pain is most noticeable around the ear lobe and can be felt in the cheek or the scalp around the affected ear. Episodes of red ear syndrome may occur without provocation, but can also be triggered by heat, exercise, and rubbing the ear. It can occur strictly on one side, either side, or in both ears. The burning pain is usually described as annoying rather than excruciating. Most of the time, the episodes last between 30 minutes to an hour, but shorter and longer attacks have been reported in the medical literature. The frequency of the attacks is also variable; some report one attack per day, while some suffer multiple attacks per day.

Brain Fog

Vestibular input plays an important role in many cognitive processes, including attention, visuospatial skills, memory, object recognition, motivation, and social cognition. Vestibular information is essential for visuospatial abilities, the skills that help us understand, interpret, and remember the spatial relationship between objects. These are abilities used for navigating, estimating distance, and measuring. These skills are not only important for performing tasks but are also vital to help us imagine and mentally manipulate objects and directions.

Visuospatial skills are vital for fields like art, sports, engineering, physics, mathematics, medicine, geography, and meteorology.

Research into the effect of vestibular input on cognition has also produced some fascinating results. For example, vestibular information influences how the brain processes information that is represented in specific spatial orders. Going up stairs or elevators improves one's ability to perform additions; likewise, going down stairs or elevators enhances the ability to perform subtractions. Moving the body forward improves one's ability to generate future-oriented words, while tipping the body backward impairs this ability.

Brain fog is a common symptom both during and in between vestibular migraine attacks. It makes it difficult to think, focus, find the right words, and come up with the right answers. When you want to say "hummingbird", brain fog makes you say "needle-nosed vibrating dwarf birdie". Brain fog can also affect processing speed, which slows the thinking processes (like trying to think through mud). In addition, brain fog may also affect attention, decision-making, and memory. Brain fog can adversely impact job performance, and activities of daily living; many of my vestibular migraine patients tell me that after dizziness and vertigo, brain fog is the most disruptive and disabling symptom they experience.

Sleep

Insomnia is common in vestibular migraine. It is more frequent in those with anxiety and depression (which themselves are common in vestibular migraine). Poor quality of sleep often leads to worsening of vestibular migraine attacks, which in turn exacerbates mood disorders that impact sleep quality, resulting in a vicious cycle that robs patients of their quality of life. Interestingly, people with migraine tend to need more hours of sleep per day compared to those without migraine; unfortunately, almost half of people with migraine do not get sufficient sleep [Kim, 2017]. In some of my patients, vestibular migraine attacks seem to exclusively occur during sleep, causing insomnia as they become terrified of sleeping and experiencing vertigo attacks.

Sleepwalking (somnambulism) and talking (somniloquy) are more common in children with migraine. Bruxism (teeth grinding) is more common in migraine as well; it can lead to TMJ dysfunction which in turn may worsen migraines.

Interestingly, sleep can stop a migraine attack. Many vestibular migraine patients try to "sleep off an attack", and awaken refreshed and symptom-free. My personal experience is similar. When I have a migraine attack, I take a nap after taking analgesics and awaken feeling 100% better.

How sleep terminates a migraine attack remains unclear. One possibility is that sleep resets the hypothalamus, shutting down the cascade of migraine activity in the brain. An exciting new discovery is the glymphatic system, our brain's very own "de-toxification" system. It consists of a series of spaces around the small blood vessels (arterioles, venules, and capillaries) of the brain, made up of astrocytes which are the connective cells of the brain. These spaces are spread extensively in the brain, reaching every neuron, and are connected to the cerebrospinal fluid spaces.

During sleep, our brains very dramatically increase glymphatic flow, sending rivulets of cerebrospinal fluid flowing through these channels to clear the brain of the toxins and waste generated during our waking hours. Sleep may terminate migraine attacks by using the glymphatic system to clear away all the toxins that triggered it in the first place.

Pain

Headache

Chronic Migraine

Chronic migraine is defined as having a headache for at least 15 days out of each month, with migraine attacks for at least 8 days out of the month. Migraine transformation or chronification refers to episodic migraine attacks that increase in frequency to the point that headaches do not go away.

Women and young adults are at higher risk of developing chronic migraine. High caffeine intake is a risk factor for developing chronic migraine. Obesity and poor sleep quality also elevate the risk of developing chronic migraine. The presence of other chronic illnesses, like asthma, metabolic syndrome, cardiovascular disease (e.g., stroke, angina, hypertension), sleep apnea, depression, anxiety, and pain disorders (e.g., fibromyalgia, back pain, neck pain) increase one's risk of migraine chronification.

A person's risk of developing chronic migraine begins to increase if he/she experiences at least 3 headache days per month. Inadequately treating migraine attacks also increases the risk of chronic migraine. This is why my advice for rescue treatments is "hit early and hit hard", rather than trying to tough out a migraine attack. However, it is also important to note that excessive use of rescue medications like analgesics, can result in medication overuse headache.

The presence of cutaneous allodynia predicts that a person will develop chronic migraine. Cutaneous allodynia refers to a neurological condition where a person perceives normally innocuous tactile stimuli (e.g., light touch, brushing hair, wearing tight clothes, wearing glasses) as being painful. Cutaneous allodynia results from central sensitization, a state where the nervous system becomes so focused on the pain that neuronal circuits amplify pain signals way beyond the level of the original stimuli, and perceive non-painful stimuli as being painful.

Tension-Type Headache

Tension-type headache is the most common type of headache, affecting practically everyone at least once in their life. The headache is a dull, vise-like pain that wraps around the head. The episodes may last between 30 minutes to 7 days. Some scalp muscles may feel sore to the touch. Unlike migraine headache, tension-type headache is not aggravated by routine activity (e.g., climbing stairs, or house chores). This means that you can "power through" a tension-type headache without making it worse. On the other hand, migraine headaches are aggravated by routine activity. In addition, while mild nausea can occur with tension-type headache, severe nausea and vomiting indicate migraine. Light or sound sensitivity may also be present; the presence of both light and sound sensitivity points to migraine.

Episodic tension-type headache occurs no more than 15 days per month. Infrequent episodic tension-type headache occurs no more than 12 days per year (which most people have). Frequent episodic tension-type headache occurs more than 12 days but less than 180 days per year. If tension-type headache occurs at least 15 days out of a month, it is classified as chronic tension-type headache. Triggers for tension-type headache may be similar to migraine, and cannot reliably differentiate the two conditions. These include stress, sleep deprivation, dehydration, and missing meals. Alcohol and menses have been reported to trigger tension-type headache as well.

For most people, tension-type headaches occur infrequently and can easily be treated with a simple over-the-counter analgesic. Combining an analgesic with caffeine increases the efficacy. Of course, beware of medication overuse headaches. If tension-type headaches are frequent, preventive treatment(s) should be considered. Amitriptyline has the most evidence to support its use. Other potential treatments include topiramate, propranolol, newer antidepressants (SSRIs and SNRIs), muscle relaxants, nerve blocks, or Botox. Non-pharmacologic interventions like relaxation therapy, exercise, cold or hot compresses, massage, biofeedback, and cognitive-behavioral therapy.

Medication Overuse Headache

Medication overuse headache arises from excessive use of analgesics (acetaminophen, NSAIDs, opioids), triptans, or ergotamines. It is also called a rebound headache.

In medication overuse headache, drugs that were supposed to relieve headache paradoxically cause and aggravate the headache. This is a state where the brain becomes "addicted" to these analgesics and needs higher and more frequent doses just to feel no pain. Using certain rescue medications more than 10 days per month for more than 3 months can lead to medication overuse headache.

Preparations that contain caffeine (e.g., Excedrin), and butalbital (e.g., Fioricet, Fiorinal) increase this risk even more. As such, it is very important to limit the usage of these medications. As a rule of thumb, I advise my patients to use triptans, acetaminophen, NSAIDs, and ergotamines no more than 3 days per week. I also advise very strongly against using opioids and any medication containing butalbital and/or caffeine.

Medication overuse headache is a miserable state to be in because the sufferer must stop all analgesics while the brain "detoxifies" and resets. During this time, headaches often worsen, lasting for up to 7 to 14 days, before they get better.

Mary had just delivered her baby and was experiencing more migraine headaches. Her gynecologist prescribed Fioricet and told her it was safe to take as needed for headaches. She found that it worked well, but as her headaches grew more frequent, she began taking it around the clock. If she missed a dose, her headaches returned with a vengeance. After several months, she saw me and I explained what medication overuse headaches were, and advised her to stop Fioricet completely. I gave her a course of prednisone to help ease her headaches. She had terrible headaches almost daily (and must have hated me, I'm sure), but by the end of 2 weeks, they lifted, and instead of constant daily headaches, she had the usual episodic migraine headache about once every 2 weeks.

Fibromyalgia

Fibromyalgia is a chronic pain condition that results in persistent widespread pain, brain fog, fatigue, and mood disorders. It typically affects women between the ages of 20 to 60. Migraine and fibromyalgia are often co-morbid and result in greater levels of disability, headache severity, and depression.

Interstitial Cystitis

Interstitial cystitis (bladder pain syndrome) manifests with urinary frequency (needing to urinate often), nocturia (the need to wake up to urinate), urgency (needing to urinate as soon as the urge is felt), dyspareunia (painful sexual intercourse), burning pain when urinating, with pelvic pain that builds as the bladder fills and diminishes with urination. Certain food triggers (e.g., caffeine, spicy food, chocolate, alcohol) can aggravate interstitial cystitis. It tends to affect middle-aged women. Interstitial cystitis often coexists with irritable bowel syndrome, fibromyalgia, depression, and migraine, indicating possible overlapping pathophysiology.

Temporomandibular, Neck, Shoulder, & Back Pain

Musculoskeletal neck, shoulder, and back pain are common in vestibular migraine. The most common cause is the abnormally stiff head and neck posture adopted to avoid head motion-induced dizziness. In some cases, positional vertigo from vestibular migraine or benign paroxysmal positional vertigo leads some patients to sleep in very uncomfortable positions, either with too many pillows under the neck or in recliners, causing neck and shoulder pain over time.

Temporomandibular joint disorder (TMD) is also associated with higher migraine risk. TMD refers to a collection of disorders related to dysfunction of the temporomandibular joint, the muscles for chewing, and related structures. TMD causes central sensitization and lowers the threshold for migraine attacks. Irritating the jaw muscles of lab rats by keeping their jaws open results in higher levels of pro-inflammatory cytokines and trigeminal sensitization [Hawkins, 2016].

There is a strong correlation between TMD and neck, shoulder, and lower back pain with migraine. Pain in these locations is more common in those with chronic migraine. In fact, the presence of low back, neck and shoulder pain predicts the evolution from episodic to chronic migraine, and the persistence of chronic migraine [Scher, 2017]. Neck and shoulder muscle inflammation increases the vulnerability to migraine attacks. In lab rats, inducing inflammation in the shoulder muscles sensitizes the trigeminal system and causes the rat equivalent of a migraine attack when they are exposed to pungent odors [Cornelison & Woodman, 2020]. Furthermore, neck muscle inflammation increases the sensitivity of the trigeminal system to TMJ pain, increasing the likelihood of migraine attacks from jaw pain [Cornelison & Chelliboina, 2020].

Chronic muscle tension causes persistent muscle contraction, resulting in ischemia (insufficient blood supply) and the release of pro-inflammatory molecules that sensitize pain neurons, including those in the trigeminal system. In addition, chronic pain alters the brain in ways that increase its sensitivity to pain. Chronic pain causes depression which increases a person's perception of pain, and a higher risk of developing migraine and other pain disorders.

Worsening migraine symptoms and dizziness also lead to physical inactivity, resulting in muscular deconditioning and pain. A vicious cycle can ensue: more migraine attacks lead to less activity, which weakens muscles and causes more pain, resulting in more migraine attacks. Depression only exacerbates this vicious cycle by increasing pain perception which only worsens depression.

Gastrointestinal Disorders

There is a growing body of research into the interactive relationship between the gut and the brain, referred to as the gut-brain axis (Chapter 13). The co-existence of a variety of gastrointestinal symptoms and disorders with migraine has long been recognized, and we are just beginning to understand some details of this fascinating relationship.

Nausea

The link between nausea and migraine is undeniable and extends beyond the nausea that accompanies migraine attacks.

Cyclical vomiting syndrome is a childhood variant of migraine, and in rare cases, can persist into adulthood. People with migraine are more prone to nausea (e.g., motion sickness, post-operative nausea). Furthermore, children with motion sickness, migraine, or who have a family history of migraine are more prone to nausea and vomiting following concussions.

Persistent and frequent nausea is not an uncommon interictal symptom in migraine and vestibular migraine. Persistent nausea tends to occur in people with more severe migraine and may predict risk for conversion to chronic migraine. In vestibular migraine, persistent dizziness worsens this propensity to frequent nausea. Constant nausea can be a very disabling symptom in some people with vestibular migraine.

Gluten-Related Disorders

Gluten is a protein found in wheat, rye, and barley. Gluten molecules give the dough a sticky, stretchy property that forms a net that traps bubbles of carbon dioxide produced by yeast. When the dough is baked, gluten becomes coagulated and its final shape is stabilized. Gluten is also used to create vegetarian imitations of meat products. Gluten may be an unexpected additive to stabilize some foods (e.g., ice cream), cosmetics, or hair products.

In genetically predisposed people, consuming gluten can trigger a reaction when consumed. Celiac disease is an autoimmune disorder caused by a reaction to gluten in genetically predisposed people. It is characterized by diarrhea, foul and pale feces, fatigue, skin disorders, depression, anxiety, anemia, weight loss, and joint pains. The diagnosis of celiac disease can be made with certain blood antibody tests and intestinal biopsies. The prevalence of migraine among people with celiac disease is higher compared to the general population [Dimitrova, 2013; Gabrielli, 2003]. In people with both celiac disease and migraine, a gluten-free diet improves both migraine and celiac disease [Burk, 2009; Gabrielli, 2003]. This is because eliminating gluten stops the inflammation that drives both disorders.

Non-celiac gluten sensitivity is a milder intolerance to gluten. Sufferers may experience diarrhea, constipation, bloating, abdominal discomfort, headaches, fatigue, mood changes, and brain fog. It is believed to affect up to 10% of the population, but is difficult to diagnose. People who suspect they have non-celiac gluten sensitivity can simply eliminate gluten from their diets to see if their symptoms improve and then recur when they reintroduce gluten into their diet.

Gastroparesis

Gastroparesis refers to abnormally slow emptying of the stomach (without any clear obstructions), resulting in nausea, vomiting, bloating, and weight loss. Gastroparesis may occur with migraine attacks or during the interictal period. During migraine attacks, autonomic dysfunction may explain why gastroparesis occurs. Gastroparesis has been proposed as the underlying reason for cyclic vomiting syndrome, and abdominal migraine. The reason gastroparesis occurs in some people during the attack-free period, however, is less clear.

Helicobacter pylori infection

Helicobacter pylori (*H. pylori*) is a bacterium found in the stomach. It causes peptic ulcers and gastritis, and can increase the risk of stomach cancer in some. There is emerging research that links *H. pylori* infection to a variety of neurological conditions including migraine, Alzheimer's disease and Parkinson's disease.

Research suggests *H. pylori* infection is more prevalent among those with migraine [Hosseinzadeh, 2011; Pinessi, 2000; Tunca, 2004; Yiannopoulou, 2007]. Eradicating *H. pylori* can result in migraine improvement in some patients [Gasbarrini, 1998]. Several explanations may explain why this occurs. *H. pylori* may induce an inflammatory state that aggravates migraine activity. It may also alter the gut microbiome in a way that induces inflammatory changes within the body and/or affects gut production of serotonin and other chemicals that play an important role in migraine.

Irritable Bowel Syndrome (IBS)

IBS is a common disorder that is estimated to affect 10-15% of the population. It manifests with abdominal pain, and irregular bowel movements; IBS can be classified according to the bowel symptoms: diarrhea-predominant (IBS-D), constipation-predominant (IBS-C), or mixed (IBS-M). A person may switch between IBS types during their lifetime. IBS is up to 40% more frequent among people with migraine. Likewise, the likelihood of having migraine is almost three times higher among those with IBS.

There are several similarities between IBS and migraine. Both affect women more than men and are associated with depression and fibromyalgia. Like migraine, people with IBS tend to be vitamin D deficient and improve with vitamin D supplementation [Abbasnezhad, 2016; El Amrousy, 2018; Nwosu, 2017; Tazzyman, 2015]. Most fascinating of all, vitamin D supplementation appears to reverse the genetic markers of IBS [Dussik, 2018]. Serotonin plays an important role in gut motility. Just like migraine and depression, IBS is associated with decreased serotonin levels.

Vestibular Symptoms

Constant, chronic dizziness is a common complaint in vestibular migraine and migraine. Like all symptoms, it can vary from very mild and annoying, to severe and life-altering. Many of my patients often tell me that this constant, chronic dizziness affects their lives more significantly than the attacks of vertigo that characterize vestibular migraine.

While most people with migraine and vestibular migraine are more prone to dizziness, interictal dizziness is much worse in some compared to others. One reason for this is the frequency of vestibular migraine attacks. Each vestibular migraine attack typically leaves a person feeling disoriented, off-balance, and dizzy for some time after an attack, similar to how a speedboat leaves waves in its wake that ripple across a calm lake. If a person suffers a vestibular migraine attack once every 4 to 6 months, these ripples dissipate long before the next attack occurs. On the other hand, if a person experiences an attack every 4 to 6 days, the brain does not have time to recover from each attack. It is much worse if a person experiences an attack every 2 days. Imagine how turbulent the waters of a lake are if speedboats are constantly zipping across its surface.

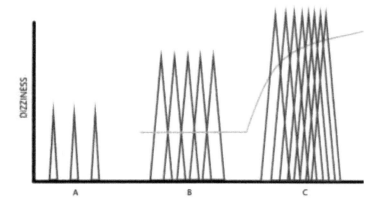

This diagram illustrates how frequent vestibular migraine attacks result in worsening interictal dizziness. Patient A experiences infrequent attacks and the brain returns to a dizzy-free state between attacks. Patient B has more frequent attacks, and before the brain returns to a dizzy-free state, another attack occurs. This keeps Patient B's brain in a constant state of low-level dizziness. Patient C suffers from much more frequent attacks compared to B; the brain remains on a high level of interictal dizziness. For patient C, this state of dizziness predisposes him/her to even more vestibular migraine attacks, leading to a spiral of deteriorating interictal dizziness and more attacks.

To understand why you have this horrible constant dizziness, we need a brief understanding of the balance system. To maintain an upright posture and balance, our brains integrate information from three sources: the visual system, the vestibular system, and the proprioceptive system. The visual system provides information based on what we see; cues in the visual environment help our brain maintain a sense of balance. The vestibular system begins in the inner ear, and travels throughout different brain regions; the vestibular system helps maintain balance by detecting motion and gravity. The proprioceptive system consists of specialized receptors in muscles and joints that tell our brain where our body parts are in space and in relation to our surroundings. The visual and vestibular systems are equally important in maintaining balance, while proprioception plays more of a supporting role.

Visually-induced dizziness refers to dizziness that is provoked by visual stimuli. In people who suffer from vertigo and dizziness, the brain eventually tries to ignore information from the vestibular system and relies a lot more on visual information. This over-reliance on visual information to maintain balance makes the brain very vulnerable to visual stimuli that produce a false sense of motion and complex, busy visual scenes. This is why looking at Venetian blinds, ceiling fans, highly patterned rugs, and moving objects causes dizziness. People with visually-induced dizziness also cannot bear to watch 3D, IMAX, or action movies.

Space and motion discomfort is a form of dizziness that is brought on by navigating more complex environments, like moving through crowds, grocery stores, and spaces with busy visual patterns and/or a lot of movement. Moving through our environments requires our vestibular systems to seamlessly integrate visual, vestibular, and proprioceptive information to accurately build a representation of motion. People with vertigo and dizziness become overly reliant on visual information, disrupting this integration, and resulting in space and motion discomfort. We typically navigate our world in a two-dimensional frame; we move forwards, backward, right and left. This 2D navigation relies on visual information. When you introduce a 3D aspect with vertical navigation (e.g., moving up/down stairs, bending over or looking upwards), our brains require more vestibular information.

This is why many people with vestibular migraine and migraine have so much trouble in grocery stores. The many objects on the shelves, and our need to visually search for groceries both horizontally and vertically whilst pushing a cart forward, overwhelms the brain's ability to integrate visual and vestibular information.

Driving also poses a significant challenge for many. Driving over bridges and overpasses produces visual information that one is high above the ground. Driving past a row of trees, concrete barriers, or picket fences creates a distorted sensation of motion. Similarly, large vehicles (e.g., trucks) passing, or crossing traffic can be very disorienting.

Head motion-induced dizziness refers to dizziness caused by head movements. Many people with vestibular migraine and migraine find it discomforting to quickly move their heads. Looking up and down is usually the most uncomfortable. Quick side-to-side head movements can also be quite problematic.

Head motion-induced dizziness is most likely the result of over-prioritization of visual input, and the brain's difficulty in integrating visual, vestibular, and proprioceptive information. When we move our heads quickly, our visual system has to shift focus. This briefly alters visual information and causes disequilibrium if we depend too much on our visual systems to maintain balance. Furthermore, head movements also alter vestibular information (by stimulating the inner ears) and proprioceptive feedback (from the neck muscles).

In normal people, the body sways slightly to attempt to correct inaccurate visual information. In those with visually- and head motion-induced dizziness, the body's fear of losing balance causes the muscles to stiffen. Many people with vestibular migraine subconsciously tighten their neck muscles to avoid turning their heads. Some even do it consciously to avoid feeling dizzy. Instead of turning their heads naturally to look at something, they will often move their upper bodies together with the head and neck as a unit. Over time, this unnatural, Frankenstein-like way of moving about can lead to neck and shoulder problems, making the head motion-induced dizziness worse.

Unsteadiness and a feeling of disequilibrium are not uncommon. People with vestibular migraine often describe walking as though they are drunk, not being able to walk a straight line, and getting dizzy if they turn corners. Some may describe feeling like they are being pulled or pushed in a particular direction while walking. Even though their balance is good, vertigo and dizziness can cause people to become afraid of losing balance, aggravating their dizziness, or falling. This fear drives them to overthink the mechanics of walking which is a normally subconscious process. They essentially succumb to what is called "choking under pressure" (or "the yips") by professional athletes, a well-known phenomenon where great athletes sabotage their performance by allowing anxiety to make them overthink the processes that should be automatic. This often leads to very maladaptive and dysfunctional walking styles, typically very stiff postures with the head and neck stuck in a rigid position and the eyes focused on the ground or looking at a distant object. This abnormal robotic gait actually increases the risk of falling.

Paroxysmal vestibular symptoms refer to brief, transient vestibular symptoms that occur without warning. A variety of vestibular symptoms may occur. The most common complaint I hear is a feeling of the ground moving or dropping, which is often called "elevator drops", "mini earthquake", or "ground shifting". Quick spinning, falling, floating, lightheaded, and tumbling sensations have also been described by my patients. It is important to note that these are interictal, meaning that they do not occur during a migraine attack and are not accompanied by the usual migraine features (headache, photophobia, phonophobia, or visual aura).

Visual height intolerance (VHI) is colloquially known as a fear of heights. This fear of high places was recognized by the ancient Greeks, Romans, and Chinese. Humans are born with an inherent ability to perceive and avoid heights, an obviously important characteristic for our survival as a species. Babies instinctively avoid going near edges where they perceive a "visual cliff". VHI is a preferable term to fear of heights because it distinguishes it from acrophobia. There is a spectrum to VHI. Some degree of VHI is natural, but some have more prominent VHI. About one-third of the general population experiences VHI. On the far end of this spectrum, acrophobia causes marked fear, incapacitating anxiety, and avoidant behavior; some acrophobics can't even go above two floors.

As discussed earlier, the visual system is one of the three pillars that maintain our balance. Part of the visual system's way of detecting motion is by perceiving "retinal slip" – the motion of visual images on the surface of the retina. If we stand on a high ladder, platform or the edge of a cliff, the objects we see become so small that our visual system cannot detect retinal slip. This interferes with our visual system's ability to help us balance, resulting in the dizziness and symptoms of VHI.

VHI is more common in people with migraine, vestibular migraine, anxiety, and depression. Many people with migraine are overly reliant on visual input to maintain balance and are more sensitive to conflicts (mismatch) between sensory channels. The concept of sensory mismatch is discussed in the section on motion sickness.

Motion Sickness

In terms of evolution, motion sickness is an ancient and conserved physiologic response. Many animal species can develop motion sickness, even fish (imagine being a seasick fish!). Motion sickness served a protective function in our animal ancestors. It compelled our ancestors to re-calibrate their bearings or movements if there was conflicting sensory information. If our fish ancestors didn't know which way was up or where the current was taking them, they wouldn't have survived for very long.

Everyone can develop motion sickness under the right conditions. Even the toughest astronaut or Navy seal can be motion-sick if the trigger is powerful enough. It's all a matter of thresholds. In migraine and vestibular migraine, this threshold is lower than that of the general population. It is predominantly driven by genetic predisposition. vulnerability to motion sickness begins in childhood, the earliest sign of the hot migraine brain, and long before any signs of migraine or vestibular migraine manifest. Parents with motion sickness are more likely to have offspring with motion sickness. Motion sickness studies in twins show a high concordance rate [Reavley, 2006]. Hormones also play a big role. Motion sickness is more common in women, and is more severe during menstruation and pregnancy.

The parts of the brain involved in motion sickness (the trigeminal, vestibular, and vagus systems) are the same parts of the brain that are involved in vestibular migraine and migraine. In fact, people with bilateral vestibular failure (a rare condition that causes the loss of function of both inner ears) are immune to motion sickness. Migraine brains are much more susceptible to the ill effects of the sensory conflict underpinning motion sickness.

Serotonin deficiency has a large part to play in this vulnerability to motion sickness as well. Low serotonin levels are found in both migraine and motion sickness. In an elegant study that placed people in a rotating drum to induce motion sickness [Drummond, 2005], tryptophan (used by our bodies to produce serotonin) depletion in people without migraine made them as susceptible to motion sickness as people with migraine. Surprisingly, tryptophan depletion did not worsen motion sickness in people with migraine, possibly because migraine brains are already low in serotonin.

Histamine may play an important role in triggering vomiting in motion sickness. In lab animals, histamine levels in the brain and inner ear rise with motion sickness. Foods high in histamine can also aggravate motion sickness. Furthermore, antihistaminergic medications like meclizine are often used to mitigate motion sickness.

Most people with migraine have some degree of motion sickness throughout life and only experience it when they try to read in a moving car or when they get on boats. In some, motion sickness is more bothersome and they must always be in the front seat or drive, or have to medicate for flights. In others, motion sickness improves in adulthood, but worsens after the onset of vestibular migraine. In another population, motion sickness only begins after vestibular migraine rears its ugly head.

When severe, motion sickness can cause sopite syndrome (from the Latin word *sopire*, which means "to lull to sleep"), which is characterized by excessive yawning, drowsiness, fatigue, apathy, depression, irritability, lack of motivation, sleep disturbances, and a preference to be left alone, which can last for hours to days afterward.

The basis of motion sickness is sensory mismatch, conflict or disagreement between the sensory channels (visual, vestibular and proprioceptive). Motion sickness also arises from a discrepancy between perceived motion signals and the anticipated, internal expectations; in other words, a conflict between what your brain perceives, and what it expects, you will become nauseous.

One form of motion sickness occurs when the visual system reports motion when the vestibular and proprioceptive systems do not. For example, when you are playing a first-person shooter video game, the avatar moves rapidly and your visual system receives information that you are moving. However, the vestibular and proprioceptive systems inform your brain that you are sitting quite still and are not moving about. This sensory conflict causes motion sickness. This is also the basis for simulator or virtual reality (VR) sickness.

The more classical form of motion sickness occurs when the visual system does not report the same motion as the vestibular and proprioceptive systems. When one is in a car, the movements of the vehicle stimulate the vestibular system and the proprioceptive nerves of the skin, muscles, joints, bones, and internal organs. Visual input provides motion information to the brain. Temperature differences (i.e., warmth over the back and buttocks) inform the brain that one is seated. If one is the driver, the brain integrates all this information well, and as the controller of the vehicle, accurately anticipates its movements (e.g., acceleration, deceleration, turns). This harmony between sensory channels, and the expected and perceived motion input explains why most people with migraine or vestibular migraine have no problems driving. As a passenger, one is not able to anticipate the movements of the vehicle as accurately (especially if the driver is slightly insane), resulting in a discrepancy between the expected and perceived motion input. Furthermore, in the back seat, visual information is more limited, resulting in further mismatch between sensory channels. This is why being in the front seat causes less motion sickness than being in the back seat, and why some migraine sufferers must drive and can never be passengers. If one reads or uses the phone in a moving vehicle, the visual information is even more restricted and everything appears more static; this is why reading or using your phone in a car is so triggering for motion sickness.

Psychiatric Disorders

Anxiety & Depression

It is absolutely vital to discuss the connections between anxiety and depression, and vestibular migraine. Many people with vestibular migraine have anxiety and depression, often because of the impact of dizziness and vertigo. Unfortunately, the diagnosis of vestibular migraine is often missed by most healthcare professionals. Their symptoms are attributed to anxiety or depression instead. People are told "It's all from anxiety" or "You are just depressed" and are prescribed antidepressants, or referred to a psychiatrist.

The coexistence of anxiety and depression with migraine is associated with a higher risk of suicide [Breslau, 2012]. The link between anxiety, depression, and migraine is not just mood disturbances arising from a chronic disease. There are common genetic traits that link these conditions.

Poor sleep is a common manifestation of both anxiety and depression. As you can predict, poor sleep leads to worsening of migraine control, which in turn results in more anxiety and/or depression – a veritable vicious cycle.

Migraine control usually leads to an improvement in anxiety, and depression. However, when these mood disorders are severe and do not improve with migraine control, or if they get in the way of adequate migraine control, obtaining the proper treatment is very important. Ignoring depression and anxiety while only focusing on controlling migraine often leads to poor treatment outcomes.

Anxiety

Anxiety is common in children and adults with migraine, and even more so in vestibular migraine. The brain centers responsible for processing balance are closely associated with those mediating fight-or-flight responses. This explains why vertigo causes so much distress, leading to a heightened state of fear and resulting in PPPD and mood disorders. Anxiety causes hypervigilance, increasing one's awareness of dizziness, and leading to even more perceived dizziness. This results in a vicious feed-forward cycle of ever-increasing dizziness and anxiety. Making matters worse, many people with vestibular migraine do not receive a clear diagnosis or explanation for their symptoms, inflaming their burgeoning levels of anxiety with the fear of the unknown.

Anxiety is associated with worsening and chronification of migraine. On the other hand, more frequent attacks of migraine lead to worsening anxiety. Among those with migraine, the presence of depression increases the likelihood of developing anxiety as well. Dysfunctions of the brain's serotonin, dopamine and GABA systems are believed to underlie both conditions.

Often, this subconscious anxiety creates an undercurrent of worry, fear, and symptom hypervigilance. Most say no if you ask them if they are anxious even though they suffer from many symptoms consistent with an anxiety disorder. Symptoms like nervousness, a sense of something bad about to happen, irrational fears, muscle tenseness, being very self-conscious about how others may judge you, elevated heart rate, rapid breathing, fatigue, irritability, trouble sleeping, difficulty concentrating, repetitive and persistent intrusive and upsetting thoughts, and fidgeting behavior can often indicate an underlying anxiety disorder.

Compared to people without migraine, panic attacks are almost 10 times more common among people with migraine.

Panic attacks are 2-3 times more common among people with chronic migraine, compared to episodic migraine. Phobias are also more frequent among those with migraine. Social phobia (now called social anxiety disorder) results in fear/anxiety in social situations, arising from fear of being negatively perceived by others. Agoraphobia (literally fear of the marketplace) refers to anxiety and fear of being in public places where the person has little control.

Some with more severe migraine experience a type of anxiety called *cephalalgiophobia* (literally, fear of headaches) [Gianini, 2013; Peres, 2007]. This fear leads to avoiding anything that could trigger a headache, as well as overusing rescue medications to ward off even the slightest hint of a headache. Similarly, patients with vestibular disorders (especially vestibular migraine) often develop dizzy-phobia, a fear of experiencing even the slightest hint of dizziness. This dizzy-phobia in and of itself can be extremely debilitating. I have seen people who are utterly terrified of leaving their homes, or fearful of sleeping on either side. A significant number of people with migraine also experience anxiety sensitivity, a fear of experiencing anxiety and its related symptoms. This causes many to assiduously avoid circumstances that could possibly provoke migraine, or social situations where embarrassment could potentially occur.

Depression

Depression is twice as common in migraine, compared to the general population. Migraine begets depression and depression begets migraine, which is unsurprising since both conditions are associated with low serotonin levels. Inflammation may also play an important role in both conditions; circulating pro-inflammatory chemicals from your immune cells are the reason you feel down and crummy when you have a cold.

Interictal light sensitivity is worse in people with depression and migraine. Furthermore, depression is linked to subjective cognitive dysfunction, a condition sometimes referred to as pseudo-dementia. People with depression also are more sensitive to pain; those with frequent migraine attacks can find

86

themselves in a vicious cycle where headaches lower their mood, and depression makes them even more vulnerable to headaches.

Similar to anxiety, many deny being depressed when asked "Are you depressed?". However, they display many symptoms of depression. Depression can manifest as a lack of motivation, fatigue, hopelessness, appetite changes, sadness, loss of pleasure in activities that used to make you happy, menstrual abnormalities, and trouble staying asleep. In addition, the negative impact of migraine and all its associated symptoms on quality of life can cause depression; this is referred to as reactive or situational depression (or adjustment disorder). Some of my patients describe being depressed and sad at how vestibular migraine has ruined their lives, and express how much they miss their old lives.

Bipolar Disorder

Bipolar disorder is characterized by fluctuating periods of depression and elevated mood. Over half of people with bipolar disorder have a history of migraine. Bipolar disorder also tends to be more severe in those who have migraine. An underlying genetic predisposition most likely links both conditions. Parental migraine increases the chances of a child developing bipolar disorder. Similarly, a family history of bipolar disorder is a risk factor for migraine [Dresler, 2019].

Bipolar disorder and migraine share several pathophysiological similarities, including higher levels of inflammation, impaired cell energy metabolism, increased levels of oxidative stress, as well as abnormalities in the serotonin, dopamine, and glutamine systems.

Post-Traumatic Stress Disorder (PTSD)

The incidence of PTSD is higher among people with migraine, particularly chronic migraine. Interestingly, a single traumatic event without PTSD does not increase the risk of migraine, and in those without PTSD recurrent trauma is required to elevate migraine risk [Dresler, 2019]. The PTSD prevalence among people with migraine is almost 4-times higher than that of the general population. People with PTSD and migraine tend to have more frequent and severe migraine headaches, compared to people with migraine but not PTSD. One potential reason for this is HPA axis dysfunction in those with PTSD. The most common traumatic events associated with worsening migraine activity include experiencing the loss or injury of a friend or family member, witnessing someone being injured/killed, experiencing a violent attack, vehicular accidents, and natural disasters. If you have both PTSD and migraine, specialized treatment for PTSD could help improve migraine control.

Eating Disorders

There is considerable overlap between migraine and eating disorders. Both typically affect young women, are associated with a high prevalence of depression and anxiety, tend to affect type A personalities, are characterized by altered brain serotonin metabolism, and demonstrate changes in similar brain regions. Three-quarters of people with eating disorders suffer from migraine, and some studies suggest that migraine may precede the onset of eating disorders in vulnerable people.

There are two main eating disorders: anorexia nervosa and bulimia nervosa. Anorexia nervosa is characterized by a driving desire to be thin and avoid gaining weight, as well as food restriction. Some use laxatives, exercise excessively, or force themselves to vomit. Bulimia nervosa is characterized by binge eating followed by purging (either by vomiting or laxative use); most people with bulimia have normal weight.

People with, or at high risk of eating disorders should avoid topiramate (Topamax) for migraine prevention because the appetite-suppressing properties of the drug may worsen the eating disorders.

Neurological Conditions

Alice In Wonderland Syndrome

This unusual neurological phenomenon was discussed in detail in a previous chapter. It can also occur independently of migraine attacks. Most of the Alice in Wonderland symptoms occur spontaneously, without warning, and usually last for a few minutes. For example, I had a patient who would suddenly feel like she was growing taller and taller, and another one who would suddenly see the TV shrink and return to normal size. A few patients of mine find that their Alice in Wonderland Syndrome symptoms are triggered by bright lights; one described how the glare of oncoming headlights would provoke episodes of feeling like he was shrinking behind the steering wheel.

Epilepsy

Migraine and epilepsy share some interesting similarities. Both conditions are essentially due to abnormal excitation of specific regions of the brain. Auras can precede both seizures and migraine. Like migraine, some forms of epilepsy are triggered by menstruation and flashing lights. Finally, anti-epileptic drugs are also effective in controlling migraine.

The prevalence of epilepsy among people with migraine is slightly higher than that of the general population. About 50% of people with both conditions experience a migraine attack following a seizure, but the migraine attack is often overlooked because of the dramatic nature of the seizure. A post-ictal headache refers to a tension-type or migraine headache that develops within 3 hours of a seizure, and usually lasts no more than 72 hours.

Hemicrania epileptica is a headache that lasts seconds to minutes, accompanied by migraine features, that occurs synchronously with a seizure. The headache is on the same side of the brain as the origin of the epileptic discharge, and stops when the seizure ceases.

Migralepsy refers to a very rare condition where a migraine is followed by a seizure within one hour. Some of the visual auras of migraine can be difficult to distinguish from the epileptic aura.

Epileptic vertigo (aka vestibular epilepsy/seizures, or *epilepsia tornado*) is a very rare type of epilepsy that usually affects children. It causes attacks of vertigo that usually last less than a minute, and can be associated with odd sensations in the head, hallucinations, convulsive movements, or transient impairment of consciousness.

Osmophobia

Do you hate the perfume section at department stores? Do you loathe the detergent section? How about your co-worker's cloying perfume? Does cigarette smoke bother you? Do I need to mention the sickening air fresheners in taxis and ride-shares? Are you able to smell something before anyone else can? If you were nodding as you read that, you likely suffer from migraine, or have a predisposition to it. The hot migraine brain is sensitive to lights, sounds, and smells.

Many people with migraine have remarkably sensitive olfactory senses. Some of my patients can smell almost anything before other people. Some can even detect when milk is about to go bad! More than half of people with migraine describe sensitivity to odors or osmophobia (an intolerance of smells). Children with osmophobia have a higher risk of developing migraine later in life. Similar to light and sound sensitivity, osmophobia occurs both during and in between migraine attacks. Odors can trigger attacks as well.

In migraine brains, the olfactory (odor-processing) system and brainstem pain processing centers are abnormally well-connected. These shared network connections can explain why migraine patients suffer from osmophobia during attacks, are sensitive to smells between attacks, and find that odors trigger their attacks. In fact, functional MRI studies in people with migraine show that the parts of the brain that respond to pain also react to odors. The olfactory system is also very closely related to the limbic system, the part of the brain that controls emotions, behavior, motivation, and memory, explaining why people with migraine who suffer from osmophobia are at higher risk of depression, anxiety, and even suicidal tendencies.

Sensory Symptoms

It is not uncommon for people with migraine to experience sensory symptoms like numbness, tingling, electrical sensations, heat, or cold even when they are not experiencing an attack. It is important to be evaluated by a neurologist to ensure that other conditions (e.g., neuropathy, spinal cord problems) are not causing these symptoms.

Vascular Disorders

There is a link between migraine and vascular disorders. At this time, there is only limited research regarding vascular disorders and vestibular migraine and as such, data has to be extrapolated from migraine studies.

Raynaud's Phenomenon

Raynaud's phenomenon is a condition characterized by constriction of blood vessels in the extremities, resulting in reduced blood flow. The hands are typically affected. When exposed to cold or with stress, the fingers or hands become numb and pale, then bluish. Pain often accompanies these changes. As blood flow returns, a burning sensation occurs, and the affected area turns red. It can occur in isolation, or be part of autoimmune conditions like systemic lupus erythematosus (SLE) or scleroderma. Sometimes, Raynaud's may occur following injuries to the hand, prolonged use of vibrating tools, and smoking.

Compared to unaffected people, those with Raynaud's are three times more likely to have migraine, and people with migraine are four times more likely to have Raynaud's. People with Raynaud's and migraine are more likely to experience chest pain compared to those with Raynaud's without migraine. It is important to avoid medications that constrict blood vessels if you have Raynaud's phenomenon, which may narrow the vessels even further. Of particular concern in migraine is the rescue medication dihydroergotamine (DHE). Other medications that may worsen Raynaud's include triptans and beta-blockers.

Stroke & Cardiovascular Disease

People with migraine appear to be twice as likely to be at risk of long-term ischemic stroke, compared to those without migraine [Spector, 2010]. A slightly higher risk of long-term cardiovascular disease is also present in migraine [Mahmoud, 2018].

In women below the age of 45, The risk of stroke is twice as high in migraine with aura (compared to those without migraine). The stroke risk in migraine without aura, and in men is much less clear. A higher number of migraine attacks (more than 12 per year) is linked to a higher risk of stroke [MacClellan, 2007]. Smoking increases the risk of stroke and cardiovascular disease significantly [Monteith, 2015]. Contraceptives with higher estrogen levels also elevate the stroke risk significantly in women with migraine with aura.

The exact reason the risk of stroke and cardiovascular disease is higher in people with migraine is not clear. One theory suggests that cortical spreading depression is associated with changes in blood flow to the brain; as the wave spreads, the brief increase in blood flow is followed by a reduction in blood flow, which may result in strokes in vulnerable brain regions. Other theories suggest a possible link to increased "stickiness" of platelets, genetic predisposition to strokes, or an enhanced tendency for blood clot formation caused by inflammation.

Since people with migraine are at higher risk of stroke and cardiovascular disease, it is imperative to take proactive measures to lower that risk. The first (and most obvious) step is to stop smoking. The second is to screen for high cholesterol and hypertension. If you have high cholesterol or blood pressure, work with your primary care doctor to control them. Higher estrogen levels may also increase the risk of strokes and cardiovascular disease since estrogen increases the blood's propensity to clot. As such, women prescribed contraceptive therapies may need to avoid using high-dose estrogen pills. Low-dose (25 micrograms or less of ethynyl estradiol) does not appear to increase the risk of stroke or cardiovascular disease [Martin, 2006]. With particular cardiovascular or stroke risks, daily antiplatelet medications (e.g., aspirin, clopidogrel) may be required (and interestingly, can lead to reduced migraine attacks); such medications should be managed by your primary care physician due to the risk of bleeding. Regular exercise, stress management, and a healthy diet are vital to mitigating cardiovascular disease and stroke risk.

Chapter 6: Misdiagnoses & Mimics

Better a murder than a misdiagnosis
House, MD

This chapter will help clear up some confusion about conditions that have similar symptoms to vestibular migraine, overlap, or even co-exist with vestibular migraine. These conditions often cause confusion for both physicians and patients. Vestibular migraine may be misdiagnosed as one of these conditions, or missed completely if one of these conditions is present. On the other hand, these conditions may be mistaken for vestibular migraine.

At times, investigations and tests like MRI or CT scans may reveal incidental findings that are erroneously blamed for a person's symptoms, even though the person has vestibular migraine. Understanding the salient features of these disorders can help illuminate the differences between them and vestibular migraine, and avoid the pitfalls of misdiagnosis.

Benign Paroxysmal Positional Vertigo (BPPV)

BPPV is the most common cause of vertigo among adults. It typically affects people over the age of 60, but anyone can develop BPPV. This condition results from displaced otolith crystals from the utricle of the inner ear that wander into the semicircular canals, causing bursts of vertigo when the head is moved in the direction of the affected canal. The vertigo is typically short-lived, lasting less than a minute, and can be accompanied by nausea but very rarely vomiting.

In most, this loose crystal often rolls into the posterior semicircular canal, which detects movements that tilt the head backward or forwards. As a consequence, vertigo occurs when a person engages in activities that cause the head to move backward or forwards. Lying down and getting out of bed are the most typical triggers for vertigo – patients often note that the attacks of vertigo are most severe when getting out of bed in the morning.

Other activities that trigger vertigo include turning in bed, lying down in a dentist's or hair stylist's chair, looking upwards, and bending over.

BPPV is more common in people with migraine and vestibular migraine. One hypothesis is that migraine results in microscopic inflammatory damage to the inner ears. Causing diagnostic confusion, vestibular migraine can sometimes cause positional vertigo.

There are several features that can help differentiate the two conditions. Firstly, BPPV causes a brief burst of vertigo when the head is moved. Vestibular migraine usually causes vertigo as long as the triggering position is maintained. Secondly, BPPV episodes are not usually accompanied by migraine features like a headache, light and sound sensitivity, or visual aura. Attacks of positional vertigo accompanied by these migraine symptoms are more characteristic of vestibular migraine.

It is important to distinguish both conditions since the treatment for either is different. If the cause of your vertigo is BPPV, the treatment consists of maneuvers to get rid of the loose crystal (Chapter 17). If the cause of your positional vertigo is vestibular migraine, the treatment is usually a rescue medication. Using migraine rescue meds for BPPV wouldn't accomplish much.

Annie's vestibular migraine had been superbly controlled for two years on nortriptyline. She called my office one day, extremely upset because she had violent spinning vertigo as she got out of bed that morning. "The vestibular migraine is back!" she exclaimed. I was mystified as to why it would suddenly reappear and arranged for her to see me the following day. As we spoke, I realized that it was most likely BPPV. I performed the Dix-Hallpike maneuver which caused the typical vertigo and nystagmus, confirming my suspicion. I then treated her by performing the Epley maneuver to dislodge the loose otolith crystal. It turned out that her vertigo was due to BPPV and not a recurrence of vestibular migraine.

As discussed before, many people with dizziness develop neck and shoulder problems related to the stiff posture adopted to reduce their dizziness. Often, vestibular migraine is misdiagnosed as cervicogenic dizziness (literally "dizziness originating from the neck"). This is because a patient often undergoes extensive testing, which often includes a neck MRI. Since most people have some degree of neck arthritis (especially older adults), their vestibular symptoms are erroneously blamed on the neck since everything else is normal.

Cervicogenic dizziness is a somewhat controversial entity, but there is evidence to support dizziness and vestibular symptoms caused by neck disorders. It typically occurs in patients with a history of neck injury (e.g., whiplash), and degenerative cervical spinal disease. Cervicogenic dizziness is due to disturbances of proprioceptive input from neck muscle receptors [Devaraja, 2018]. In other words, damage or injury to the nerves that detect movement and neck position results in erroneous information being conveyed to the brain regarding head and neck movements, causing dizziness. Patients with this condition usually describe dizziness when the head and neck assume certain positions.

Confusion with vestibular migraine arises when a person experiences both neck pain and dizziness. Neck pain can be a manifestation of migraine, and neck pain from non-migraine causes (e.g., degenerative spine disease) can aggravate migraine attacks. As discussed before, positional vertigo/dizziness may occur in vestibular migraine as well. Differentiating both conditions is important because the treatments are different.

In cervicogenic dizziness, there is usually a history of neck pain or injury preceding the onset of dizziness [Magnusson, 2016]. There are tender points on the neck, and pain can radiate to the shoulders and head [Devaraja, 2018, Magnusson, 2016]. The dizziness is episodic and is triggered by neck movements [Devaraja, 2018]. Usually, the dizziness is not accompanied by migraine features. Examination and vestibular testing in patients with cervicogenic dizziness are normal [Devaraja, 2018;

Magnusson, 2016]. Cervicogenic dizziness, in my experience, is much less common than vestibular migraine, and BPPV; however, it should be recognized to ensure timely and appropriate treatment.

Treatment for cervicogenic dizziness consists of neck therapy (a specialized form of physical therapy to address disorders affecting the musculoskeletal system of the neck), dry needling, massage, or trigger point injections. Sometimes, injecting a mixture of steroids and lidocaine (or a similar agent) around small cervical joints under X-ray guidance may be considered. In some cases, surgery may be considered.

Chiari I Malformation

People with Chiari malformations are born with a smaller, tighter space in the back of skull, causing part of the cerebellum to protrude through the bottom of the skull. Type I Chiari malformation is the most common of the Chiari malformations; it is defined as the descent of the cerebellar tonsils at least 5 mm past the foramen magnum (the opening of the skull to the spine).

Symptoms are caused when the cerebellum, brainstem, or structures in the back of the skull are squished. These symptoms typically appear insidiously in the late teens and 20s. Patients commonly describe occipital and neck pain provoked by physical activity or maneuvers that increase pressure inside the skull. For example, coughing or straining (i.e., bearing down like when you are constipated or lifting a heavy object) can trigger headaches and vertigo. Patients with Chiari I malformation can also experience imbalance, vertigo, nystagmus, hearing loss, ear fullness, and tinnitus. Rarely, drop attacks (suddenly falling due to loss of muscle tone without any loss of consciousness) may occur. Infrequent symptoms include hoarseness, difficulty swallowing, tongue weakness, arm pain, arm tingling or arm numbness.

People with symptomatic Chiari malformations should be referred for neurosurgical evaluation for posterior fossa decompression surgery (where the back of the skull is removed to allow more room). However, it is important to note that Chiari type I malformations may also be asymptomatic, and discovered incidentally when the patient undergoes MRI for dizziness or vertigo arising from an unrelated disorder.

A careful history is essential to determine if the Chiari malformation is truly symptomatic, or if another disorder is causing a person's dizziness and vertigo. The lack of headache, neck pain, or vestibular symptoms provoked by straining or maneuvers that increase intracranial pressure argues against symptomatic Chiari malformation. Generally, such patients should not be subjected to the risks of surgery.

I cannot emphasize this enough. I have seen several patients with vestibular migraine, who have asymptomatic Chiari I malformations on MRI but underwent posterior fossa decompression surgery. Unfortunately, their vertigo and dizziness did not improve after the surgery because the Chiari malformation was not the cause of their symptoms. This is a serious surgery that can result in significant complications.

Robert was one such person. He saw another neurosurgeon for a second surgery because the first was apparently unhelpful. Unfortunately, the second surgery caused serious damage to his cerebellum, resulting in permanent gait imbalance. When he saw me, I diagnosed him with vestibular migraine, and with the right medications, his vertigo episodes subsided. However, there was no fix for his balance problems. Imagine how his quality of life would have been if he hadn't undergone unnecessary surgery!

Concussion & Postconcussive Syndrome

A concussion is a mild traumatic brain injury that disrupts brain activities without causing detectable structural damage on conventional imaging. Headache and dizziness are very common symptoms of concussion. Other symptoms include light and sound sensitivity, nausea, tinnitus, cognitive dysfunction (including trouble with memory and attention), problems with visual focus, sleep changes, depression, anxiety, and irritability.

These symptoms are often aggravated by alcohol use. As you can see, there is a huge overlap with vestibular migraine.

The symptoms of a concussion resolve within 14 days in about three-quarters of patients and within 3 months in 90%. If symptoms persist beyond 14 days, it is called postconcussive syndrome. The majority of postconcussive syndrome symptoms are gone within 3 months. The term persistent postconcussive syndrome applies to symptoms that continue beyond this 3-month mark. If a concussion causes a person to lose consciousness, it increases the risk of postconcussive syndrome.

Of course, following a concussion, a brain CT and MRI are very important. Remember that the goal of the CT and MRI are not to diagnose a concussion, but to rule out potentially emergent or urgent injuries. A CT helps detect acute bleeding or skull fractures. A brain MRI helps evaluate for injury to the brain tissue. If the MRI is "normal" or "unremarkable", it does not mean that a concussion did not occur. After a concussion, the direct injuries to the brain are often invisible and undetectable on conventional MRI. This is because the injury occurs on a cellular and tissue level (e.g., microscopic tears to nerves, disruption of the cell protein architecture, and breaking of connections between neurons). In people who are predisposed to migraine, a concussion often leads to the development of migraine.

If a person develops vestibular migraine following a concussion, treatments aimed at migraine will be useful. However, if a person has postconcussive syndrome *and* vestibular migraine, care will often need to include specialists in traumatic brain injury and concussion to optimize the outcome. This may include cognitive therapy, psychological counseling, physical therapy, vision therapy, and the appropriate medications.

Mal De Débarquement Syndrome (MDDS)

MDDS is a fairly uncommon neurological condition characterized by a pervasive rocking, swaying and/or bobbing sensation (as if one is on a boat in choppy waters). People with MDDS often describe feeling that they are constantly in motion.

The hallmark and most unusual feature of this condition is that the continuous sensation of motion improves when a person is in a moving vehicle (car, boat, plane, etc.) but almost immediately returns when the vehicle stops or when the person disembarks. There are two types of MDDS. *Motion-triggered MDDS* is the classic form of MDDS, where the sensation of motion begins after one has been on a cruise, boat ride, long car ride, or flight. *Non-motion triggered MDDS* is sometimes called "spontaneous onset MDDS" but I find that to be a bit of a misnomer since there is usually an identifiable trigger. Many non-motion triggers have been described in MDDS including virtual reality, stress, pregnancy, medical illness, and other vestibular disorders. In my experience, the most common cause of non-motion-triggered MDDS is vestibular migraine.

MDDS typically affects women after the age of 50; it is less common in men and younger women. It can be associated with other symptoms, including brain fog, difficulty with busy visual scenes, blurry vision, feeling off balance, heaviness in the legs, and unsteadiness when walking (sometimes called trampoline walking). The pervasive rocking sensation of MDDS can be aggravated by stress, menses, moving around too much, or darkness. It can be more pronounced when a person lies down, leading to significant trouble with insomnia; I have even seen patients who have nightmares of being tossed around in the ocean.

There is a strong relationship between MDDS with migraine and vestibular migraine. Up to half of people with MDDS have a history of migraine. As you can see, the symptoms and factors that aggravate MDDS are similar to those for vestibular migraine, which can lead to some confusion between the two entities. In my experience, people with vestibular migraine and MDDS tend to have more severe dizziness and suffer a greater impact from it initially, but remarkably, tend to have a much better response to treatment compared to people with MDDS without vestibular migraine. I discuss MDDS in much more detail in my book, *Disembark*.

Mast Cell Activation Syndrome (MCAS)

Mast cell activation disorders are a constellation of disorders that are characterized by the accumulation of dysfunctional mast cells, and/or the abnormal release of chemicals produced by mall cells. MCAS is a mast cell activation disorder.

It is characterized by flushing, hives, easy bruising, itchiness, burning sensations, diarrhea and/or constipation, feeling faint, nasal congestion, chronic coughing or wheezing, and dermatographism ("skin writing" - an allergic-like reaction that causes a red wheal to form when the skin is scratched).

It can occur in people with migraine and vestibular migraine; the link between mast cells and neurogenic inflammation certainly supports this relationship. However, it is not clear if people with MCAS have a higher incidence of migraine or vestibular migraine. The diagnosis can be challenging to make and may require consultation with an immunologist.

Menière's Disease

Vestibular migraine is often misdiagnosed as Menière's disease. This is not unsurprising since Menière's disease is the better-known of the two conditions, and medical school curricula teach Menière's disease but not vestibular migraine. Confusing matters even more, both conditions involve ear symptoms (like ear pressure, tinnitus, and muffled hearing) and vertigo attacks.

Menière's disease refers to a condition that causes endolymphatic fluid to build up, swelling up parts of the inner ear responsible for hearing and balance. This swelling results in ear pressure, tinnitus (usually a low-pitched rumble or roar), and muffled hearing. When the pressure finally causes the fluid to burst through the membrane that contains it, vertigo ensues. The breach eventually heals, and the symptoms start again when the fluid pressure builds up.

The cause of Menière's disease is unknown but believed to be due to a combination of genetic and environmental factors. It is not a common disease, and is believed to affect 8.2 to 157 per 100,000 individuals per year [Espinosa-Sanchez, 2016]. The attacks of Meniere's disease are typically characterized by one-sided ear pressure or fullness, muffled hearing, and a low-pitched rumbling or roaring tinnitus followed by vertigo. These vertigo attacks last between 20 minutes to 12 hours [Espinosa-Sanchez, 2016]. It is important to note that this classic triad of vertigo, tinnitus, and hearing loss only occurs in 40% of patients [Belinchon, 2012]; it is not uncommon to experience episodic vertigo without ear symptoms in the first year [Pyykko, 2013]. Hearing tests are important to identify asymmetric low-frequency hearing loss or fluctuating hearing loss – vital clues to making the diagnosis.

As you can see, Menière's disease and vestibular migraine share similar symptoms, and can often overlap. Complicating matters, there is a higher prevalence of migraine among Menière's disease patients (about one-third) [Shin, 2013]. There is also a bidirectional relationship between migraine and Menière's disease: people with migraine have a two-fold risk of developing Menière's disease and vice versa. Furthermore, migraines may be provoked by Menière's disease attacks, resulting in the appearance of episodes of vertigo accompanied by migraine symptoms. Salty foods, chocolate, alcohol, and caffeine, which are migraine triggers, also provoke Menière's disease episodes. Sometimes, a person may have both Menière's disease and vestibular migraine. In my experience, optimizing migraine treatment for people with both conditions can often lead to improvement.

How do we distinguish vestibular migraine from Menière's disease? Firstly, the ear symptoms in Menière's disease tend to be one-sided (unilateral) while those in vestibular migraine tend to be bilateral. Secondly, Menière's disease usually results in low-frequency hearing loss in one ear; the absence of any hearing loss with repeated audiograms over a few years makes Menière's disease highly unlikely. Thirdly, the presence of photophobia and phonophobia during vertigo attacks suggests vestibular migraine rather than Menière's disease. Fourthly, vestibular migraine is much more likely if the duration of the vertigo attacks is more than 12 hours.

Of course, in real life, there can be a lot of overlapping and inconsistency in symptoms. My professors often reminded me in medical school that our patients don't read and follow our textbooks. I have seen a small but growing number of patients that fit the clinical picture of Meniere's disease but remarkably improved with migraine treatment.

Multiple Sclerosis (MS)

MS is one of the diagnoses that is brought up almost every time a person presents with unexplained neurological symptoms. It is the boogeyman of neurological diagnoses. Many patients I diagnose with vestibular migraine are worried about MS, partly because they were told "it could be MS" after evaluations for their vertigo and dizziness were unremarkable.

MS is an autoimmune disease that affects the myelin (insulating covering of nerves) in the brain and spinal cord. It typically manifests as optic neuritis (painful vision loss in one eye), and sensory changes or weakness in the legs or arms. Infrequently, vertigo and imbalance may occur if MS affects certain parts of the brainstem and cerebellum.

Typically, there can be vertigo or imbalance lasting for a few days if an acute MS lesion affects certain parts of the brainstem or cerebellum. At times, a person may experience short spells of vertigo or imbalance when a "short circuit" occurs inside an MS plaque that involves vestibular structures in the brain. MS does not cause recurrent episodes of vertigo and dizziness accompanied by migraine features.

MS can be easily diagnosed with a brain and spinal cord MRI. There are characteristic lesions on the MRI that can help nail the diagnosis. Now, it is important to mention that non-specific MRI findings (which are "spots" in the white matter of the brain, called "subcortical FLAIR hyperintense lesions") can be seen in people with migraine. In people with hypertension, similar "spots" can be seen on MRI, and are referred to as "chronic ischemic microvascular disease" – the radiologic term for tiny silent strokes. These often cause confusion because radiologists often mention MS or demyelinating disease in their reports. This is because radiologists don't see the patients, and have to provide a broad interpretation of these MRI findings to help the ordering physician.

However, the MRI lesions of MS are distinct, and different from these incidental findings. A study from the Netherlands showed that the MRI "spots" of migraine do not worsen over time, or cause neurological damage. On the other hand, MS lesions almost always worsen over time.

Perilymph Fistula

Perilymph fistula is a very rare condition caused by leakage of perilymph (the fluid surrounding the membranous labyrinth of the inner ear) at the round or oval window. Symptoms include vertigo, imbalance, tinnitus, fluctuating hearing, ear pressure, and aural fullness. These symptoms may fluctuate, with good and bad days. In some cases, pressure-maneuvers like straining, can aggravate these symptoms (which may also happen in Chiari malformations). Cognitive difficulties may occur in some.

Head trauma is a common cause of perilymph fistula. The similarity of symptoms between perilymph fistula, vestibular migraine and concussion can lead to a lot of confusion and misdiagnosis. Other causes of perilymph fistula include acoustic trauma (exposure to very loud sounds), barotrauma (from flying, diving, or scuba diving), forceful sneezing or coughing, stapedectomy surgery (for otosclerosis), and congenital abnormalities.

Perilymph fistula is a controversial disorder in otolaryngology. It was over-diagnosed before vestibular migraine was more well-recognized. Some doubt its existence because of this history. I believe that it is a real but rare condition. Tests that can help with the diagnosis include the fistula test, audiometry, and electrocochleography. Surgical correction can be considered if it is present.

Persistent Postural Perceptual Dizziness (PPPD)

PPPD is a common neuro-vestibular cause of chronic dizziness. It is typically triggered by an event like severe stress, a serious medical problem, a fall, or vertigo, that throws off the brain's neurotransmitter milieu and chemistry, resulting in a constant state of dizziness.

It is not exclusively caused by vestibular migraine, but often coexists with it; over half of my vestibular migraine patients also have PPPD. PPPD is characterized by constant dizziness (e.g., lightheadedness, disorientation, discombobulation, feeling "off") that is more noticeable when upright and moving around. The dizziness is often aggravated by visual stimuli and head movements. Busy visual environments, driving in heavy traffic, walking in crowds, walking on uneven surfaces, moving the head around too much or too quickly, bending over, and looking up usually aggravate the dizziness.

PPPD is often accompanied by significant anxiety, and sometimes depression. It is often responsible for the constant dizziness experienced by those with vestibular migraine. PPPD and vestibular migraine often form an unholy alliance – vestibular migraine attacks drive PPPD, and the dizziness from PPPD provokes more attacks. There can be a lot of confusion between PPPD and vestibular migraine. I have seen patients who were diagnosed with PPPD only but have both vestibular migraine and PPPD, and I have seen patients diagnosed with vestibular migraine who actually only have PPPD. The distinction between the two can be confusing, particularly if someone has both!

In PPPD without vestibular migraine, a person tends to experience fairly constant dizziness that sometimes temporarily increases when exposed to certain stimuli. In PPPD with vestibular migraine, a person tends to experience a constant baseline level dizziness with superimposed "spikes" of vestibular migraine attacks. I find it useful to distinguish PPPD *without* vestibular migraine from PPPD *with* vestibular migraine. Migraine treatments are often useful in controlling PPPD when vestibular migraine is present and driving it. More PPPD-specific treatments (e.g., vestibular rehabilitation therapy, antidepressants, benzodiazepines) are more effective for those who have PPPD not directly driven by vestibular migraine.

Postural Orthostatic Tachycardia Syndrome (POTS)

POTS is a disorder that affects the autonomic nervous system, which controls blood pressure, heart rate, breathing rate, digestion, urination, and defecation. It used to be called by many other names including mitral valve prolapse syndrome, chronic orthostatic intolerance, and neurocirculatory asthenia.

Symptoms of POTS include dizziness with standing, fatigue, palpitations, exercise intolerance, cognitive difficulties, fainting, blurry vision, trouble breathing, leg heaviness, and an unusual mottling discoloration in the legs when standing (believed to be due to poor circulation). It can be mild in some patients but in others it is severe enough to interfere with their jobs and family life.

The diagnosis of POTS requires:

• An increase in heart rate of at least 30 beats per minute within 10 minutes of going from a lying position to standing (patients aged 20 and older). For children aged 12-19, the heart rate increase should be over 40 beats per minute.

• Symptoms get worse with upright posture, and improve with lying down.

• Symptoms lasting for at least 6 months

Tilt table testing, and autonomic testing are needed to ascertain the diagnosis. Laboratory testing, imaging, and other investigations may be undertaken to evaluate for disorders that can mimic POTS.

There is a strong correlation between POTS and migraine; over one-third of patients with POTS have migraine. POTS can co-exist or be confused for other vestibular disorders, especially vestibular migraine, due to the overlap, and similarity of symptoms between the two conditions. It can be even more confusing if a person has both POTS and vestibular migraine. It can take an experienced otoneurologist and a specialist in autonomic disorders to clearly diagnose both conditions.

Spontaneous Intracranial Hypotension (SIH)

SIH, sometimes called spinal fluid leak, is an underdiagnosed and under-recognized condition. A slow, insidious leak of spinal fluid from the lower spine results in a drop in the fluid pressure inside the skull, resulting in engorgement and stretching of blood vessels surrounding the brain, traction of the pain-sensitive meninges (brain covering), and sagging of the brain.

What makes SIH extremely tricky to diagnose is that it can cause a host of symptoms, including dizziness, tinnitus, hearing loss, alterations of taste, neck pain, brain fog, a pulling sensation in the head, heaviness in the head, nausea, light sensitivity, and blurry vision. The headache and symptoms worsen when a person is upright and improve upon lying down; the longer a person remains upright, the worse the symptoms are. In serious cases, the brain sags so much due to the low pressure, that it causes double vision (from pressure on the nerves that control eye movements), and slowed breathing and heart rate (due to pressure on the brainstem). Very rarely, coma can occur.

SIH can occur in people who have undergone back surgery, lumbar puncture, or epidural anesthesia because these procedures breach the dura (covering of the spinal cord), allowing spinal fluid to leak out. Sometimes, a dural tear may occur during exercise, particularly weight-lifting exercises with fast ballistic movements (e.g., clean n' jerk). People with disorders that affect the integrity of connective tissue (e.g., Ehlers-Danlos syndrome, Marfan's syndrome) are at higher risk of developing SIH because the dura is weaker; people with these disorders are typically tall, double-jointed, and very flexible. Spinal bone spurs, which occur in degenerative spine disease, can pierce the dura and cause SIH. Tarlov cysts are spinal fluid-filled cysts located at the nerve roots where they exit the spinal cord; if a cyst ruptures, fluid leakage and SIH can occur.

The combination of symptoms can lead to misdiagnosis as migraine. It is important to recognize SIH because its treatment is very different from that of migraine. SIH is diagnosed based on a patient's symptoms, and the appropriate imaging findings. A brain MRI may show evidence of SIH, but such findings may not be present in about one-third of cases. A spine MRI, or myelography (real-time study of the movement of contrast in the spinal fluid space) can help identify where the leak is. It is very important to be evaluated by an experienced neuro-radiologist as small or fast leaks could be easily missed. Once diagnosed, a blood patch or fibrin glue can be applied to seal up the leak.

Superior Canal Dehiscence Syndrome (SCDS)

SCDS is a rare but distinct and fascinating condition. It is characterized by abnormal thinning or loss of a small area of skull bone that covers the superior semicircular canal of the inner ear resulting in abnormal transmission of sound and pressure to this canal. Symptoms include pulsatile tinnitus (hearing one's heartbeat in the affected ear), vertigo triggered by certain sounds (not just a sensitivity to all noise), and vertigo provoked by straining.

Despite having low-frequency hearing loss on audiological testing, people with SCDS are extra sensitive to specific noises. For example, a patient of mine described being able to hear the electrical humming of lamps and lights. A physician I know had a patient who could other people's stomachs growling. Another interesting symptom is an increased sensitivity to self-generated noises. Some describe their voices, breathing, and chewing as being too loud. Others can hear their joints creak, and their footsteps stomping on the ground while walking. Perhaps the most fascinating example of this sensitivity to self-generated noises is hearing one's eyes move, described to me by a patient as a "swoosh" like a race car zipping by.

Vestibular tests can provide important clues about the presence of SCDS. A temporal bone CT (not a general brain CT or an MRI) helps identify the area of abnormally thin or absent temporal bone. Surgical repair can be pursued if the symptoms cause significant problems.

Vestibular Neuritis

Vestibular neuritis (sometimes called vestibular neuronitis) is caused by a viral infection of the vestibular nerve, which is the nerve that conveys balance information from the inner ear to the brain. The most common virus that causes vestibular neuritis is Herpes Simplex Virus type 1 (HSV-1), the same virus that causes cold sores. It is uncommon in children, and makes up about 6% of adult emergency department admissions for vertigo [Tarnutzer, 2011]. The term labyrinthitis is used when hearing loss occurs with vertigo.

Typically, people with vestibular neuritis will experience symptoms of an upper-respiratory illness (cough, fever, runny nose, etc.) a few days before, or at the onset of vertigo or severe imbalance. The vertigo usually lasts for about 2-3 days, before it subsides and is followed by a period of feeling off balance, and disoriented which can last for several weeks.

Vestibular neuritis does not cause repeated attacks of vertigo over months or years. It is typically a single attack of vertigo followed by a period of dizziness (and sometimes triggers PPPD). Vestibular migraine, however, causes recurrent attacks of vertigo (accompanied by migraine features) over months or years.

The treatment for vestibular neuritis is a course of steroids. A short treatment of anti-nausea agents can be considered. A person may use benzodiazepines or meclizine to reduce the vertigo, but it is vital to remember NOT to use such medications for more than 2-3 days. After vestibular neuritis, the brain needs to adapt to the loss of inner ear function and reorganize the balance system (a process called central compensation). These medications impede central compensation and will cause a person to feel off balance and dizzy for a very long time. On the other hand, vestibular rehabilitation therapy enhances central compensation and should be started as soon as possible after vestibular neuritis.

Vestibular Schwannoma

Vestibular schwannomas are benign tumors arising from the cells that form the covering of the vestibular nerves. It used to be called acoustic neuroma, but the term vestibular schwannoma is more accurate and preferred.

Most cases are diagnosed in people aged between 30 and 60. The typical history is a slowly progressively one-sided hearing loss and tinnitus. It can be accompanied by vestibular symptoms, usually imbalance and dizziness, but may include vertigo infrequently. Larger tumors may affect surrounding structures, and cause facial weakness, and headaches. Very rarely, if the tumor grows unchecked and compresses the brainstem, more severe and potentially life-threatening manifestations may occur; such situations are extremely rare since most people will get an MRI long before the condition progresses that far. In rare situations, it is an emergency if there is bleeding into the tumor.

Vestibular schwannomas usually arise sporadically but can be associated with a genetic condition called neurofibromatosis type-2. Some have suggested a link to prior radiation, and possibly frequent cell phone usage but there is not strong scientific evidence to support the connection.

Hearing tests may indicate unilateral hearing loss, which then prompts further evaluation with a brain MRI that confirms the presence of a vestibular schwannoma. In people with vestibular migraine, small vestibular schwannomas are usually found incidentally when they undergo brain MRIs.

The treatment for vestibular schwannoma varies, due to their somewhat unpredictable nature. Most are slow-growing and can remain dormant for many years. In rare cases, they may grow at a faster rate. Due to the slow-growing and benign nature of the tumor, most are observed with serial MRIs (repeated every 6 to 12 months). In older adults, this approach is best, especially for very small tumors because they may not grow at all. Surgery can be considered to control tumor growth to preserve hearing and the function of other cranial nerves. Stereotactic radiation can also be considered to control tumor growth. You should consult a neuro-otologist to decide which treatment approach is best.

Chapter 7: COVID-19

We were standing on one side of a massive river of uncertainty and hardship... We're now seeing the other side of the river.

Christine Lagarde, European Central Bank President

The first edition of this book was written and published at the beginning of the COVID-19 pandemic in 2020. At that time, very little was known about what vestibular symptoms occurred in COVID-19 or the impact of SARS-CoV-2 infection on vestibular disorders. Since then, we have learned more about how COVID-19, long COVID, and the COVID vaccination may affect vestibular and migraine disorders.

As you probably understand, there are many, many symptoms that can occur in COVID-19 and it will take another book to just cover the neurological manifestations of this disease. In keeping with the theme of this book, I will focus on vestibular, otologic, and headache symptoms of COVID-19. We will divide this chapter into sections that discuss acute COVID-19 infection, long COVID, and COVID-19 vaccination.

Acute COVID-19

Headaches are very common in acute COVID-19 infection with evidence that the virus attacks the trigeminal nerve endings in the oral cavity, scalp, eyes, ears, and meninges. Interestingly, headaches during acute infection may predict a less severe disease course [Caronna, 2022]. The headaches are usually frontal and bilateral, and often described as a pressing sensation. It can be associated with light and noise sensitivity, or nausea. Some patients also experience neck pain. The headache of acute COVID-19 infection is typically due to meningeal inflammation and irritation. It can be aggravated by coughing, sneezing, bearing down, or bending over. This headache usually lasts for several days to two weeks. In about half of patients, acetaminophen and non-steroidal anti-inflammatory drugs are enough to relieve it.

Other treatment options include nerve blocks. People with migraine often experience an increase in migraine attacks with acute COVID-19 infection.

Vestibular symptoms in acute COVID-19 are also common during the acute infection. About 50% of patients describe dizziness an average of 3 days into the illness. In most, it is a non-specific dizziness that occurs during any acute viral infection; most people feel somewhat "off" when they are sick. This lasts a few days and improves as the infection subsides. Those with vestibular migraine often experience worsening of their symptoms during acute COVID-19 infections. This is similar to how vestibular migraine symptoms may flare up from any acute infection (e.g., common cold, flu, urinary tract infection) or physical stress (e.g., surgery) and is most likely the consequence of systemic inflammation. Using your migraine rescue medications during this time can be helpful but if the flare-up is severe, other medications (e.g., benzodiazepines) may be considered.

Other vestibular disorders may also be caused by COVID-19. There is emerging evidence that benign paroxysmal positional vertigo (BPPV) may occur following the infection [Picciotti, 2021], most likely because of inflammation in the inner ear. BPPV usually occurs within 1-2 weeks of the infection and can be treated using the relevant maneuvers (see Chapter 17). At times, SARS-CoV2 has been known to cause vestibular neuritis or labyrinthitis. Very rarely, COVID-19 may result in cerebellitis (cerebellar inflammation), labyrinthine hemorrhage (bleeding in the inner ear), or strokes involving the brainstem or cerebellum. If you experience vertigo or loss of balance that is atypical of your usual vestibular migraine attacks, or any new neurological symptoms, go to the nearest emergency department immediately.

Autonomic involvement in acute COVID-19 is not uncommon and can cause dizziness, typically a lightheadedness, a feeling of faintness, or fainting. Tachycardia (rapid heart rate) can be persistent, episodic, or provoked by certain triggers (e.g., exercise, standing up). Orthostatic hypotension refers to drops in blood pressure with standing or getting up from a seated or lying position. Checking your heart rate and blood pressure if you feel these symptoms, especially comparing your readings while seated and standing, can be useful. If present, you should contact your family doctor or cardiologist immediately. If severe, go to the nearest emergency department immediately.

Long COVID

About 30% of people go on to develop long COVID (also called post-acute sequelae of COVID-19, chronic COVID, post-COVID-19 syndrome, or post-COVID-19 condition). This is not unique to COVID-19. Other viral infections known to cause persistent symptoms beyond the acute infection include the Spanish Flu, Epstein-Barr, and Ebola. Those at higher risk for long COVID include women, older adults, asthmatics, diabetics, obese individuals, and people who suffer more severe acute symptoms. The time frame to define long COVID has not been clearly defined yet, ranging from one to three months after the onset of acute COVID-19. Furthermore, there is no clear consensus yet about what symptoms constitute long COVID; as such, any persistent symptoms following confirmed or suspected COVID-19 infection may be considered long COVID.

A large number of symptoms may occur in long COVID. The most common and debilitating symptoms include fatigue, brain fog (including impaired memory, processing speed, and attention), headache, dizziness, psychiatric disorders (e.g., depression, anxiety, post-traumatic stress disorder), sleep changes, cardiovascular disorders (e.g., POTS, tachycardia, orthostatic hypotension), persistent cough, shortness of breath, and gastrointestinal symptoms (e.g., diarrhea, bloating, pain, constipation). There are a myriad of less common symptoms including altered smell/taste, tinnitus, ear pressure, muscle fasciculations, and neuropathy.

As you can see, many of these symptoms overlap with those seen in people with vestibular migraine. We will explore some of the overlapping symptoms here with a focus on vestibular migraine.

The Pathophysiology of Long COVID

Why long COVID develops remains a mystery but there are several potential possibilities. Firstly, SARS-CoV-2 can remain hidden in immunologically-privileged organs (e.g., brain, testicles, ovaries and eyes) long after the acute infection is over. These organs are normally protected from most immune cells, which shields them from the ill effects of systemic inflammation. However, when a pathogen like SARS-CoV-2 manages to infiltrate such organs, it is also protected from the attacks of the immune system. This reservoir of SARS-CoV-2 may provoke a chronic, low-level inflammatory state that drives the symptoms of long COVID. Secondly, the acute infection may trigger changes in the immune system that result in a chronic state of inflammation. In other words, the immune system is stuck in a perpetual state of ongoing inflammation. Thirdly, the acute infection may weaken some components of the immune system and allow the reactivation of dormant viruses. Epstein-Barr virus (EBV) is the top viral suspect in long COVID. EBV infection (infectious mononucleosis) is well-known for causing severe fatigue and brain fog.

Fourth, COVID-19 infection may cause a state of redox imbalance, characterized by high levels of free radicals (reactive oxygen and nitrogen species) which damage healthy cells. Fifth, SARS-CoV-2 can invade and damage the mitochondria, the powerhouses of the cells responsible for generating energy. Depleted of their fuel source, cells are unable to function optimally. This can clearly cause symptoms like fatigue and brain fog, but may also aggravate or trigger migraine (remember that one of the causes of migraine is bioenergetic dysfunction).

Sixth, COVID-19 infection appears to alter the gut microbiome negatively (dysbiosis), resulting in diminished microbial diversity, reduction in good bacteria, and proliferation of negative microbes. This dysbiosis can skew the immune system towards inflammation, alter the production of neurotransmitters (e.g., serotonin) and vitamins, and even alter brain activity. Seventh, it is possible that one's nutritional state at the time of infection affects the risk of developing long COVID. This is an area that needs more research but there is emerging evidence of a link between low vitamin D levels and long COVID. Finally, COVID-19 appears to damage the endothelium (inner lining of blood vessels) and cause micro-clots to form. This deprives tissues (including the brain) of oxygen and nutrients needed for optimal functioning.

Neurological & Audio-Vestibular Effects of COVID19

We will start with a discussion about how the previously discussed long COVID pathophysiological mechanisms may specifically affect the brain and inner ear. This will provide a framework for understanding how long COVID may cause certain symptoms.

Direct viral infection and damage can occur in the brain and inner ear. The virus can infect the brain by several routes: by direct invasion of the olfactory nerve (the cranial nerve that detects odors), by breaching the blood-brain barrier, or by traveling along infected nerves to the brain via a process called trans-synaptic transfer. Viral persistence in the brain and inner ear can trigger an ongoing inflammatory response in these areas as the body attempts to eradicate it. SARS-CoV-2 may also invade the endolymphatic sac (a pouch that produces the endolymphatic fluid inside the inner ear organs), the stria vascularis (a blood vessel network that controls electrolyte levels in the endolymphatic fluid) or by creeping into the middle ear via the Eustachian tubes. Once inside the inner ear, the virus and the inflammatory response it provokes can damage these sensitive organs. This may explain why BPPV appears to occur shortly after acute COVID-19; damage to the otolithic organs causes disintegration of the crystals that subsequently wander into the semicircular canals. In addition, damage from viral invasion may also explain why some people with Meniere's disease experience a worsening of attacks following COVID-19.

A chronic inflammatory state in the body results in higher levels of circulating pro-inflammatory molecules (e.g., interleukin-g, tumor necrosis factor). These enter the brain and affect many of the brain regions that control functions relevant to long COVID. For example, the amygdala (which controls fear and threat response) is stimulated by such inflammatory molecules, resulting in increased anxiety, feelings of social isolation, and threat. The microglia are specialized immune cells that serve as the brain's guards, moving around the brain, scanning for infection or pathology, and then multiplying to fight off any pathogens or kill off diseased cells. Circulating inflammatory cytokines that seep into the brain can trigger and activate the microglia as well. Microglia are of special interest in long COVID as they can serve as viral reservoirs, drive chronic inflammation, and even cause neurodegeneration by damaging healthy neurons. This increased inflammatory state may explain why some people with well-controlled autoimmune inner ear disease experience an increase in disease activity following COVID-19.

Altered neurotransmitter states following COVID-19 infection are the most important driver for neurological manifestations, especially vestibular migraine, migraine, PPPD, and MDDS. Inflammatory molecules affect the levels of neurotransmitters many neurotransmitters. Inflammatory states diminish acetylcholine production in the hippocampi [Dunn, 2006], which may explain why brain fog is so problematic in long COVID. Dopamine and norepinephrine levels are also adversely impacted by inflammatory cytokines [Dunn, 2006]. A fascinating study from the University of Pennsylvania [Wong, 2023] showed that in long COVID, viral RNA, and inflammatory molecules depleted serotonin levels through several mechanisms, including diminishing tryptophan levels (by decreasing uptake and increasing its breakdown in the gut), altering platelet physiology and numbers (which store serotonin), and increasing the metabolic degradation of serotonin. This serotonin depletion affects neurological function by altering the activity of the vagus nerve. Serotonin deficiency correlates with many long COVID symptoms including fatigue, brain fog, headache, sleep problems, and vestibular symptoms.

Recall the excitatory and inhibitory systems of the brain. COVID-19 causes changes in the brain networks and function that favor the excitatory system. Inflammatory states elevate the levels of glutamate in the central nervous system. These changes are likely responsible for worsening many conditions that are already characterized by overly-excitable brains, like migraine, PPPD, MDDS, and vestibular migraine. The previously discussed long COVID pathophysiological mechanisms can also result in central sensitization.

One fascinating complication of COVID-19 is autoimmune disease. In susceptible individuals, SARS-CoV-2 appears to trigger the body's immune system to attack its own cells, mistaking them for viral proteins. Following COVID-19 infection, up to 50% of people test positive for autoantibodies that target a wide variety of cells and organs, accounting for the persistence of symptoms seen in long COVID in the absence of the virus. There have also been many reports of new autoimmune diseases (e.g., rheumatoid arthritis, Sjogren's syndrome, lupus erythematosus, Hashimoto's thyroiditis, Grave's disease, hives), and allergies emerging following COVID-19 infection. There is a possibility that COVID-19 triggers the production of autoantibodies that can attack inner ear proteins, damaging the vestibular and cochlear cells. This may explain why some patients develop autoimmune inner ear disease following COVID-19.

Endothelial damage and micro-clots are the most likely reasons why some people experience sudden hearing and vestibular loss with COVID-19. The cochlear and vestibular cells are supplied by a delicate network of capillaries and a small artery (called the audio-vestibular artery) without any collateral supplies. As such, any disruption of this critical network will cause an infarction (i.e., stroke) of these cells, often resulting in permanent loss of function.

Without a doubt, our collective stress levels were heightened by the pandemic. There was health anxiety surrounding the potential of being infected and suffering the severe complications of the disease. Images of bodies stacked in hospital hallways and freezer trucks filled the news cycles. There was also fear over the lack of any clear treatments or vaccinations in the early days of the pandemic. Furthermore, financial and job insecurity weighed heavily on almost every adult on the planet. On top of that, parents were forced to adapt to caring for and teaching their children at home daily. These stressors caused vestibular migraine, PPPD, and even MDDS in some patients, and exacerbated the symptoms in those with pre-existing conditions.

Some of the protective measures needed to curb the spread of COVID-19, especially in the early days of the pandemic, also affected many people with vestibular & migraine disorders. Consistent use of masks helped control infections by reducing the amount of droplets released. It was a necessary step but also had a few drawbacks. They were uncomfortable to wear for long periods. Half to over 80% of healthcare workers respondents reported developing a headache after using masks, especially the tighter N95 type [Ong, 2020; Ramirez-Moreno, 2020; Toksoy, 2021]. People with migraine and allodynia had a hard time wearing them for prolonged periods. Masks also made it difficult for people with hearing difficulties to others' lips during conversations.

Social distancing measures were a mixed blessing for many with vestibular disorders and migraine. The ability to avoid crowds, limit driving, and get things done online was a plus for many. People found more time to care for themselves and organize their lives. In fact, in both adults and children, the lockdown actually improved migraine control [Caronna, 2022]. Unfortunately, the lockdown also restricted the ability to exercise in many. Furthermore, the increased use of computers, smartphones and tablets worsens the symptoms in many who are sensitive to electronic screens. The pandemic also spurred the adoption of telemedicine, which was lagging for years (thanks to insurance companies' recalcitrance). Telemedicine has been a great advantage for many patients, negating the need to travel far and waste precious time but at the same time, potentially aggravating symptoms related to electronic screen use. Finally, social isolation diminished the warmth and closeness of human contact, worsening loneliness, depression, and anxiety in many.

Fatigue & Brain Fog

Fatigue is more than just a state of tiredness. It is a persistent and disabling deficit of physical, mental, and emotional energy that interferes with one's ability to function in a normal capacity. Fatigue affects a person's self-esteem, quality of life, and employability; in fact, many people with multiple sclerosis and traumatic brain injury blame fatigue as the most challenging and distressing symptom they have to deal with.

Fatigue is the most common and often the most debilitating long COVID symptom. Approximately 60-90% of long COVID patients report fatigue. It is more common in women, especially those with a prior history of depression or anxiety [Augustin, 2021], and not affected by the severity of acute illness. Over two-thirds of people with long COVID-related fatigue report it adversely affects their job, family, social, or recreational activities [Ceban, 2021]. Almost half of COVID-19 survivors are not able to return to their previous jobs because of is disabling fatigue [Ceban, 2021].

Fatigue and brain fog are common in vestibular migraine but are much more severe in those with long COVID. The fatigue and brain fog of long COVID resembles a much older condition known as myalgic encephalitis/chronic fatigue syndrome (ME/CFS), a post-infectious chronic disorder characterized by fatigue, post-exertional malaise, brain fog, unrefreshing sleep, and orthostatic intolerance.

Post-exertional symptom exacerbation (PESE) is experienced by more than half of long COVID patients and is similar to post-exertional malaise in ME/CFS. Other terms for PESE include exercise or exertional intolerance. It refers to worsening of fatigue and brain fog after minimal physical, emotional, or mental exertion. Other symptoms that may occur include joint pain, muscle pain, or flu-like symptoms. In the ME/CFS world, this is commonly called "crashing". Not infrequently, trivial physical activity like house chores, grocery shopping, or even being upright for too long can trigger it. PESE may occur immediately after the triggering activity, or take anywhere from an hour to 3 days afterward. It typically lasts between 12 to 48 hours but can last for days. Many people require complete rest with minimal sensory stimulation to recover. PESE is not a feature of vestibular migraine.

Brain fog is a colloquial term that encompasses cognitive dysfunction in many conditions. Almost 75% of long COVID sufferers report some degree of brain fog. The characteristics of brain fog in vestibular migraine are similar but usually less severe. These include confusion, an inability to clearly articulate thoughts ("my brain knows what to say but my mouth can't say it"), difficulty multitasking, impaired attention ("I just can't focus"), slowness of thought or impaired processing speed ("thinking through pea soup"), poor memory ("I can't remember things clearly"), dysfluency ("can't find the right words"), and cognitive fatigue ("I don't have the mental stamina"). As there are many different cognitive domains, long COVID affects each domain differently in each person, accounting for the variable symptoms that fall under the "brain fog" umbrella. Ongoing long COVID symptoms do not predict or correlate with any specific cognitive deficits. Interestingly, however, a British study [Guo, 2022] suggested that some acute COVID-19 symptoms correlate with specific cognitive effects. Headache severity was associated with slower reaction time, associative memory, and fluency, while dizziness severity predicted perseverative errors [Guo, 2022]. Just like PESE, strenuous mental tasks can result in worsening or relapse of brain fog. Brain fog and fatigue are often lumped together in long COVID, but one study indicated that both symptoms evolve independently [Woo, 2020]. This is similar to my observation of people with migraine. Brain fog affects many vestibular migraine sufferers, regardless of the presence or magnitude of fatigue.

Headache

Headaches are also common long COVID symptoms; about one-third of patients experience headache a month after infection. In 80%, the headaches resolve within 2 months; it appears unlikely that headaches will spontaneously remit if they do not resolve at the 2-month mark. Loss of smell during the acute infection appears to increase the risk of long COVID headache [Tana, 2022]. The headache is often associated with fatigue, brain fog, and insomnia.

Similar to vestibular symptoms after the acute infection, headaches can also be classified under several categories i.e., new daily persistent headache (NDPH), tension-type headache, or migraine. Tension-type headache is the most common type of headache in long COVID. Medication overuse headache may occur in those who use analgesics or triptans excessively. A previous history of migraine increases the likelihood of developing long COVID headache [Tana, 2022] and fatigue [Caronna, 2022]. In fact, those with pre-existing headache disorders often experience a worsening of these headaches with COVID-19. About 60% of people with migraine continue to have increased headaches seven months after COVID-19 infection [Caronna, 2022].

Vestibular Symptoms

While the presence of vestibular symptoms following COVID-19 infection is clearly documented in published medical reports, there is a lack of information about the cause. There does not appear to be a uniform "long COVID dizziness/vertigo" condition. Instead, vestibular symptoms in long COVID may be classified under several diagnoses.

Infection or strokes of the brainstem or cerebellum can damage the brain regions responsible for balance and processing vestibular information. This can result in permanent imbalance or ataxia. Some unsteadiness may be the result of labyrinthitis or vestibular neuritis; central compensation helps this improve over time and can be promoted with vestibular therapy.

Other vestibular disorders that may be triggered by COVID-19 include vestibular migraine, PPPD, MDDS, Meniere's disease, or BPPV. In many, these conditions may not start immediately with the acute infection but may manifest a few weeks after the infection. People with these pre-existing vestibular disorders often experience a worsening of their symptoms following COVID-19. Many of my patients with vestibular migraine, PPPD, and MDDS experience a significant worsening of their symptoms with COVID19 infections. In my experience, pre-Omicron variants of SARS-CoV-2 often caused long-term exacerbation of these conditions but thankfully, Omicron and subsequent variants are much less likely to do so.

Ear Symptoms

Ear symptoms in long COVID are also being increasingly recognized. Some studies have shown an increase in the number of people presenting with hearing loss and tinnitus to ENT and audiology clinics since the pandemic started. They are usually bilateral but may be unilateral in some. The hearing loss is usually sudden and occurs within a month of the infection in the majority of cases. Men seem to be at higher risk of sudden hearing loss after COVID19 infections. People with pre-existing hearing loss may suffer further hearing loss following COVID19 infection [Mustafa, 2020]. Hearing loss and tinnitus may also occur as a result of some drugs used to treat COVID-19 that are toxic to the inner ear, including hydroxychloroquine and azithromycin.

Ear pain may also occur following COVID-19 [Kokoglu, 2021; Lechien, 2020]. In acute COVID19, most cases appear to be due to acute otitis externa and media (bacterial infection of the outer and middle ear, respectively). Ear pressure can be highly distressing in long COVID; it is almost always bilateral. The cause of this remains unclear. Migraine is one possible hypothesis but ear pressure often fails to respond to migraine treatment in my experience. Inflammation or damage to the trigeminocervical branches that supply the ear may also be possible. Another potential explanation for ear pressure is Eustachian tube damage or dysfunction.

COVID-19 Vaccination

It is essential to separate politics from the science of the COVID-19 vaccination. The vaccination is not a protective talisman that will stop the virus from infecting you. It also does not make you magnetic, infertile, insane, or turn into a virus-shedding zombie. The COVID-19 vaccination helps reduce the chances of severe illness, hospitalization, and long COVID. It does not prevent infection; rather, it decreases the risks of the infection becoming severe and/or developing into long COVID. As with everything in medicine, it is not 100% effective and side effects are possible.

Headache is a common symptom after COVID-19 vaccination, occurring in about 40% to two-thirds of recipients [Skarzynska, 2022; Caronna, 2023]. It is usually a pressing, bilateral headache. Light and noise sensitivity, or nausea are infrequent. This headache starts within a day of receiving the vaccination and typically lasts no more than a few days.

Dizziness has been reported in about 8.3% of healthcare workers after vaccination, while 2.5% report vertigo [Kadali, 2021; Kadali, 2022]. An Italian study reported that 21% of recipients reported dizziness [Gianfredi, 2021]. In Germany, only 0.1 to 0.2 of 1000 vaccine recipients reported dizziness [Gerb, 2022]. A German study [Gerb, 2022] of 4137 patients presenting to a vestibular disorders center identified 72 people who reported vestibular symptoms following vaccination. In 22, the symptoms occurred within 24 hours of vaccination, 1 week in 23 patients, and 2-4 weeks in the rest. One-third were diagnosed with PPPD, 19.4% with vestibular migraine, and 18.1% with both vestibular migraine and PPPD. BPPV was diagnosed in 12.5%, while unilateral vestibular weakness and Meniere's disease occurred in 4.2% each, and vestibular paroxysmia in 2.8%. One patient had pre-existing diabetic neuropathy, one had mild cerebellar ataxia, and another had oscillopsia from an eye muscle paresis. This is also quite consistent with my observations. Most of the vestibular syndromes in my patients following the COVID-19 vaccinations (Pfizer, Moderna, and J&J in my patients) tend to be vestibular migraine, PPPD, or a combination of both. I've seen some cases of MDDS and BPPV following vaccination as well.

There have been rare instances of hearing loss following COVID-19 vaccinations. A House Clinic study of several thousand clinic visits found 25 patients who experienced hearing loss on average 10.5 days after receiving the COVID-19 vaccine; about one-third had pre-existing ear disease (including Meniere's disease and autoimmune inner dear disease) [Wichova, 2021]. However, the incidence of hearing loss after COVID-19 vaccination does not exceed that of unvaccinated people and the general population before the availability of the vaccines [Ciorba, 2021; Formeister, 2022; Michael, 2023]. As such, in those without prior hearing impairment, there does not appear to be a higher risk of hearing loss with the vaccines. In my experience, other symptoms that have been reported by some patients following vaccination include ear pressure, fatigue, and brain fog.

Since vaccines work by inducing an inflammatory response that activates the immune system to recognize a particular pathogen, these post-vaccination symptoms are most likely a result of inflammation. Just like how inflammation may be responsible for some long COVID symptoms following infection, it is likely that the immune response triggered by vaccination drives some of the abovementioned symptoms. However, it is important to point out that vestibular migraine, PPPD, and MDDS can be triggered by any inflammatory response, not specifically by COVID-19 vaccination. Inflammation can be caused by many conditions, including infection, surgery, stress, and even allergies.

It is important to note that the risk of persistent symptoms following vaccination is much lower than that of COVID-19 infection. As with many things in life and medicine, we have to weigh the potential benefits and risks. The Moderna vaccine (Spikevax) appears to have a slightly higher chance of side effects compared to Pfizer's (Cominarty) but also induces a more robust immune response that helps the body fight SARS-CoV-2 more effectively.

Chapter 8: Acceptance

So, you've been diagnosed with vestibular migraine. You're pretty confident in the diagnosis. Now, it is time for acceptance. Acceptance is an important psychological process that will help prepare you for the next steps in your journey.

Acceptance helps you deal with illness uncertainty & intrusiveness

Illness uncertainty refers to a person's perception of the ambiguities surrounding an illness; in chronic conditions like vestibular migraine, illness uncertainty can exact a heavy emotional toll. Accept that vestibular migraine attacks are unpredictable, but there is much you can do to prevent and treat these attacks.

Illness intrusiveness refers to how an illness and its treatment(s) interfere with one's valued activities and interests. It is more severe in unpredictable diseases, like vestibular migraine. A study found that vertigo is more intrusive than 33 out of 37 chronic illnesses, including laryngeal cancer, multiple sclerosis, rheumatoid arthritis, and kidney failure [Arroll, 2012]. Vertigo was only surpassed by HIV, fibromyalgia, anxiety, and chronic fatigue syndrome [Arroll, 2012]. Accept that vestibular migraine is an incurable chronic illness. It will be an unwelcome companion for life but it can be controlled. Accept that vestibular migraine can cause persistent and bothersome symptoms for life and you may need to make certain adjustments to help control it. Accept that sheer force of will, diet, or supplements alone may not be enough to control your symptoms, and accept that medications are sometimes needed.

Acceptance gives you psychological flexibility, the ability to live life to as full a degree as possible while accepting that some symptoms may be present. Psychological flexibility enables you to live your life without being discouraged that some level of dizziness and migraine symptoms may be present. The opposite of this concept is psychological inflexibility, a state of mind that says, "I cannot live my life unless I feel completely well". Psychological flexibility is beautifully summarized in the serenity prayer: *God, grant me the serenity to accept the things I cannot change, the courage to change the things I can, and the wisdom to know the difference.*

Acceptance frees you from struggling to appear ok

Acceptance frees you from the constant need to hide your struggles, and from that awful fear of how others judge you. You don't have to work so hard to appear "normal".

The philosophy of Tao refers to the harmonious approach to the natural order of the universe. *Wuwei* refers to an understanding and conformation to this natural order, not fighting against it. A Ferrari is designed for speed, not muddy and rocky terrain. It would not last very long if pushed into such conditions. A Land Rover, on the other hand, is made for such terrain but is quite useless in a race. In the same way, you must learn to listen to your body. You must learn what your brain and body are designed to handle, and how to improve those abilities.

Accepting that you have vestibular migraine helps you acknowledge that your brain and body have certain unique requirements and limitations. Acceptance allows you to discover your individual traits, and to stop forcing your body to fit your and others' expectations of "normal".

Acceptance helps you process medical trauma

Accepting that you have vestibular migraine and that your trauma is real starts the process of healing. Is it possible to be unaware of trauma? Traumatic experiences, especially subtle ongoing ones, may be encoded as fragments in the memory. These fragments exist on a subconscious level but still affect a person's emotions, personality, and outlook.

Unprocessed trauma refers to trauma that has been suppressed, ignored, and/or denied. Many symptoms experienced by vestibular migraine patients overlap with those of unprocessed trauma, including anxiety, fatigue, gastrointestinal upset, headaches, poor self-esteem, sleeping problems, and irritability. Unprocessed trauma can have real physical effects and may lead to maladaptive changes in the brain's fear network and HPA axis, as well as a pro-inflammatory state. Coming to terms with the diagnosis of vestibular migraine and confronting the possibility of medical trauma allows you to process and seek treatment for these experiences. Processing these experiences helps integrate the trauma in a way that restores the brain's sense of security, safety, predictability, and control.

Acceptance allows room for self-compassion

Instead of mercilessly judging and criticizing yourself for various inadequacies or shortcomings, self-compassion means that you are kind and understanding when confronted with personal failings – after all, who ever said you were supposed to be perfect?

Dr. Kristin Neff

We are often told to be kind to others, especially the less fortunate. We don't look at a stroke victim limping down a grocery aisle and think, "Why don't you just walk like a normal person?". We feel compassion for the person's difficulty, and empathize – we feel a desire to help the person. We take action if we see the person struggling to get a large can from a high shelf, offering to retrieve it for them, and instantly feel the warm glow of altruism. We would never judge or shame the person. We would never tolerate someone who judges or shames another less fortunate person.

If we can be kind to others, why do we find it so hard to be kind to ourselves? Why are we so hard on ourselves? Why do we mentally bully, shame, and judge ourselves for our perceived failures? We have to learn the art of self-compassion. Don't guilt or condemn yourself if vestibular migraine makes it tough for you to use a computer for 8 hours a day, unload the dishwasher, run an hour on the treadmill, or teach a class of middle school children. Don't say "Why can't I be normal?". Don't look at the co-worker or friend who doesn't have vestibular migraine and think "Why can't I be like them?".

Be kind to yourself. Don't judge yourself as inadequate, or a failure. It's ok to be vulnerable and acknowledge that you need help. Self-judgement suppresses negative thoughts and emotions but like a hidden termite nest under your house, these negative elements slowly eat away at your mental health, confidence, and well-being and eventually sweep you away in a tide of negativity. Acknowledging your limitations and shortcomings removes the poison from such negative reactivity and allows you to be kind to yourself and focus on healing.

Acceptance allows you to focus on the journey ahead.

Learning how your brain works and how vestibular migraine affects you is be a journey. Acceptance opens the gate for you to embark on that journey and allows you to focus your precious energy and resources on conquering vestibular migraine. Your journey will not be a straight highway with clear signposts. It is a river, with rapids and waterfalls early in its course, unexpected swirls and turbulence, and a meandering course later in the journey. Like a river, your journey moves onward constantly. Learn to go with the flow and enjoy the ride, even the unexpected turns and storms.

The Greek philosopher Heraclitus' principle of *panta rhei* (everything flows) can be summed up as "No man ever steps in the same river twice". The journey of people with chronic invisible illnesses like vestibular migraine is as unpredictable as a river. No one experiences the same journey, even though we can learn lessons from others. Accepting and even embracing this unpredictable river helps us avoid becoming depressed, anxious, and stressed out. Swimming and fighting against the flow will exhaust us. Better to learn how to swim with the flow, using it to our advantage, and prudently making adjustments to avoid rocks and obstacles in our way.

I have seen the effect of acceptance in many patients' journeys, particularly those with multiple sclerosis (MS). I have seen patients in their 20s who only have mild numbness from MS but are consumed by the "Why me?" resentment and constantly worrying about how MS may handicap them, losing all joy and becoming hollow, depressed shells. I have seen patients who utterly refuse to accept that they need proper treatment, choosing to "fight" MS by sheer force of will and "healthy living" and end up completely disabled by the ravages of the disease. The most amazing and happiest patients were a few elderly ladies in wheelchairs. They were diagnosed with MS before any treatments were available and by the time effective therapies could be prescribed, they had already suffered significant disability from MS. However, they started the right treatments and continued to live life as fully as they could. They accepted they had MS, did what was needed to control the disease, and carried on living. They recognized but never surrendered to their disabilities. They were happy, always smiling, and thankful that they could continue doing everything they did. They found ways to continue taking care of their families and enjoying life to its fullest.

That is the ideal mindset and attitude to this journey. One day, there will be a cure for vestibular migraine but until then, we must prepare for our journey. We accept the diagnosis of vestibular migraine, accept that it may place certain limitations on our lives, make the appropriate life changes, start the right treatment plan, and embrace the ride ahead, no matter how wild it may be.

Acceptance prepares you for **ACTION**.

Ever-never waters flow on those who step into the same rivers... We both step and do not step in the same rivers. We are and are not.
Heraclitus of Ephesus

Part II:
The **ACTION** Plan

A: *Alternative* non-drug therapies

C: Life *Changes*

T: *Therapeutic* options

I: *Interictal* & Co-morbid Disorders

ON: *Onward!*

A

Alternative drug-free therapies
Explore the healing powers of nutraceuticals, complementary medicine, & exercise

Chapter 9: Nutraceuticals & Acupoints

Herbs are the friend of the physician and the pride of cooks
Charlemagne (748-814)

The term "nutraceutical" refers to foods or components of food that provide specific medicinal benefits. Other terms used include functional foods, designer foods, medical foods, and dietary supplements.

Nutraceuticals play an important role in drug-free migraine control. However, the nutraceutical market is massive and awash with purported cures for every health problem known to humanity. Charlatans spout all kinds of pseudo-scientific nonsense to separate desperate people from their hard-earned cash. Count how many online ads you encounter for products that claim to improve memory, reduce body fat, and enhance energy. How does one wade through the swamp of misinformation and get real scientific, evidence-based information about nutraceuticals?

In this chapter, we will discuss the nutraceuticals that have scientific evidence to support their use in vestibular migraine. You will get only the solid, real information to help you make the right choice about which nutraceutical is right for you. The goal of this chapter is to summarize the important features of each supplement, by briefly discussing the biological role they play, recommended dosage for vestibular migraine, safety for use in pregnancy, and precautions.

Before we proceed, there are a few important points to remember about supplements. **Always** consult your physician(s) before starting any supplements. Vitamins and mineral supplements are generally safe but may be harmful in some circumstances. For example, B6 can cause toxicity if taken in excess. Some caution is required with herbs. Many herbs are metabolized by the liver. Some herbs may affect the same liver enzymes that metabolize certain medications, leading to increased medication levels (which may be toxic), or decreased levels (which may impair the efficacy of the medication).

Furthermore, some herbs can be toxic to the liver, particularly in people with liver disease. In rare cases, some people have suffered liver failure from using certain herb supplements. Be sure to check for these interactions, and discuss them with your treating physician.

Because the supplement market is unregulated, the purity of some products may be questionable. Unscrupulous manufacturers may sell minuscule amounts of the advertised supplement. Worse, some may just sell you inactive filler while claiming that they are giving you the real thing! For example, in 2015, the New York Attorney General filed suit against four major retailers (look it up on Google) after finding that only 21% of the products actually had DNA of the plants advertised on the label. Some of the products were contaminated with other substances including rice, beans, pine, citrus, and... wait for it... house plants! Some of the crooks (ahem, retailers) of course, claimed to stand by the "quality" of their products.

The Food and Drug Administration (FDA) is the federal agency responsible for regulating products that affect public health, including food products, medications, cosmetics, medical devices, and tobacco products. For supplements, the FDA is an enforcement agency that defines the claims companies can make about their products. It also enforces its Current Good Manufacturing Practices (CGMP) which requires manufacturers and retailers to establish and follow certain standards to ensure the quality of the dietary supplement, its packaging, and its labeling. The FDA is tasked with detecting and removing adulterated and misbranded supplements from the market. Because supplements are not regulated as drugs, pre-approval is not required before they are sold. The FDA monitors supplement manufacturing and labeling to ensure compliance with regulations.

Other regulatory bodies have similar roles in other regions. For example, the Natural and Non-Prescription Health Products Directorate (NNHPD) is responsible for regulating supplements (called natural health products) in Canada. In the European Union (EU), the European Food Safety Authority

(EFSA) assesses the risks of food products and supplements but member states have final regulatory power.

There are independent organizations that verify the purity, identity, and potency of supplements as well. The United States Pharmacopeial Convention (USP) grants the "USP Verified" seal to brands that meet their standards. The National Sanitation Foundation (NSF) is another organization that certifies supplements. Consumer Lab (consumerlab.com) and Lab Door (labdoor.com) test dietary supplements and charge a fee to access their reports.

This chapter is subdivided into four sections. In the first section, we will discuss the various nutraceuticals and their potential benefits for migraine. In the second section, we will discuss the role of medical cannabis and psychedelics – substances that are not quite legal yet, but which may be useful for migraine. In the third section, we will discuss how to put together a nutraceutical plan for yourself. In the final section, the role of acupuncture and acupressure will be discussed.

Section I – The Nutraceuticals

Vitamin B2

Vitamin B2 (riboflavin) is a vital constituent of cofactors (flavin mononucleotide and flavin adenine dinucleotide) that are essential to cellular energy production, cell protein production, metabolism of other vitamins (A, B6, B12, niacin, and folate) and iron, as well as glutathione reduction (an important antioxidant).

Food sources of vitamin B2 include milk, unprocessed grains, cheese, eggs, liver, kidneys, mushrooms, almonds, legumes, and leafy vegetables. Polishing grains like rice and wheat removes most of the riboflavin; enriching these products replaces some of the lost B2. Vitamin B2 is continuously lost in the urine. Alcoholism, hypothyroidism, adrenal insufficiency, and oral contraceptive use increase B2 loss. As such, an adequate intake is important.

Vitamin B2 supplementation significantly reduces migraine attack frequency [Thompson, 2017]. Note that this is typically seen three months after supplementation. Taking a vitamin B2 supplement is a sure way of guaranteeing adequate intake for migraine prevention. B2 supplementation also promotes eye health (improving corneal health and reducing cataract risk), cardiovascular health, and the body's ability to withstand the oxidative stress of chemotherapy.

For vestibular migraine control, aim for 400 mg daily. You can take it once a day, with a meal. It is very safe and has no significant side effects. One harmless side effect is bright yellow urine. There is no risk of "overdosing" on vitamin B2. Vitamin B complex supplements and multivitamins contain some vitamin B2, but usually not at the dosages needed for migraine control. Because stomach acids improve the bioavailability of riboflavin, it should be taken with food. Riboflavin can be degraded by ultraviolet and blue light, and should always be stored in a dry, dark place.

An interesting study [Di Lorenzo, 2009] showed B2 supplementation was only half as effective for migraine control in people with the H haplogroup in their mitochondrial DNA. This genetic trait is found in about 40% of people of European ancestry. These findings may explain why some medications work for some, but not others. One's genetic makeup not only predicts migraine risk but also determines how one metabolizes and responds to certain medications.

Vitamins B6, B9 & B12

Vitamins B6 (pyridoxine, pyridoxal, or pyridoxamine), B9 (folate or folic acid), and B12 (cyanocobalamin) play certain roles together, and individually. Together, they control the level of a protein called homocysteine; lowering the level of homocysteine reduces the risk of cardiovascular disease, osteoporosis, certain cancers, macular degeneration, and dementia.

Folate and B12 are important in DNA and amino acid metabolism, and many other biochemical reactions critical for cell health. B6 plays a vital role in serotonin and dopamine production, building cell receptors that respond to sex hormones like estrogen and testosterone, red blood cell production, and tryptophan metabolism. B6 may reduce the risk of depression, morning sickness, and pre-menstrual symptoms. B12 is one of the most important vitamins for neurological health. Low B12 levels often lead to a host of neurological problems, ranging from depression and dementia, to peripheral nerve damage and spinal cord dysfunction.

Good folate sources include green leafy vegetables, legumes, asparagus, enriched pasta, enriched grain products, and enriched bread. Certain medications like methotrexate, anti-epileptic medications (phenytoin, primidone, and phenobarbital), and large doses of NSAIDs lower folate levels.

Great sources of B6 include poultry, meat, garbanzo beans (chickpeas), and potatoes. B6 levels are lower in older people, those with autoimmune disorders, and with medications like isoniazid. Of note, too much Ginkgo biloba can deplete B6 levels.

B12 is made by bacteria. Foods naturally rich in B12 include dairy, eggs, and meat. This is why vegans need to supplement with B12. B12 absorption is impaired in disorders of the gut, including atrophic gastritis, pernicious anemia, malabsorption syndromes (e.g., celiac disease), and gastric bypass surgery.

Medications that lower stomach acidity (proton pump inhibitors like omeprazole, and histamine-2 receptor antagonists like ranitidine) also reduce B12 absorption. Nitrous oxide (laughing gas) can inactivate vitamin B12, leading to a drop in B12 levels.

Higher homocysteine levels correlate with greater migraine disability. Lower B12 levels are associated with higher migraine headache frequency. Similarly, increased folate intake improves migraine frequency and severity. Studies investigating folate supplementation alone in migraine control have produced mixed results. On the other hand, supplementing with a combination of folate, B6 and B12 reduces homocysteine levels and improves migraine control. For vestibular migraine prevention, I recommend taking 400 micrograms of folate, and 250 micrograms of B12 daily. There are no known side effects or toxicities with high doses of folate or B12.

However, high B6 consumption (i.e., above 100 mg daily) can cause peripheral nerve damage. Since it is not difficult to obtain B6 from food, a B6 supplement is not necessary; if you would like to try it, I do not recommend taking more than 50 mg of B6 daily. People who have undergone bariatric surgeries or have gastrointestinal disorders that impair B12 absorption require B12 intramuscular injections to ensure proper levels.

Vitamins C & E

Vitamins C (ascorbic acid) and E (tocopherol) play important antioxidant roles, as well as maintain healthy immune function and cardiovascular health. Vitamin C is important in wound healing, collagen production, and immune function. It also has many essential functions in brain health, including myelin formation, neuronal development, and neurotransmission. Vitamin C regulates the formation and release of neurotransmitters (particularly GABA, serotonin, and norepinephrine) as well as their binding to their respective receptors. It is involved in the formation of collagen, which is important in the integrity of brain blood vessels, and connective tissue. Vitamin E decreases the effects of diabetes, lowers the risk of dementia, and improves liver function in non-alcoholic fatty liver disease.

Unfortunately, the vast majority of Americans do not consume enough vitamins C and E daily. Fresh vegetables and fruit are the best sources of vitamin C, but most people do not consume enough of such foods. Vitamin E-rich foods include seeds, nuts, avocados, leafy greens, asparagus, and vegetable oils. Smoking and inflammatory diseases deplete vitamin E levels. Vitamin C restores vitamin E levels, by helping our cells recycle oxidized vitamin E.

While no studies show vitamin C mitigates migraine, it can help with complex regional pain syndrome as well as shingles-related pain, presumably through antioxidant activity. Interestingly, because vitamin C is essential in the formation of collagen (the building block of ligaments, tendons, and joints), patients with back pain and arthritis have lower vitamin C levels [Dionne, 2016]. Furthermore, vitamin C may improve the effect of antidepressants, which are often used as migraine preventives. In addition, vitamin C can increase levels of diamine oxidase (see later), which breaks down histamine. Because it is very safe, helps restore vitamin E levels, and may control pain, it is reasonable to supplement with 1000 mg of vitamin C daily for migraine prophylaxis.

Vitamin E supplementation may be useful in women who experience migraine attacks during menstruation, possibly because it inhibits the release of arachidonic acid and its conversion to prostaglandins. For women with menstrual migraine, taking 400 IU of vitamin E during menstruation can be helpful [Ziaei, 2009]. There are no studies regarding the daily usage of vitamin E in migraine at this time. It is reasonable to take 400 IU daily to help with migraine control. High doses of vitamin E can interfere with vitamin K's role in blood clotting. Be sure to avoid vitamin E supplementation 2-4 weeks before any elective surgery to minimize the risk of bleeding.

Vitamin D

Vitamin D is not really a vitamin but a hormone that is extremely important to health. Calcitriol or D3 (the active form of vitamin D) binds to vitamin D receptors that control 200 different genes. We obtain vitamin D from our diet and it is manufactured in our skin when it is exposed to ultraviolet light. Over a billion people worldwide have low vitamin D levels. This is not surprising since most activities are indoors nowadays, and excessive sunlight carries a risk of melanoma. People with darker skin are at higher risk of low vitamin D because the melanin pigment in the skin (which acts as a shade to protect against ultraviolet damage) reduces vitamin D production. People with migraine often avoid being out in the sun because of light sensitivity, leading to lower vitamin D levels.

Vitamin D may improve cognition, stress levels, depression, anxiety, and sleep quality. Vitamin D has a Goldilocks effect on the immune system, keeping it at optimal function - not too aggressive and not too weak. It boosts immune function to lower the risk of infections but regulates it to reduce the likelihood of autoimmune processes. Adequate vitamin D levels also confer protective effects on bone, muscle, and cardiovascular, health, and may even reduce the risks of certain cancers (breast, colon, prostate, pancreas, skin, and ovary). As icing on the cake, vitamin D supplementation reduces the risk of premature death from all causes. Fibromyalgia and IBS, which frequently coexist with migraine, improve with vitamin D supplementation.

The role of vitamin D in migraine is intriguing. Vitamin D has antioxidant, anti-inflammatory, and neuroprotective properties, and influences the levels of many neurotransmitters. Low vitamin D levels are linked to more frequent and severe migraine headaches [Ghorbani, 2019; Hussein, 2019; Song, 2017; Togha, 2018]. This may be because of several reasons. Firstly, low vitamin D may lead to increased neurogenic inflammation. Secondly, vitamin D deficiency can lead to higher levels of nitric oxide, which increases the release of CGRP and dilates meningeal blood vessels. Thirdly, lower vitamin D levels are associated with lower magnesium levels (see Magnesium section) because magnesium absorption requires vitamin D. Vitamin D stimulates the enzyme tryptophan hydroxylase, which is essential in the production of serotonin [Kaneko, 2015]. Finally, vitamin D deficiency is associated with lower dopamine levels. Vitamin D supplementation improves migraine frequency [Mottaghi, 2015; Gazerani, 2019], and reduces serum CGRP levels [Ghorbani, 2020].

The amount of vitamin D we get from food is limited. Fatty fish and fish liver oils are a rich natural source of vitamin D. Mushrooms (shiitake and portobello) exposed to ultraviolet light produce some vitamin D. Dairy products are enriched with vitamin D but you will need to eat a huge amount for optimal vitamin D levels. Unsurprisingly, the vitamin D intake of most people is too low, barely meeting the Recommended Dietary Allowance of 400 International Units (IU) daily (which is the minimum intake needed to prevent rickets, a bone disease that causes bow legs).

Two vitamin D supplement forms are available: D2 (ergocalciferol) and D3 (cholecalciferol). D2 is derived from fungi that are exposed to ultraviolet light. D3 is derived from sheep and is the form of vitamin D naturally produced by our skin. Some D3 supplements are derived from lichens. D3 is more bioavailable and has a longer shelf life than D2

There is no clear consensus on the best goal for daily intake. For healthy people with no kidney problems, I advise taking 5000 IU every day for migraine prophylaxis. Toxicity can occur in healthy people who consume levels above 40,000 IU (1000 micrograms) per day, an enormous amount. People with kidney disease should consult their nephrologists before starting vitamin D supplementation.

Boswellia

Boswellia serrata (Indian frankincense) resin contains phytochemicals called pentacyclic tripertene acids (of which boswellic acid is the major bio-active compound) that have anti-inflammatory, antioxidant, and analgesic properties. Interestingly, Boswellia also appears to suppress the growth of certain cancers.

While there are no specific studies of Boswellia in migraine, it could potentially help. Boswellia extract improves cluster headache by reducing headaches and enhancing sleep quality. Of particular interest in migraine, Boswellia can decrease glutamate toxicity (one of the main excitatory neurotransmitters in the brain). Furthermore, Boswellia helps with asthma, irritable bowel disease, and arthritic pain. A typical dosage for Boswellia is 300 mg three times a day. Side effects are uncommon, but gastrointestinal symptoms may occur. There is no pregnancy data; as such, Boswellia should be avoided by women who are trying to be, or who are pregnant.

Butterbur

Butterbur (*Petasites* sp) is a marsh shrub found in Europe, North America, and Asia. The large leaves were used in Europe to wrap butter, hence the name. It has been used in traditional medicine for a variety of conditions, including asthma, and allergic rhinitis.

The butterbur species *Petasites hybridus* is an effective preventive treatment for migraine [Diener, 2004; Diener, 2005; Lipton, 2004; Pothmann, 2005] These migraine studies used a specific proprietary brand called Petadolex®, made in Germany. Petasin and isopetasin are the bio-active agents in butterbur that help with migraine.

Children, pregnant women, and breastfeeding women should avoid butterbur. It is usually well-tolerated but may cause gastrointestinal upset. If not properly purified, butterbur extract contains toxic pyrrolizidine alkaloids that may cause liver damage and cancer.

Unfortunately, many commercially-available butterbur products are contaminated with pyrrolizidine alkaloids, and do not contain enough petasins to be useful in migraine. The brand Petadolex® was felt to be the safest preparation. However, it was banned in Germany and Switzerland. The American Academy of Neurology has withdrawn its recommendation for butterbur and the American Headache Society cautions against its use. Because of the potential risks of butterbur, I recommend against its use at this time. There are many other equally effective and much safer nutraceuticals for vestibular migraine.

Coenzyme Q10

CoQ10 (ubiquinone) is an important cofactor in the mitochondria, the powerhouses of the cells. Unsurprisingly, organs that require lots of energy (like the brain) contain high levels of CoQ10. In addition, CoQ10 helps maintain the health of lysosomes, the cellular organelles that help clear waste. Working with vitamin E, CoQ10 has important antioxidant functions, protecting cell membranes from oxidative damage.

Tissue levels of CoQ10 decrease with age. Statins (cholesterol-lowering medications) may reduce the body's CoQ10 levels which is why people on statins should supplement with CoQ10. Diseases that reduce CoQ10 levels include diabetes and cancer. Up to one-third of people with migraine suffer from CoQ10 deficiency.

CoQ10 is found in naturally high levels in meats and fish, especially in organs like the heart and liver. Soybean, grapeseed, canola, and olive oil, as well as parsley, sesame seeds, and pistachios are also good sources. Frying foods in grease can reduce the CoQ10 content by about 25%.

CoQ10 supplementation significantly reduces the number and severity of migraine attacks [Rozen, 2002; Hershey, 2007; Sandor, 2005; Shoeibi, 2016]. Supplementing with CoQ10 increases the number of brain mitochondria, suggesting it enhances the brain's bioenergetic processes. CoQ10 supplementation also reduces CGRP levels and inflammatory markers. Furthermore, CoQ10 can help improve cardiovascular health, cholesterol levels, and blood sugar control.

For vestibular migraine, I recommend taking between 300 to 400 mg daily. You can take it once a day with a meal, or take 100 mg with breakfast, lunch, and dinner. CoQ10 is fat-soluble; consuming it with meals that contain some fat improves its absorption. Taking CoQ10 in capsules made with an oil suspension improves its absorption and bioavailability. There are newer, water-soluble forms of CoQ10 but little evidence to support their superiority.

CoQ10 is very well-tolerated. Taking too much may cause gastrointestinal upset but otherwise no other side effects. It should be avoided in those taking the blood thinner coumadin (warfarin), because CoQ10 may interfere with its therapeutic levels, and increase the risk of blood clots.

Diamine Oxidase (DAO)

DAO is an enzyme produced by the kidneys, thymus gland, and lining of the gastrointestinal tract. DAO breaks down histamine to keep the levels in check. People with DAO deficiency suffer from histamine intolerance which is characterized by allergy-type symptoms (e.g., hives, itching, runny nose) due to the excessive circulating levels of histamine.

DAO deficiency is linked to gluten sensitivity, irritable bowel syndrome, lactose intolerance, and carbohydrate malabsorption. One small study showed low serum DAO activity levels in some people with migraine [Izquierdo-Casas, 2018]. The same research team then found that DAO supplementation in migraine sufferers who were DAO deficient resulted in a small improvement in migraine attack duration after one month [Izquierdo-Casas, 2019]. DAO supplements also help those with allergies.

DAO supplements derived from pig kidneys are commercially available but rather pricey. Research into supplementing with DAO in migraine remains scarce and the price tag for DAO supplements makes it rather unappealing. Limiting dietary histamine intake, and using anti-histaminergic migraine preventives would be preferable and potentially more effective.

However, if you have gluten sensitivity, and other gastrointestinal disorders as well, DAO supplements could be worth trying. Ensure that the supplements are enteric-coated; this will ensure that they are released in the small intestine and not degraded by stomach acid. Sprouted legume seeds (e.g., pea sprouts) are a rich natural source of DAO. More research is needed to determine if legume seedlings can improve DAO function in the body.

Feverfew

In 1978 the British Health Magazine wrote about a 68-year-old woman with severe migraines since she was a teenager.

After 10 months of eating 3 feverfew leaves a day, her migraines completely stopped.

Feverfew (*Tanacetum parthenium*) has been used in traditional medicine since the time of the ancient Greeks for fevers (hence the name), arthritis, gynecological disorders, toothache, insect bites, and inflammation. The most important bioactive agents in feverfew are sesquiterpene lactones, the principal one being parthenolide. Feverfew has anti-inflammatory effects, most likely because it inhibits prostaglandin synthesis, and/or kills certain pro-inflammatory immune cells. Feverfew also relaxes vascular smooth muscle, which may prevent migraines by interfering with the effect of trigeminal activation on vascular walls. It may also improve migraine by preventing platelet granule secretion and mast cell histamine release.

Several studies have confirmed that feverfew is a safe and effective migraine preventive [Diener, 2005; Johnson, 1985; Murphy, 1988; Pfaffenrath, 2002]. For migraine prevention, take 100 mg (standardized to 0.2 to 0.4% parthenolides) two to three times a day. It has few side effects at this dose. Feverfew should not be used during pregnancy or lactation.

Post-feverfew syndrome is characterized by headaches, insomnia, nervousness, muscle stiffness, and aching joints; this occurs in people who abruptly stop consuming feverfew after using it for several years. If you have been taking feverfew for some time, it is prudent to wean off rather than stopping it cold turkey.

Ginger

Ginger's uniquely sweet, peppery, and pungent aroma has a unique place in Asian cuisine. It was one of the first spices exported from Asia to ancient Greece and Rome. Ginger's most well-known attribute is its anti-nausea properties. Ginger root oleoresin contains a rich diversity of bioactive compounds. Gingerols are the main phytochemical believed to be responsible for ginger's distinct odor and health benefits, which include anti-nausea, anti-inflammatory, and antioxidant effects. Besides its well-known anti-nausea benefits, ginger may confer protection against cancer, cardiovascular disease, dementia, and diabetes.

Ginger is available in many forms, including candied, dried, crystallized, pickled, powdered, ground, or as a tea. Consuming ginger can prevent motion sickness [Schmid, 1994; Grontved, 1988], and may even be superior to dimenhydrinate (Dramamine) [Mowrey, 1982]. Ginger is safe to use in pregnancy and is often used for morning sickness.

Ginger has been shown to prevent motion sickness [Grontverd, 1988; Holtmann, 1989] and postoperative nausea and vomiting [Bone, 1990; Phillips, 1993]. It can relieve hyperemesis gravidarum (morning sickness) [Fischer-Rasmussen, 1990] and chemotherapy-induced vomiting [Crichton, 2019]. Two studies showed that a sublingual ginger/feverfew preparation relieves acute migraine attacks [Cady, 2005; Cady, 2011]. One study showed that combining 400 mg of ginger extract with intravenous ketoprofen was more effective at terminating a migraine attack, compared to administering intravenous ketoprofen alone [Martins, 2019]. One study indicated that ginger was not effective for migraine prevention [Martins, 2020].

There are several ways to use ginger root in vestibular migraine. For acute vestibular migraine attacks, take 1000 to 1500 mg as soon as you feel an attack coming. For motion sickness, take about 1000 to 1500 mg before traveling. If you suffer from nausea, non-caffeinated ginger tea, or crystallized ginger can be useful. While it has not proven to be effective in migraine prevention, I know a few patients who take a ginger root supplement once or twice a day for vestibular migraine control. Try taking 1000 to 1500 mg of ginger root twice a day with meals, or incorporating ginger into meals.

Ginkgo Biloba

Ginkgo biloba is the oldest living tree species in the world and has been around for almost 300 million years. Some trees in

China and Japan are over 1000 years old. Ginkgo has been used in traditional medicine and food. The bioactive components consist of flavonoids, terpenoids, and terpene lactones (ginkgolides and bilobalide). The extract from its leaves may possess antioxidant and anti-inflammatory properties, and promote cardiovascular health, cognition, as well as mood.

Several studies have shown that ginkgo is an effective migraine preventive [D'Andrea, 2009; Esposito, 2011; Usai, 2011]. One small study suggested that ginkgo helps treat acute migraine aura [Allais, 2013]. Ginkgo reduces blood viscosity and enhances blood flow, including inner ear circulation. Three studies [Schwerdtreger, 1981; Hamann, 1985; [Haguenauer, 1986] show possible benefits for people with vertigo and dizziness but the disorders treated in these studies were not clear. Ginkgo may improve dizziness and tinnitus in elderly dementia patients [Spiegel, 2018]. An Italian study in a small group of patients with various vestibular disorders showed that Ginkgo improved vertigo, dizziness, balance, and eye movement abnormalities [Cesarani, 1998]. In a study of chronic vertigo patients, ginkgo supplements improved subjective symptoms and response to balance training [Decker, 2021]. A study in Meniere's disease showed that ginkgo improved the number of vertigo attacks and quality of life [Sokolova, 2014].

Most studies used a standardized ginkgo extract called EGb 761 (containing 6% terpenoids and 24% flavonoid glycosides) which is commercially available. Some migraine studies used MigraSoll® which is only available in Italy. When selecting a ginkgo supplement, choose one that contains a standardized extract with 24% flavonoid glycosides, and 6% terpenoids. The standard dosage is 80 mg twice a day, or 40 mg three times a day. Do not exceed 240 mg per day. Possible side effects include headache, palpitations, gastrointestinal upset, constipation, and skin allergies.

Ginkgo is allergenic and should be avoided if you have severe allergic reactions to poison ivy, mango, and cashew nuts. You should take vitamin B6 50 mg daily if you use ginkgo supplements. There is an increased bleeding risk and hence, ginkgo should be avoided in people taking on anti-coagulants (like warfarin and rivaroxaban), and anti-platelet medications (like clopidogrel and aspirin). Stop taking ginkgo two to four weeks before any elective surgical procedures. Ginkgotoxin can cause seizures and should be avoided in people with epilepsy. Ginkgotoxin is found in high concentrations in raw ginkgo seeds; consuming raw ginkgo nuts can cause acute B6 deficiency resulting in seizures and loss of consciousness.

L-Carnitine

L-carnitine (or acetyl-L-carnitine) is an essential part of the cell's energy production system. Almost all of the body's L-carnitine stores are found in muscle tissue. It is produced by the cells, and requires adequate levels of vitamin C. Most dietary L-carnitine comes from meat, not plants. L-carnitine supplementation may improve cognition in some degenerative diseases, cardiovascular health, as well as blood sugar control. Despite the hype, there is very weak evidence for L-carnitine being a "fat-burning" supplement.

The results for migraine are somewhat mixed. A small study showed that a combination treatment of L-carnitine and CoQ10 improved migraine symptoms [Hajihashemi, 2019]. Another small study indicated some benefit in migraine control [Esfanjani, 2012]. A larger, placebo-controlled study showed no benefit with L-carnitine supplementation [Hagen, 2015]. L-carnitine supplementation can improve fatigue levels in people with multiple sclerosis, and as such, may be useful if you suffer from fatigue. The main side effect of L-carnitine supplementation is gastrointestinal upset. Taking 1-2 grams a day appears to be safe. Doses above 3 grams a day can cause a fishy body odor.

Lipoic Acid

Alpha lipoic acid (ALA), also known as thioctic acid, is produced in the mitochondria. It is an antioxidant that can slow aging, reduce weight, improve blood sugar levels, and optimize nerve function. ALA is produced in small amounts in cells. Meat and organs are a rich source of ALA. Good plant sources of ALA include yeast, broccoli, tomatoes, Brussels sprouts, and spinach. Two studies suggest a potentially beneficial role for ALA in migraine [Magis, 2007; Cavestro, 2018]. ALA may also improve tinnitus. Doses of between 200 to 400 mg twice daily can be taken. ALA should be taken on an empty stomach; this means taking it 30 minutes before, or 2 hours after a meal.

Magnesium

Magnesium is the most common trace element in the human body and plays a huge metabolic role, serving as an enzyme cofactor in over 300 biochemical reactions. Calcium gets all the attention for bone health, but magnesium plays an equally important role by regulating the cells that build bone tissue and controlling blood calcium levels by acting on parathyroid hormone. In fact, more than half of your body's magnesium supply is stored in bones. Higher dietary magnesium intake is associated with improved bone density. Magnesium may also help regulate blood pressure, lipid levels, and blood sugar levels thus reducing the risk of diabetes, hypertension, and cardiovascular disease.

Low magnesium levels are strongly associated with depression and anxiety, common comorbid conditions in those with vestibular migraine Magnesium helps stabilize nerve and muscle cells and prevent abnormal excitation. Recall that abnormal excitation in the trigeminal system is responsible for migraine attacks. Half of those with migraine are magnesium deficient! Low blood magnesium levels are associated with more frequent and severe migraines. Migraine attacks also occur when blood magnesium levels are lower. Magnetic resonance spectroscopy imaging confirms that brain levels of magnesium (not just blood levels) are lower in people with migraine.

Supplementing with magnesium has been shown to improve migraine frequency and severity. In fact, intravenous magnesium is an effective treatment for patients suffering from bad migraine attacks.

James is a patient of mine who discovered that magnesium supplements worked wonders for vestibular migraine. He actually found that his vestibular migraine attacks started shortly after he was prescribed esomeprazole (Nexium) for heartburn. One of the less known side effects of this drug is low magnesium levels! James also found that taking an extra magnesium dose at the onset of a vestibular migraine attack was an effective rescue treatment.

Unfortunately, magnesium gut absorption decreases with age, alcoholism, gastrointestinal diseases (like Crohn's), and medications (e.g., diuretics, stomach acid reducers). Stress depletes magnesium reserves (and may be one reason, it is such a potent migraine trigger). Cold clammy hands, palpitations, brain fog, and muscle cramps may indicate low magnesium levels. Magnesium-rich foods include nuts (almonds, peanuts, cashews), seeds, beans, soy products, dark leafy greens (spinach, chard), whole grains, beef, fish, bananas, and raisins. However, for migraine, getting enough magnesium to prevent attacks may be difficult to achieve through diet alone. Magnesium supplements are probably the best way to ensure adequate intake.

There are many forms of magnesium. To understand which are most beneficial, it is important to first define the term bioavailability: the fraction of any administered drug or substance that reaches the circulation.

Inorganic Magnesium Salts

Magnesium oxide has a high magnesium content per weight but has the least bioavailability of magnesium supplements. It can be used to relieve heartburn. While the cheapest magnesium supplement, it is the least useful for migraine prevention.

Magnesium sulfate is found in Epsom salt and can be absorbed through the skin (albeit poorly). In an intravenous form, it is administered to treat pre-eclampsia, torsades de pointes (a dangerous cardiac arrhythmia), asthma, and yes, for acute treatment of migraines. In oral form, it can be used as a laxative but is not useful for migraine prevention.

Magnesium hydroxide (Milk of Magnesia) is a laxative and antacid and is not useful for migraine prevention.

Magnesium chloride is very effective for migraine prevention when administered topically. It is well-absorbed through the skin as a topical preparation like magnesium oil, lotion, or gel (not taken orally!). Topical magnesium chloride can be a great way to supplement magnesium without having the gastrointestinal side effects of oral magnesium. When applied to sore muscles, magnesium chloride can also relieve pain.

Organic Magnesium Salts

Magnesium citrate has decent bioavailability but due to its laxative properties, may be difficult to use for migraine prevention. It can be useful if you suffer from constipation or taking medications that cause constipation.

Magnesium lactate has decent bioavailability and fewer gastrointestinal side effects. However, there is a possibility that higher lactate levels may worsen migraines.

Magnesium (or di-magnesium) malate has good bioavailability. As an added benefit, malic acid may improve pain levels in fibromyalgia.

Magnesium L-aspartate has good bioavailability. It should be noted that aspartate is an excitatory neurotransmitter, and higher levels have been found in people with migraine. While aspartate is found naturally in food, it is not clear if supplements with aspartate will increase blood levels and aggravate migraine.

Magnesium taurate has good bioavailability. Taurine may have the added benefit of improving blood sugar and blood pressure control.

Magnesium pidolate has good bioavailability. It may have an additional benefit of reducing red blood cell dehydration in people with sickle cell disease.

Magnesium glycinate (also called di- or bis-glycinate) has good bioavailability. Glycine may be helpful for sleep in those with insomnia. Furthermore, the incidence of diarrhea and gastrointestinal upset is low. I typically recommend using magnesium glycinate for vestibular migraine.

Magnesium orotate has good bioavailability. Orotate has some potential heart health benefits.

Magnesium gluconate has good bioavailability. Furthermore, gluconic acid may help improve energy metabolism in the mitochondria, an added benefit for migraine control.

Magnesium L-threonate is often said to treat brain fog because it is the best form for improving brain levels of magnesium. This idea is a bit of an exaggeration of two studies involving lab rats [Abumaria, 2011; Slutsky, 2010]. To date, migraine studies involving magnesium have utilized other forms of magnesium, not L-threonate. While it is certainly safe, magnesium L-threonate may not be worth the extra expense.

So many magnesium choices!!

Which one is best for migraine control? If you prefer an oral supplement, start with an organic magnesium salt – I usually recommend either glycinate or gluconate. If one preparation causes gastrointestinal upset, try a different preparation. If all oral magnesium supplements cause gastrointestinal side effects, use topical magnesium chloride. The goal for migraine control should be approximately 500 mg daily. A slightly higher intake is not harmful but may cause gastrointestinal upset. Toxicity is very rare from magnesium supplements. Since it is excreted by the kidneys, people with renal disease should exercise caution when supplementing with magnesium and should only do so under a nephrologist's supervision.

Melatonin

Melatonin is the "clock neurohormone" secreted in the pineal gland of the brain that helps with sleep. Its secretion is controlled by the suprachiasmatic nucleus in the hypothalamus. The suprachiasmatic nucleus is controlled by light signals from the retinal ganglion cells. Exposure to bright light (more specifically, the blue spectrum of light) suppresses melatonin release, which is why we are not sleepy during the day. As darkness settles, the suprachiasmatic nucleus signals the pineal gland to release melatonin, causing us to feel sleepy. This system's role in migraine is intriguing. Light sensitivity in people with migraine is predominantly driven by blue light and insomnia is more common in migraine, indicating a possible problem in the nerve pathways that control melatonin release.

Melatonin is as effective as some pharmacologic medications for migraine prevention, including amitriptyline [Goncalves, 2016; Peres, 2004], and sodium valproate [Ebrahimi-Monfared, 2017]. Melatonin may help control migraine by suppressing CGRP release, normalizing the sleep-wake cycle, activating endorphins, reducing anxiety and depression, raising serotonin levels, decreasing excitatory neurotransmitter levels, diminishing nitric oxide release, and enhancing the activity of the GABAergic system (the "relaxation" neurotransmitter of the brain). Other benefits of melatonin include helping irritable bowel syndrome, depression, anxiety, and fibromyalgia.

For migraine, I recommend taking 5 mg in the evening. If you feel hungover or tired the next day, take 3 mg instead. Melatonin could also be used as a rescue medication; taking 5 mg and going to sleep can abort a migraine attack. It is very safe and well-tolerated in general. Infrequent side effects include headaches, muscle cramps, and mood swings. Melatonin supplements do not appear to affect your body's natural melatonin production. Tart cherry juice contains a high amount of melatonin. Drinking 8 ounces twice a day can help insomnia and improve sleep quality [Losso, 2018]. The melatonin and high amounts of antioxidants in tart cherry juice can also help with migraine control. Be sure to look for products that do not contain too much sugar.

N-Acetyl-Cysteine (NAC)

Before delving into the role of NAC, let us discuss free radicals. A free radical is an unstable molecule that contains an unpaired electron in its orbit. Because electrons must exist in pairs, free radicals rob stable molecules to obtain the electron they lack. Free radicals are molecular homewreckers, stealing spouses from happy marriages.

In the body, reactive oxygen species and reactive nitrogen species are the predominant free radicals. Free radicals are usually waste products of cellular metabolism and energy production. Exposure to agents that damage cells, like UV light, pollutants, and tobacco smoke results in excessive free radical production as well. However, free radicals have an important role to play in cellular function, inflammation, and immunity. For example, our immune system uses free radicals to destroy microbes. Macrophages and neutrophils swallow up microbes that invade the body; once inside, the immune cell produces a burst of free radicals that kill the pathogens. Conditions like stress that shift the body towards an inflammatory state and elevate the production of free radicals.

Free radicals damage cells, particularly the DNA. This is the underlying cause of degenerative diseases, aging, and cancer. As such, limiting exposure to agents that increase free radical production can slow aging and reduce the risk of many diseases. Our bodies' defense against free radicals is antioxidants. Antioxidants neutralize free radicals by providing the missing electron, sparing healthy cells the ravages of these unstable molecules. Glutathione is one of the most potent antioxidants in our bodies; it is made from cysteine, an amino acid found in founds like turkey, chicken, eggs, legumes and seeds.

NAC is the supplemental form of cysteine. It is used to protect the liver from the toxic effects of medications, like acetaminophen. According to some studies, it reduces mucus viscosity and improves respiratory function and reduces flare-ups of asthma and chronic obstructive pulmonary disease. NAC also may protect the cochlear cells from noise damage. Interestingly NAC may help psychiatric disorders like obsessive-compulsive disorder, anxiety, depression, addiction, and cravings, as well as delay the deterioration in neurodegenerative diseases like Alzheimer's disease and Parkinson's disease. Furthermore, NAC may improve fertility in men and women, reduce insulin resistance in fat cells, and decrease cardiovascular disease risk.

An Australian study showed that a combination of NAC, vitamin C, and vitamin E improved migraine control [Visser, 2020]. NAC also helps improve symptoms of traumatic brain injury [Hoffer, 2013] and post-traumatic headache [Chen, 2008; Eakin, 2014]. An indirect benefit of NAC in those with migraine is protecting the liver against potentially toxic effects of medications like valproic acid.

The dose for migraine control is 600 mg twice a day. For the best antioxidant benefit, combine it with vitamin C 500 mg and vitamin E 200 IU. It is generally quite safe when taken orally. Common side effects include gastrointestinal upset, which may occur if one consumes more than 1200 mg per day. Anaphylaxis and severe allergic reactions have been reported with intravenous NAC administration. There is a possibility of low blood sugar when used with diabetic medications; if you are on diabetes treatment, check with your physician before starting NAC. Its safety in pregnancy and breastfeeding has not been established and as such, should be discussed with your gynecologist.

Essential Oils

Menthol is naturally found in mint plants like peppermint and spearmint. It produces a cooling sensation when applied to the skin and can relieve pain, and muscle spasms. Peppermint has a high menthol content, and can be useful for people with migraine. Peppermint oil has been shown to help reduce the severity and duration of a migraine attack.

For acute vestibular migraine episodes, one should apply a few drops of peppermint oil to the forehead or temples, or put a few drops of peppermint oil in a bowl of hot water and inhale the steam. Eating peppermint candy, drinking peppermint leaf tea, or smelling peppermint oil can help relieve nausea. Be sure to purchase peppermint oil from a reputable manufacturer. Use peppermint oil topically and smell it, rather than consume it orally. Before applying peppermint oil, make sure you do not have an allergy to it by applying a very small amount to an inconspicuous area of the skin.

Lavender oil may be helpful for anxiety. Lavender oil inhalation increases brain alpha waves, a marker of a relaxed state [Diego, 1998]. The topical application of lavender oil is often used for massage, but high concentrations (above 0.125%) may cause skin damage and irritation; approximately 14% of users develop contact dermatitis [Sugiura, 2000]. There are reports that lavender has estrogenic activity, with case reports of prepubertal boys developing enlarged breast tissue (gynecomastia). Women with breast cancer (or a previous history of it) should consult their gynecologist and oncologist before using lavender. French lavender (*Lavendula stoechas*) can induce abortions and should be avoided if you are pregnant, or trying to get pregnant.

Omega-3 Fatty Acids

Long-chain omega-3 polyunsaturated fatty acids like eicosapentaenoic acid (EPA) and docosahexaenoic acid (DHA) have strong anti-inflammatory and antioxidant properties and are important for brain and cardiovascular health. The key to the anti-inflammatory benefits is a higher omega-3 to omega-6 fatty acid ratio in one's diet. A typical diet contains a lot of omega-6 fatty acids because of the high content of vegetable oils. If the proportion of omega-6 is too high, a pro-inflammatory state is produced by its metabolites.

A diet higher in omega-3 fatty acids favors an anti-inflammatory environment in the body. Omega-3 fatty acids may improve anxiety and depression, blood sugar control, lipid levels, and asthma. Omega-3 fatty acids may also reduce the risk of dementia. Some small studies suggest that a higher omega-3 fatty acid intake may help reduce the duration and frequency of migraine attacks. Omega-3 fatty acids may help control migraines by reducing nitrous oxide levels, increasing serotonin levels, and decreasing inflammation.

Because of the benefits of an omega-3 fatty acid-rich diet, fish oil supplements were promoted as being great for heart health, improving memory, and reducing inflammation. Americans fork out over $1 billion every year for fish oil products that promise these health benefits. Unfortunately, the evidence for such supplements is mixed, without any clear health benefits. This may be because manufacturing processes used to extract omega-3 fatty acids from natural sources oxidize and damage these molecules. Furthermore, some fish oil supplements may contain heavy metals (particularly mercury) and contaminants (e.g., dioxins).

The best way to increase omega-3 fatty acid intake is by consuming foods like fatty fish (anchovy, mackerel, salmon, tuna, sardines, trout, cod, halibut), chia seeds, flaxseed, and walnuts. Albacore tuna intake should be limited because of its higher mercury content. Pregnant women or women trying to get pregnant should limit their intake of larger fish like tuna to minimize mercury exposure.

Pycnogenol

Pycnogenol® is a proprietary extract from the bark of the French marine pine (*Pinus pinaster*). The main bio-active phytochemicals in this extract are procyanidins (biopolymers of catechin and epicatechin), and phenolic acids (derivatives of benzoic and cinnamic acid). The commercially available is standardized for 70% procyanidins.

Interestingly, the benefits of Pycnogenol require a mixture of all these phytochemicals and not one specific compound. It is a potent antioxidant in and of itself, and also helps in regenerating antioxidant vitamins C and E. Pycnogenol acts on endothelial cells (that line blood vessels) to improve blood pressure, circulation, hemorrhoids, and erectile dysfunction. Its anti-inflammatory effects may potentially help with arthritis pain, asthma, and autoimmune disorders. In animal studies, Pycnogenol prevents chemotherapy-related toxicity and is neuroprotective following traumatic brain injury. Some suggest that it could help improve attention deficit hyperactivity disorder (ADHD) in children and relieve perimenopausal symptoms.

Several small studies indicated that pine bark extract (including *Pinus radiata*, not just Pycnogenol) significantly reduces migraine attacks [Chayasirisobohn, 2006;

Chayasirisobohn, 2013; Cesarone, 2020]. Of particular interest for those with vestibular migraine, and tinnitus, a small study in Ménière's disease showed that it improved cochlear artery blood flow, attacks of vertigo, and tinnitus severity [Luzzi, 2014]. Another interesting small study in patients with one-sided tinnitus showed that Pycnogenol improved cochlear artery blood flow in the affected ear and reduced tinnitus severity [Grossi, 2010].

Given its potential benefit in migraine, it is quite reasonable to try it for vestibular migraine prophylaxis. Take between 100 to 150 mg of Pycnogenol daily. There are very few side effects, the most common being gastrointestinal upset. It should not be taken during pregnancy or when breastfeeding.

Tryptophan

Tryptophan is the amino acid in turkey that makes you sleepy after Thanksgiving dinner. Tryptophan is found in many other foods, including eggs, cod, chia seeds, sesame seeds, oats, sunflower seeds, parmesan cheese, cheddar cheese, milk, garbanzo beans, chicken, beef, pork, lamb, and quinoa. It is an essential amino acid (meaning our bodies cannot produce it), that is converted to 5-hydroxytryptophan (5HT), which is transformed into serotonin and melatonin. We already know that low serotonin levels increase the risk of migraine attacks. Low tryptophan levels worsen nausea, headache, and light sensitivity in people with migraine [Drummond, 2006]. Consuming foods rich in tryptophan, or supplementing with L-tryptophan or 5HT can raise plasma levels.

Tryptophan supplements improve depression, anxiety, and insomnia; and can augment the effects of antidepressants. Two studies from the 70s showed that L-tryptophan supplementation significantly improved headaches [Kangasniemi, 1978; Steardo, 1977]. One clinical study showed that 5HT improved migraine control [Titus, 1986]. These supplements also reduce the brain's susceptibility to cortical spreading depression during the menstrual cycle [Chauvel, 2018].

Eating more turkey is certainly a delectable and healthy option. If you prefer, take L-tryptophan 500-2000 mg with dinner or at bedtime. My patients who feel hungover with melatonin often find that L-tryptophan works just as well for sleep and does not cause drowsiness the following day.

If you prefer to supplement with 5-HT, slow-, timed- or extended-release preparations are better tolerated and superior to immediate-release forms. For migraine, take between 100 to 300 mg at bedtime. 5-HT and L-tryptophan are generally safe and well-tolerated. However, in 1989, a condition called eosinophilic myalgia syndrome was traced to a contaminant called Peak X found in some tryptophan supplements. Poor quality tryptophan supplements contain small amounts of Peak X and as such, it is important to purchase your supplement from a reliable manufacturer. Taking L-tryptophan or 5-HT with carbidopa (a Parkinson's disease drug) may cause scleroderma, a rare dermatologic condition that causes thickening of the skin.

Turmeric (Curcumin)

Turmeric (*Curcuma longa*) is a ginger species with a distinct but mild flavor. Turmeric is responsible for the distinct golden orange color of curry. Curcumin is the main bioactive phytochemical found in turmeric. Curcumin has antioxidant, anti-inflammatory, and pain-relieving properties. Curcumin also influences brain levels of serotonin and dopamine. As an adaptogen, curcumin helps the body and brain cope with stress. Curcumin can improve cognitive function, fatigue, and mood [Cox, 2015]. There is evidence that curcumin can improve migraine control, most likely via its antioxidant, anti-inflammatory, and antidepressant properties.

However, curcumin alone has very poor bioavailability; consuming curcumin with piperine (found in black pepper) increases its absorption by 2000%. It should also be consumed with fat for better absorption. Dishes that require cooking turmeric with black pepper and oil are best. If regularly cooking curry dishes is not feasible, turmeric supplements can be considered. Remember to choose one with piperidine, and to take it a meal with some fat. A curcumin-phospholipid complex improves the absorption even further. Several enhanced curcumin preparations (e.g., Meriva, CurcuWin, LongVida) are used in commercially available supplements. Doses above 500 mg can cause diarrhea, rash, and yellow stool [Hewlings, 2017].

Turmeric powder is sometimes adulterated with various additives, including dangerous substances like lead chromate. Turmeric root may even be dyed to make it look brighter. Do not purchase suspiciously cheap turmeric. Two simple home tests can also help you identify adulterated turmeric. Rub a small amount of turmeric powder on your palm; real turmeric will stain and adhere to your skin but adulterated turmeric will mostly fall off. You can also drop a teaspoon of turmeric into a glass of water. Real turmeric powder does not dissolve and will sink to the bottom leaving the water very slightly yellow. While some adulterated turmeric will sink, partially dissolve, and turn the water into a stronger and brighter yellow.

Vitex

Vitex (*Vitex agnus-castus*) is also known as chaste tree, chaste berry, monk's pepper, Texas lilac, and Abraham's balm. It is the sacred tree of the virginal goddess Hestia (Greek) or Vesta (Roman), hence the name "chaste". Pliny, in *Historia Naturalis*, wrote that it "cooled the heat of lust" and could control the libido. It has traditionally been used to treat gynecologic ailments. Some studies suggest that vitex supplements improve premenstrual syndrome, cyclic mastalgia, and premenstrual dysmorphic disorder [Cerqueira, 2017; van Die, 2013]. One study showed that vitex extract improved migraine attack frequency and premenstrual syndrome [Ambrosini, 2012]. Vitex berry extract contains flavonoids (vitexin, casticin), irinoids, neolignans, diterpenoids, essential oils, and terpenes. It lowers follicle stimulating hormone levels and increases luteinizing hormone production, thereby lowering estrogen and increasing progesterone levels. It also binds to and stimulates dopamine receptors. Its ability to lower prolactin levels may also explain its positive effects on the aforementioned gynecologic disorders, as well as possibly improving female fertility.

The exact dose to use for migraine is difficult to ascertain due to differences in preparations used in studies and those that are commercially available. Most commercial preparations are 400 mg capsules, with recommendations to take one capsule two to three times per day for 8-12 weeks, then one capsule daily thereafter. Many clinical studies used a Swiss preparation (Prefemin – Ze 440) with 20 mg dry extract from the Vitex fruit dosed once daily.

Side effects are infrequent, but may include headache, nausea, gastrointestinal upset, rash, acne, menstrual irregularities, and itching. It should be avoided in women who are, or planning to get, pregnant as well as those who are breastfeeding. Do not take Vitex if you are using contraceptive pills or hormone replacement therapy. Due to its hormonal effects, males should avoid taking Vitex.

Section II –Marijuana & Psychedelics

Marijuana

Marijuana has enjoyed a long history in human civilization and culture. The plant was used to make ropes in Neolithic China and Japan, and traces of hashish have been detected in Egyptian mummies. Medicinal use of cannabis and its euphoric effects stretches back thousands of years, in China, Egypt, Assyria, and India. The ancient Aryans showed Scythians and Assyrians how to get high. The Assyrians called it *qanab* (to produce smoke). The Greeks called it *kannabis*, which was later adapted to the Latin *cannabis* [Brucki, 2021]. Cannabis' primary active compounds are tetrahydrocannabinol (THC) and cannabidiol (CBD). It also contains many other active compounds, including cannabinol (CBN), cannabitriol (CBT), cannabi-no-diol (CBND), cannabidiverin (CBDV), terpenes (e.g., myrcene, limonene), cannaflavin, apigenin, and bioflavonoids.

Cannabinoids (or endocannabinoids) are molecules produced within the body that bind to and activate cannabinoid (or endocannabinoid) receptors on cells. This endocannabinoid system dates back over 100 million years. When researching the effects of THC, scientists found that it binds to certain proteins, which they subsequently named cannabinoids. Endocannabinoid receptors are found throughout the brain, including the trigeminal and vestibular systems. Marijuana has analgesic, anti-nausea, anti-inflammatory, anti-anxiety, and nerve-stabilizing properties, which are desirable effects in people with migraine.

Cannabinoid signaling increases dopamine and serotonin receptor expression. THC can enhance the effect of GABA on their receptors; however, prolonged THC exposure leads to tolerance. THC and cannabinoids enhance the activity of the glycinergic system, another inhibitory neurotransmitter pathway. Cannabis also suppresses the excitatory pathways of the brain, particularly glutamate and NMDA; this effect is more pronounced with regular use. Both THC and CBD suppress inflammatory changes in the brain. THC is associated with many of the unwanted (usually) effects of cannabis use, including reduced mental clarity and feeling high. CBD does not have any significant side effects. The psychoactive effects of THC are reduced when combined with CBD. As such, it would be preferable to select products with higher CBD content for migraine treatment.

CBD is effective in controlling seizures. Migraine has a lot in common with epilepsy, which is why anticonvulsant medications work for migraine. There are many anecdotal accounts of CBD's benefits in migraine. Some small studies suggest that CBD may reduce headache frequency in migraine. Other studies suggest that the CBD-THC combination works better for migraine headache. Most indicate that the efficacy of cannabis decreases over time, leading to a need for higher doses. I wonder if this may be similar to medication-overuse headache and could be mitigated by "drug holidays" – using medical cannabis for a few days out of the week, and taking other days off. A few case reports describe the beneficial effects from cannabis on nystagmus and vestibular disturbances, suggesting that cannabis acts on the vestibular system as well. Some of my patients have also found that marijuana helps both as a preventive and rescue treatment in vestibular migraine. This is unsurprising since the vestibular system is full of cannabinoid receptors [Ashton, 2006; Breivogel, 1997].

The acute effects of marijuana are well-known, including eye redness, mouth dryness, impaired motor skills, memory difficulties, euphoria, increased appetite, and difficulty thinking clearly. High doses may cause psychosis, anxiety, and paranoia. Cannabinoid hyperemesis syndrome is a rare adverse effect, characterized by nausea, vomiting, and abdominal cramps; it can be relieved by a hot shower. THC impairs driving skills for about 6-8 hours after use. There is some evidence that cannabis has estrogenic activity and may lower testosterone levels. It is also important to point out that marijuana can cause dizziness and vertigo as well; a few patients I've seen developed vestibular symptoms after using cannabis products.

Stopping cannabis after heavy, long-term, regular use can cause withdrawal symptoms, including insomnia, irritability, gastrointestinal upset, sweating, chills, headache, appetite loss, strange dreams, restlessness, and cravings for marijuana. Smoking and vaping may be associated with respiratory adverse effects (e.g., airway irritation, lung injury). Because CBD is metabolized in the liver, it may alter the serum levels of medications that use the same pathway.

While marijuana is being used more widely, there are several points to consider. Firstly, the cannabis plant has a complex cocktail of phytochemicals, and studies suggest that a synergistic combination of the compounds may be responsible for the benefits. Merely reducing cannabis to THC and CBD, and labeling THC "bad", and CBD "good" is far too simplistic. In fact, a large Canadian study showed that eating the cannabis flower was more effective for migraine control than inhaling concentrates with more potent levels of CBD and THC [Cuttler, 2019]. Just like how we need an optimal ratio of omega-3 to omega-6 fatty acids in our diet, the best results from cannabis may be derived from a specific ratio of THC, CBD, and other phytochemicals, including terpenes like limonene, and pinene. Nature has created a unique cocktail of phytochemicals in the cannabis plant that work synergistically for our health. Using one or two compounds while ignoring the other phytochemicals will most likely lead to disappointment and suboptimal results.

Secondly, product purity is problematic given the lack of uniform regulations. Selective breeding has led to an ever-growing number of species, each with its own unique proportion of THC and CBD. As such, it has become more complicated and challenging to scientifically determine the benefits of cannabis. Unscrupulous scammers even try to sell cooking oil labeled as "CBD oil". While most CBD products have a tiny amount of THC, some may be contaminated with higher THC concentrations and may cause possible psychoactive effects or (worse) result in a positive THC result on mandatory drug tests. Don't forget that cannabis remains illegal at the federal level and the Supreme Court has ruled that employers can fire employees with positive marijuana drug tests even though they work in states where cannabis is legal. Other contaminants that may be potentially dangerous, include solvents (e.g., butane, propane), pesticides, molds, bacteria, and heavy metals.

Thirdly, the optimal dose range and route of administration of cannabis in migraine are not clear. Smoking cannabis causes too many lung problems and can increase the risk of cancer. Vaping has been linked to severe lung disease due to vitamin E oil used in the vaping liquid. Ingestion, nasal sprays or topical application (skin creams, lotions, etc.) are much safer ways to administer it. However, more research is needed to determine the best route of administration and dose for migraine.

Fourth, drug interactions with cannabis are important to consider. One relevant example is the liver's CYP3A4 enzyme, which metabolizes CBD, and several migraine medications including ubrogepant, rimegepant, and verapamil. As such, CBD may alter the levels of these medications and affect their efficacy.

Cannabis is certainly a very interesting and potentially promising migraine treatment. Compared to opioids and butalbital, I believe that cannabis has more benefits and a superior safety profile. Our understanding of the role of marijuana in migraine is in its infancy, and more studies are needed to help elucidate the precise role and doses needed for optimal migraine control. If you decide to use a CBD product, you should research the brand as much as possible, and determine what safety and quality control measures and certifications are in place. Of course, do not break any laws and always discuss it with your physician(s).

Psychedelics

Psilocybin is a naturally occurring psychedelic found in multiple fungi. Lysergic acid diethylamide (LSD) was created by Albert Hofmann in 1938 from lysergic acid, derived from fungi. Mescaline is a psychedelic found in peyote and some cacti species; mescaline is less potent than psilocybin and LSD.

Psychedelics act by stimulating the serotonin receptors. Psilocybin and LSD are considered illegal drugs according to US federal law (and in most countries), although Oregon voted to legalize the therapeutic use of psilocybin in 2020. Mescaline is permitted for religious ceremonies in some states in the US and Colorado decriminalized the use of synthetic mescaline (but not cacti-derived) in 2022. As with cannabis, the legal status of psychedelics has hampered research into their medical applications.

Psilocybin and LSD are emerging as potential treatments for migraine in people who have failed conventional therapies [Andersson, 2017; Sicuteri, 1963] Some studies indicate low, subhallucinogenic, doses of psilocybin and LSD are beneficial for migraine [Schindler, 2021]. Compared to migraine, there is a much larger body of research into psychedelics and psychiatric disorders. There is promising potential for these substances to help depression, anxiety, substance abuse, and post-traumatic stress disorder. As discussed before, depression and anxiety are frequent in people with migraine; comprehensive migraine control requires adequately addressing these mood disorders.

Micro-dosing psychedelics is gaining attention as a way of "brain hacking" or improving one's neurological functioning. Some have blogged and written about their experience with psychedelic micro-dosing in migraine. There are some ongoing studies into the benefits of micro-dosing psychedelics in migraine, but no data is available at the time of writing.

Section III - Creating Your Nutraceutical Plan

As you can see, you can choose from many supplements. Taking all of them may not make much sense and would be expensive. Here are my recommendations to help you plan your supplements for migraine prevention. Of course, you can feel free to add or subtract supplements according to your preference.

Your starting migraine prevention stack should be vitamin B2 400 mg, magnesium 500 mg, vitamin D3 2000 IU, B12 250 micrograms, and coenzyme-Q10 300-400 mg daily, as well as melatonin 3-5 mg at bedtime. Vitamin B2, magnesium, and coenzyme-Q10 have the best evidence for migraine prevention. If you choose, you can also take folate.

a. If you have migraine attacks around the time of menstruation, also take L-tryptophan 1000-2000 mg at bedtime, vitamin E 400 IU daily, and vitamin C 1000 mg daily for a week around the time of menstruation (see Chapter 18).

b. You may also take L-tryptophan 2000 mg at bedtime if you have insomnia and find no benefit with melatonin.

c. If you have Meniere's disease and/or tinnitus, you can also take Pycnogenol 100 to 150 mg daily.

After 3 months, if you do not see any benefit, you can stop taking these supplements. If you notice some improvement but still have issues with migraine you may try adding pycnogenol, ginkgo, or B6. If you do not see any benefits from a supplement after 3 months, it is reasonable to stop taking it.

For migraine rescue, try taking an extra 500 mg dose of magnesium and/or ginger (about 1000 mg) at the onset of a migraine attack. Peppermint oil can be used instead, or in combination with magnesium and/or ginger. Alternately, take melatonin 5 mg and go to sleep.

For nausea, consume ginger or smell peppermint oil.

For motion sickness prevention, use ginger and vitamin C before traveling and consume some during the journey if needed. Keep peppermint oil handy during the journey, and smell it if you feel nauseous. If you find smelling other essential oils is more effective, use those instead.

Section IV – Acupoints

Acupuncture is an ancient Chinese traditional treatment that involves inserting metallic needles into specific points in the body. The biological mechanism of action is unknown. Traditional Chinese medicine believes that there are meridians through which one's life energy flows and diseases arise from disharmony or imbalance in these meridians. Inserting needles at the acupoints purportedly helps restore harmony and balance in the body. Acupuncture may help migraine headaches and vestibular symptoms. However, the studies investigating acupuncture in these conditions are small and difficult to compare due to differences in treatment protocols and strong placebo effects. Acupuncture may not be remarkably effective but it is certainly safe. Make sure that your acupuncturist is licensed by the relevant state board.

Acupressure is a form of traditional Chinese medicine based on putting pressure on the acupoints used in acupuncture. You can perform acupressure on yourself, and all you need to know is the location of the specific acupoints.

Acupoint EX-HN3 (Yintang)

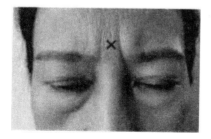

Acupoint EX-HN3 ("Hall of Impressions") is believed to help headaches and stress. It is right between your eyebrows, in the purported location of the third eye. Apply gentle pressure at this point with your thumb, moving in a slow circular motion for 30 seconds with your eyes closed. Repeat until you feel better.

Acupoint LI4 (Hegu)

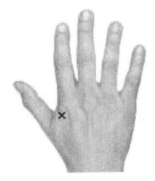

Acupoint LI4 ("Joining Valley") can be used for the treatment of headache. It is at the base of the thumb and index finger. Use your right thumb to apply firm pressure at this point while moving it in a slow circular motion for 5 minutes. You do not have to press so hard as to cause pain. Repeat this on the right hand.

Acupoint EX-HN5 (Taiyang)

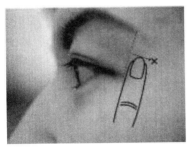

Acupoint EX-HN5 ("Supreme Yang") is believed to help soothe headache, eye pain, eye strain, dizziness, and visual symptoms. It is one finger-breadth behind the mid-point of an imaginary line between the outer edge of the eyebrow and the eye. You will feel a small depression in this area. Place your index fingers on each side and gently massage in a circular motion for one minute; repeat until you feel better. You can massage this acupoint at regular intervals while using electronic screens.

Acupoint GB20 (Fengchi)

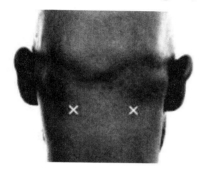

Acupoint GB20 ("Wind Palace") may be used to treat dizziness, headache, stress, and neck pain. It is at the base of the skull and top of the neck, on the outer aspect of the trapezii muscles. You will feel a small depression in this area. Apply firm pressure at this point for 30 seconds, release, then massage gently for 2 minutes. Repeat as many times as needed until you feel better.

Acupoint ST36 (Zusanli)

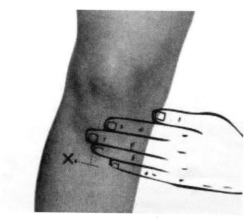

Acupoint ST36 ("Leg Three Miles") can be used for treating motion sickness, gastrointestinal upset, depression, and nausea and vomiting. It is four finger-breadths below the lower edge of the patella (kneecap) on the outer aspect of the tibia (shin). Use your thumb to apply firm pressure at this point and moving it in a circular motion for 5 minutes on one leg then the other.

Acupoint P6 (Neiguan)

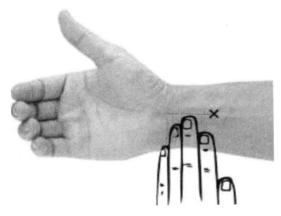

Acupoint P6 ("Inner Gate") is the most studied acupoint for nausea, vomiting, motion sickness, and vertigo. It is on the inner forearm, three finger-breadths from the wrist crease (X). The broken lines mark the two tendons that connect the forearm muscles to your fingers. Use your index finger or thumb to press firmly while moving it in a slow circular motion for 3 minutes. Repeat on the other forearm. Sea Bands are acupressure wrist bands worn at this point. Some products utilize electrical stimulation at P6 but may be pricey.

Chapter 10: Exercise

Life is like riding a bicycle. To keep your balance, you must keep moving.

Albert Einstein (1879-1955)

The number of studies demonstrating the benefits of exercise is myriad. Exercise improves both brain and physical health. It promotes brain-muscle connections thus improving the brain's ability to integrate visual, vestibular, and proprioceptive information. Exercise is also crucial to neuroplasticity, stimulating the release of various neuropeptides (e.g., brain-derived neurotrophic factor, insulin-like growth factor 1) that promote neurogenesis (formation of new neurons) and synaptogenesis (formation of new synapses).

Furthermore, exercise promotes the release of neurotransmitters like dopamine, serotonin, and norepinephrine, which are important in migraine control, PPPD, and mood. Many of my patients feel better after exercising and worse when they slack off. Exercise also reduces stress levels and regulates the HPA axis, mitigating inflammation and glucocorticoid levels. There is emerging scientific evidence in animal and human studies that exercise alters the gut microbiome, increasing the diversity and proportion of healthy microbes [Cryan, 2019].

Physical inactivity is a major cause of depression, anxiety, pain, cardiovascular disease, and dementia. Vertigo and dizziness create a lot of discomfort with movement and cause many to limit their physical activity. Unfortunately, this diminishes the brain's tolerance for movement (i.e., narrows one's comfort zone) and eventually results in more dizziness when a person tries to resume physical activity. This vicious cycle can be very harmful and in severe cases, almost paralyzes a person. I have seen patients who spend their days in bed or couches, terrified of causing any dizziness if they move about. One patient even suffered a deep vein thrombosis (a blood clot in her leg) resulting in a pulmonary embolism that almost killed her. Fortunately, she survived, and we worked on helping her get her vestibular migraine under control and getting her more active.

In this chapter, we will focus on exercises that help your brain and body heal. You will learn why exercise is so important and how to improve your activity level. We will also discuss the importance of vestibular and physical therapy.

What exercise to choose?

Different types of exercise offer different health benefits. Combining various exercise types can help in significant ways. For example, engage in stretching exercises to relieve pain and promote flexibility, aerobic exercise for cardiovascular health and migraine control, and resistance exercises for muscle and bone health.

Find exercises you enjoy. If you find something tedious, you will not be motivated to exercise. Remember to find exercises that challenge you without excessive risk of injury – don't be a couch potato, but don't be a cowboy either. If you have back problems, you may need to avoid certain exercises (e.g., rowing machines, deadlifts). Injuries will force you to stop exercising temporarily and may lead to regression.

Before aerobic and resistance exercises, it is prudent to take a few measures to prevent a migraine attack. Dehydration can trigger migraine attacks, so drink enough fluids before and during your workout. A small snack with complex carbohydrates (e.g., oatmeal, whole-grain bread, apples) and protein can help prevent a blood sugar drop that may trigger an attack. If heat triggers your migraine attacks, work out in cooler environments, drink ice water while exercising, or use cooling towels (e.g., Frogg Toggs). Crowds and noise can aggravate migraine attacks; choose a less busy gym or go at quieter times.

Exercise progression is an important principle. You need to tailor your exercise program based on what you can tolerate. Exercises that are too challenging will make you horribly dizzy, discourage you, erode your motivation, and may even trigger a vestibular migraine attack. Exercises that are too simple are unhelpful and accomplish nothing. The key is to find an activity level that challenges you but does not trigger a vestibular migraine attack. For example, if you feel dizzy when walking on a flat surface for more than 10 minutes, getting on a treadmill and sprinting for 30 minutes will be too much, and doing 5-minute stretching exercises in bed would be far too simple. You will need to aim to walk for 12 minutes, then aim for 15 minutes, then 20 minutes, and so on.

You must choose a level of intensity that is achievable but challenging. Try to test and expand your limits in steps. Take advantage of the motivation feedback loop: set challenging but achievable goals, and when you reach that target, the sense of accomplishment and reward will motivate you to set another goal.

Home Vestibular Exercises

If you experience a lot of dizziness with visual stimuli and head movements, you will need to perform some simple home exercises to reduce your dizziness, improve the coordination between your visual and vestibular systems, and relax the neck and shoulder muscles. As you find your ability to perform these vestibular exercises improves, you will be able to progress to more challenging exercise routines. These exercises will cause some dizziness or discomfort because they are designed to help your brain build its tolerance.

This is a home exercise program to help with your dizziness. You will perform these exercises in stages; each stage is designed to be progressively harder. Rate your discomfort or dizziness with each stage on a scale of 0 to 10 (0 meaning none, and 10 indicating the worst ever). Once you find that a particular stage causes dizziness/discomfort at a 0-3, you can move on to the next stage. Do not proceed if the dizziness/discomfort is more than 5. Perform the exercises more slowly if you find that the dizziness/discomfort is above 8.

Stage 1: Lying Down

While lying in bed, perform the following:

Eye movements

1. Move your eyes up and down. Repeat 10 times.

2. Move your eyes from side to side. Repeat 10 times.

3. Focus on your finger or a pen. Move it from an arm's length to within 6 inches of your nose, and back again. Repeat 10 times.

4. Now hold your left thumb in front of you at arm's length, and your right thumb about one foot to the right. Move your eyes back and forth between each thumb. Repeat 10 times.

5. Hold your right thumb in front of you at arm's length, and your left thumb about one foot to its left. Move your eyes back and forth between each thumb. Repeat 10 times.

Head movements

1. Bend your head forwards and backward with your eyes closed. Repeat 10 times.

2. Turn your head from side to side with your eyes closed. Repeat 10 times.

3. Bend your head forward and backward with your eyes open. Repeat 10 times.

4. Turn your head from side to side with your eyes open. Repeat 10 times.

5. Focus on your finger or pen at arm's length. Bend your head forward and backward while focusing on it. Repeat 10 times.

6. Turn your head from side to side while focusing on the pen/finger. Repeat this 10 times.

7. While moving your finger/pen from side to side (from about 45 degrees to the right and left), keep your eyes focused on it and turn your head so that it moves in tandem with your finger/pen. The aim is to move your head, eyes, and target together as a unit from side to side. Repeat 20 times.

Stage 2: Seated

While seated in a firm chair with a back support:

1. Perform the same eye and head movement exercises listed in Stage 1.

2. Throw a tennis ball from one hand to the other for about 30 seconds.

3. Place the tennis ball on the ground in front of you. Bend forwards to pick it up and then replace it on the ground, and sit back up. Repeat 10 times.

4. Place the tennis ball on the ground about 6 inches to the right of your right heel. Bend forwards to pick it up and then replace it, and sit back up. Repeat 10 times.

5. Place the tennis ball on the ground about 6 inches to the left of your left heel. Bend forwards to pick it up and then replace it, and sit back up. Repeat 10 times.

6. Chair squats: scoot to the edge of the chair, ensure that your heels are underneath your knees, lean forward and push yourself to a standing position. Lower yourself in a controlled manner to the seated position again. Repeat 15 times. It is ok to use your arms to help you stand and sit initially, but you should work at this until you can cross your arms across your chest while performing this exercise.

Stage 3: Standing with Support

Stand behind a chair. While you hold on the back of the chair for support:

1. Perform the same eye and head movement exercises in Stage 1.

2. Place the tennis ball about 6 inches to the right of the chair. While holding the back of the chair for support, bend over to pick it up, stand up, then bend over to replace it and stand back up. Repeat 10 times.

3. Place the tennis ball about 6 inches to the left of the chair. While holding the back of the chair for support, bend over to pick it up, stand up, then bend over to replace it and stand back up. Repeat 10 times.

4. One-legged balance: while holding the back of the chair with your right hand, close your eyes, lift your right leg off the floor, and balance on the left leg. Maintain this position for 10 seconds. Repeat by supporting yourself with your left hand, lifting the left leg off the floor, and balancing on the right leg. Perform 10 repetitions of this exercise for each leg.

5. Mini squats: with your feet shoulder-width apart and holding the back of the chair for support, slowly bend at the hips, pushing your buttocks backward (as if trying to sit) until your knees are bent to 45 degrees. Hold this position for 1-2 seconds, then slowly stand up again. Repeat 15 times.

Stage 4: Standing without Support

Find a corner of a room to stand. Do not lean on the walls but be close to walls just in case you need to support yourself. When you first start performing the exercises in this stage, have someone close by for safety.

1. Perform the same eye and head movement exercises listed in Stage 1.

2. Bend forwards to pick an object off the ground, stand back up, then replace the object on the ground.

3. Throw the tennis ball from hand to hand, with your hands about one foot apart. Do this for 30 seconds. When you can do this comfortably, try throwing the ball from hand to hand, with your hands two and then three feet apart.

4. With your eyes open, cross your arms across your chest, and stand with your heels touching each other. Maintain this position for 10 seconds. When you can do this comfortably, try it with your eyes closed. Repeat 10 times.

5. When you can comfortably stand with your eyes closed, try the one-legged balance exercise. While standing with your eyes open, lift the right foot an inch or two off the ground and balance on the left leg. Maintain this position for 10 seconds. Repeat by lifting the left food off the ground, and balancing on the right leg. Repeat 10 times for each leg. Once you can perform this exercise comfortably with your eyes open, try it with your eyes closed.

Stage 5: Moving Around

<u>Walking</u>

1. Find a flat, clear area where you can walk for about 20 to 25 feet, like a driveway. Walk from one end to the other. Repeat 10 times.

2. Try turning your head slowly from side to side while walking 20 to 25 feet. Repeat 10 times.

3. Now try moving your head up and down while walking 20 to 25 feet. Repeat 10 times.

4. Try throwing and catching a tennis ball from one hand to the other while walking 20 to 25 feet. Repeat 10 times.

<u>Tandem walking</u>

1. Walk heel to toe (like a field sobriety test) for 25 feet. It is ok to take breaks to catch your balance initially, but aim to complete 20 to 25 feet without pausing. Repeat 5 times.

2. Once you can do so, try tandem walking backward. Yes, backward. Again, aim for 20 to 25 feet. Repeat 5 times.

3. If you have hip, knee, or back problems that make tandem walking difficult, you may skip this.

Aerobic Exercises

Aerobic exercise has positive effects on migraine and vestibular migraine. Studies have shown that aerobic exercise improves vestibular migraine and migraine severity, AND lowers blood levels of pro-inflammatory compounds.

Aerobic exercise (often called "cardio") refers to low to high-intensity exercise that requires the body to use oxygen to meet energy demands. Aerobic exercise does NOT have to be a heart-pounding, sweat-drenched ordeal that takes you to the borderlands of life and death. The studies in migraine and vestibular migraine used moderate-intensity aerobic exercise, which is defined as activities that bring the heart rate to 50-70% of maximum heart rate or feel somewhere between light and somewhat heavy exertion.

Activities that count as moderate-intensity exercises include jogging, brisk walking, elliptical training, cycling under 10 mph, swimming, water aerobics, and dance classes. A leisurely stroll around the neighborhood does not count, sorry. The studies found that 30-45 minutes of such activity (not including warm up and cool down), three times per week was enough to obtain benefits for migraine and vestibular migraine. In fact, migraine improvement with such an exercise program is comparable to that achieved with topiramate or tricyclic antidepressants.

Start with brisk walking. As your endurance and tolerance improve, you can try jogging, swimming, or cycling. Stationary bicycles, treadmills, and stair-masters are good indoor options. Dance classes and water aerobics may be slightly challenging if crowds of moving people make you dizzy. The up-and-down movements of elliptical trainers can be challenging for some.

Those who are more fit can consider high-intensity interval training (HIIT) workouts. HIIT workouts are characterized by alternating short bursts of intense aerobic exercise with short periods of rest. For example, one can alternate running at 95% of maximum heart rate for 3 minutes with walking briskly for 3 minutes for 30 minutes. These workouts are challenging, but burn more calories in a shorter period compared to continuous exercise at a moderate intensity (e.g., jogging for 30 minutes), and are effective for migraine control [Hanssen, 2017].

Resistance Exercises

Resistance exercises require muscles to work against a weight or force. While aerobic exercise is great for our cardiovascular system, resistance exercises can help improve bone and muscle health. Resistance exercises also promote muscle insulin sensitivity, resulting in better blood sugar control. Resistance exercises enhance bone health (preventing or reducing osteoporosis) and range of motion. They strengthen your core and back muscles, decreasing pain and improving both posture and balance. Resistance exercises directly improve migraine control as well. Among office workers (who are relatively inactive while at work), just one hour of resistance exercises per week has been shown to improve migraine control significantly.

Resistance exercises can utilize one's body weight (e.g., push-ups), elastic bands, barbells, dumbbells, or kettlebells. Many exercises can be performed and the right program will depend on your fitness level, age, and co-morbid conditions. Young adults with no medical issues could easily start using barbells or dumbbells. Older adults, particularly those with back and joint problems, should start with light resistance bands or body weight. If you have a physical therapist, they will usually teach you some resistance exercises.

Hiring an experienced personal trainer may be a good investment. They can help design an appropriate resistance exercise program and teach you proper exercise techniques. Once you get the hang of it, you can design your own resistance exercise program. You can easily mix resistance and aerobic exercises. Start with 30 minutes of aerobic exercise then follow it with 30 minutes of resistance training (or vice versa), three times a week.

Aquatic Exercises

The hydrostatic and hydrodynamic properties of water create challenges and permit movements that cannot be replicated by exercising on dry land. For example, swimming is performed in the prone (face down) position, uses both arms and legs for propulsion through a medium (water) that provides more resistance than air and requires controlled breathing.

A major advantage of aquatic exercises is that water temperature can be adjusted. Heat and dehydration are well-known migraine triggers. Such thermal stress is avoided by exercising in cool water. Alternately, warmer water is more soothing for joint, back and muscle pain. Another advantage for people with joint and back problems is how buoyancy and hydrostatic pressure decrease the apparent body weight and weight load on joints. The magnitude of ground reaction and impact forces are lower in water compared to dry land.

While aquatic exercises provide aerobic and resistance benefits, they are typically non-weight-bearing. As such, it can help improve lean body mass, endurance, and cardiovascular health, but not bone density.

Neck Stretching

Neck pain is a major problem for many people with migraine, and neck problems can often exacerbate migraine attacks. Stretching tight muscles and strengthening weak ones improves neck, and shoulder pain, as well as scalp muscle tension.

Neck Stretching Exercises

These can help improve neck, and shoulder pain, as well as scalp muscle tension. They can be performed daily, and when the pain is more noticeable. Some stretching exercises include:

Shoulder Roll: Rotate your shoulders backward, squeezing your shoulder blades together as you do so. Hold for 3 seconds, release, and repeat 10 times. After that, repeat it but this time, roll your shoulders forward instead.

Head Roll: Tilt your head slowly to bring your right ear towards your right shoulder. Feel the muscles on the left side of your neck stretch for 3-5 seconds, and then roll your head forward. Now tuck your chin into your chest, feeling the base of your neck stretch for 3-5 seconds. Then, roll your head towards the left so that your left ear is directed towards your left shoulder, feeling the right side of your neck stretch. Hold for 3-5 seconds, then roll back towards the middle and right. Repeat 10 times.

Neck Rotations: Turn your head to the right to look over the right shoulder as far as possible without hurting yourself. Hold this for 3-5 seconds then repeat for the left side. Perform 10 repetitions for the right and left sides.

Neck Side Stretches: With your back straight, tilt your head to bring the right ear towards your right shoulder. Put your right hand on top of your head and press down lightly, feeling the muscles in the left side of your neck stretching. Hold for 3-5 seconds, then repeat for the left side. Perform 10 repetitions for the right and left sides.

Neck Strengthening Exercises

Neck pain is often related to weakness of the muscles that help maintain good posture. These are some exercises that can help strengthen these muscles.

Chin Tuck: Lie on your back, with a rolled-up towel supporting the base of your neck and occiput (back of the head). Place your tongue on the roof of your mouth, and keep your lips together with teeth slightly apart. Gently glide your chin straight back by about 1-2 inches. Don't tilt your head, or bend your neck. Hold this position for 10 seconds, and repeat it 10 times. Once you find this easy to perform, add a head lift to make it more challenging; perform the chin tuck, then lift your head one inch off the towel.

Neck Isometrics: Sit on a firm chair with both feet flat on the floor, and your back straight. Push your palm against your forehead and resist with your neck muscles; hold for 10 seconds, and repeat 10 times. Do the same with your palm pushing the right, left, and back of your head.

You can perform these simple exercises once a day. If you have a desk job, the stretches can be done every few hours to relieve muscle and joint tension from excessive sitting and poor posture. There are many more stretching exercises for neck, shoulder, scalp, and back muscle tightness, soreness, and pain. Working with a physical therapist or an experienced personal trainer can help you learn the best stretching exercises for you.

Low-impact, low-velocity balance exercises can be very helpful for those with vestibular migraine. These exercises also produce minimum stress on your joints and involve slower, more deliberate movements. Besides improving your flexibility, these exercises help reduce anxiety, stress, and sensitivity to the many head, eye, and body movements that cause dizziness.

Yoga is very popular and there are many classes available, even from the comfort of home. People with back or joint problems can benefit from chair yoga. If you have significant dizziness and disequilibrium, chair yoga can be a good place to start. Yogic breathing and certain yoga postures directly stimulate the vagus nerve. Emerging evidence shows that yoga can reduce the frequency and severity of migraine attacks. Pilates is more challenging than yoga and can be useful for people who can perform yoga with some ease.

Taichi and Qigong are ancient Chinese exercises that involve coordinated body posture, movement, and breathing. These can improve balance, posture, dizziness, and fall risk. Other benefits include improved cardiovascular health, psychological well-being, stress levels, joint pain, and cognitive function [Solloway, 2016]. Classes are a bit harder to find in some locations but a Google search may help locate classes or videos to help you get started.

Other Exercises

Certain sports are excellent for enhancing eye-head-hand coordination and are great ways of helping your balance and decreasing your dizziness. Tennis, pickleball, racquetball (squash), table tennis, and badminton are some examples of sports that can be aerobic exercises that also improve dizziness and balance.

Henry saw me because he felt a bit off balance if he moved too fast. It was not bad but it was an annoyance. To my surprise, testing showed that he had zero vestibular function in both inner ears! With such severe loss, people usually have debilitating balance problems. His secret? *Pickleball.* He played several times per week, his whole life. Pickleball is a paddleball sport that involves a lot of eye-head-neck-hand coordination. Although Henry had *zero* peripheral vestibular function, years of playing pickleball had helped his brain adapt so well that he only had mild imbalance if he moved too quickly. Through neuroplasticity, his brain re-wired his balance system despite lacking peripheral vestibular input.

Dancing is a fun way to improve balance and dizziness. Like sports, dancing incorporates head, eye, neck, and body movements and requires coordination between the visual, vestibular, and proprioceptive systems. Start with simple classes for beginners, like Zumba or line dancing, and progress to more challenging dance classes. My mentor, Dr. David Zee, is a great proponent of ballroom dancing to improve balance and dizziness.

Vestibular Rehabilitation Therapy (VRT)

VRT is a specialized form of physical therapy that focuses on disorders that cause dizziness, vertigo, and imbalance. VRT utilizes exercises that promote processes called adaptation, substitution, and desensitization, which reduce vestibular symptoms, improve stability, enhance brain adaptation to vestibular disorders, decrease the fall risk, and promote mobility.

Adaptation exercises help a person become aware of, and either ignore or improve problems related to maintaining balance. Substitution helps an individual tap into alternative sensory input or actions to improve balance; for instance, after vestibular neuritis, VRT enhances the function of other systems involved in maintaining balance. Desensitization exercises help improve tolerance for stimuli and responses that cause dizziness, vertigo, or imbalance; for example, if a person gets dizzy with head movements, a vestibular therapist will work on exercises that progressively reduce the brain's sensitivity to head motion. VRT builds on and improves neuroplasticity, which is the brain's innate ability to re-organize and repair itself. A vestibular therapist evaluates each patient to design a personalized program. There is no "one-size fits all" VRT program – it must be tailored for each unique person. Vestibular therapists can also treat benign paroxysmal positional vertigo by performing maneuvers that dislodge the misplaced crystal.

A few studies have confirmed that VRT is helpful in people with vestibular migraine. For these patients, VRT exercises focus on adaptation and desensitization. These are called habituation exercises and gaze stability training, designed to help decrease the constant dizziness, visually-induced dizziness, a sensation of vision "jumping", and head motion-induced dizziness. Such exercises stimulate mild to moderate dizziness, and over time, the brain becomes more resilient and the dizziness will decrease.

In general, in those with severe symptoms, I find that VRT works best for vestibular migraine once we start the appropriate prevention therapy to "cool" the hot migraine brain first. If VRT is performed when the brain is in a very sensitive and hyperexcitable state, even the mild dizziness produced by VRT may be too overwhelming, and could aggravate their vestibular migraine symptoms. In addition, balance training exercises can be performed for people with vestibular migraine who feel unsteady, off balance, and who are at risk for falls.

VRT is performed on an outpatient basis. In addition to the exercises performed when a person sees the vestibular therapist, there will be exercises that need to be performed at home. When you undergo VRT, you must be disciplined, diligent, and motivated to perform these home exercises to guarantee the best possible outcome.

Physical Therapy

Physical therapy encompasses a wide range of exercises and treatments designed to improve mobility, balance, joint range of motion, balance, pain control, and athletic function. While I usually refer my patients to vestibular therapy for the treatment of vestibular symptoms, physical therapy plays an important role in treating pain and musculoskeletal disorders that may occur in people with vestibular migraine.

Neck and shoulder pain are very common complications of vestibular migraine because the neck and shoulders are often tensed up to minimize head motion-induced dizziness. Neck therapy is a specialized form of physical therapy aimed at helping those with neck pain. Dry needling is performed by trained physical therapists to treat neuromusculoskeletal pain and involves inserting monofilament needles in painful regions. Transcutaneous electrical stimulation (TENS) can also be performed by physical therapists to treat musculoskeletal pain.

Physical therapy can also help treat conditions that are unrelated to, but aggravate, vestibular migraine. For example, lower back, hip, and knee pain are very common and can make it hard for people to participate in VRT or exercise; physical therapy can help address the conditions.

Chiropractic Manipulation

Chiropractic manipulation can be useful for back and neck pain. I typically caution against high-velocity neck adjustments ("neck cracking") due to the risk of causing arterial dissection (tearing of the inner lining of the arteries in the neck) which can result in strokes. People with migraine may be at higher risk of dissection, and as such, should be careful with such maneuvers. Manual soft tissue release, joint mobilization, and deep neck flexion exercises may be helpful for headache, as well as neck, back, and joint pain. Some chiropractors also perform VRT-type exercises that can help people with vestibular migraine.

Massage Therapy

Massage therapy involves soft tissue manipulation to treat pain disorders. In vestibular migraine, massage therapy can be effective at treating neck, shoulder, and lower back pain, as well as headaches. Fibromyalgia, which can be co-morbid with migraine, may also benefit from massage therapy.

C

Life Changes

Recognizing triggers, changing to your lifestyle, and understanding the relationship between your gut, diet and vestibular migraine.

Chapter 11: Vestibular Migraine Triggers

One man's windchimes are another man's migraine
Marcus Dagan

All bodies have a physiologic comfort zone. This is the range within which the body can tolerate certain changes. For example, we have different tolerance levels for changes in sleep, hydration, blood pressure, food, and stress. Variations within our personal comfort zone won't cause any problems but when we stray outside this zone, our bodies will protest. The migraine brain has a narrower comfort zone than a non-migraine brain. It is exquisitely sensitive to changes in the body's physiology and the external environment. The hyperexcitable migraine brain loves routine and loathes deviation from its metabolic comfort zone.

Migraine triggers don't cause migraine. Instead, migraine triggers are stimuli in the external environment or the body's internal physiologic milieu that push the migraine brain outside its metabolic comfort zone, resulting in a migraine attack. Vestibular migraine triggers are unique to each person. Some triggers affect many people (e.g., stress, weather), but some triggers only affect a small number of people. Some triggers are unavoidable, but many can be avoided. Now, sensitivity to triggers can also change throughout one's life. You may be sensitive to some triggers at points in your life but not others. For example, you may be more sensitive to skipping a meal during times of high stress but can easily miss a meal when you're more relaxed. You also may become much less sensitive to some triggers once you get on an effective migraine preventive treatment plan.

Keep track of your migraine attacks by recording them in a diary to help you identify your unique triggers. For example, if you notice that you have attacks consistently after eating peanuts, peanuts are your migraine trigger. Identifying your unique triggers helps you seize the initiative and reduce exposure. For instance, if you notice that sleeping less than 6 hours a night triggers a migraine attack, make the necessary adjustments to ensure you get the requisite amount of sleep. If working on your computer continuously for more than 2 hours triggers an attack, set a timer on your phone to ensure you take a 5-minute break after 90 minutes. A diary can also help you determine the most effective countermeasure to address a specific trigger.

Stress

"Do I in any way profit from this misery?" Nietzsche finally responded. "I have reflected no that very question for many years. Perhaps I do profit. In two ways. You suggest that the attacks are caused by stress, but sometimes the opposite is true – that the attacks dissipate stress. My work is stressful. It requires me to face the dark side of existence, and the migraine attack, awful as it is, may be a cleansing convulsion that permits me to continue."

Irvin D. Yalom, When Nietzsche Wept

By far, the most common vestibular migraine trigger is stress. Almost three-quarters of migraine sufferers find that stress is a definite trigger and higher stress levels increase the risk of chronic migraine. As discussed in previous chapters, stress plays a huge role in the genesis of migraine and is the top factor in triggering and worsening migraine. Stress is the most commonly reported trigger in my vestibular migraine patient population and periods of stress often cause clusters of vestibular migraine attacks.

It is difficult to define exactly what stress is. Like how Justice Potter Stewart described pornography in 1964 ("I shall not today attempt to further define the kinds of material [pornography]... but I know it when I see it"), stress is difficult to define but easy to recognize. Stress can be broadly understood as a state of being unable to cope with the demands of life events which may be related to responsibilities (both job and non-job-related), relationships, and health.

The fight-or-flight response and the HPA axis are discussed in Chapter 3. Our bodies can easily handle acute stress but chronic stress is insidious and deadly. With chronic stress, the flight-or-fight response is almost perpetually turned on. Levels of cortisol are chronically elevated, disrupting the body's metabolic state – raising blood sugar, pressure, and lipid levels; altering sleep patterns; triggering sugar cravings; unleashing pro-inflammatory processes; suppressing the immune system; and disrupting other hormones critical to our homeostatic well-being. The net result is a jittery brain vulnerable to pain, vertigo, anxiety, and depression, and a body prone to obesity, diabetes, heart disease, cancer, infertility, infections, autoimmune disease, bone disease, and stroke. Like the proverbial frog being slowly boiled alive, chronic stress can kill you without you even knowing it.

However, even though the overall level of cortisol is higher in chronically stressed people, their bodies' ability to provide a momentary cortisol boost in response to an acute stressor is blunted and the body's responsiveness to cortisol is lowered. In essence, chronic stress elevates baseline cortisol levels (causing serious metabolic harm to our bodies) but impairs the ability to react effectively to acute stress. This may explain why a sudden reduction in stress following a period of high stress, can also trigger a migraine attack (called "let-down headache"). This phenomenon is hypothesized to be due to the sudden drop in cortisol levels.

Stress is an unavoidable part of life. However, we can certainly do many things to control the level of stress, and to alter our stress response. This can help mitigate the impact of stress on vestibular migraine. From Nietzsche's perspective, could it be that a migraine attack is our brain's way of telling us that it has had enough and we need to stop and rest? We would do well to manage both stress levels and how we deal with it, thereby minimizing the need for our brains to force that "cleansing convulsion" upon us.

Weather Changes

Approaching storms, heat, and humidity are common weather-related migraine triggers. My patients often tell me that they can predict a storm front better than meteorologists. Vestibular migraine attacks often precede a storm by a day to several hours. Interestingly, Meniere's disease attacks can also be provoked by weather changes, highlighting its overlap with vestibular migraine.

How does the weather trigger vestibular migraine attacks? Drops in atmospheric pressure, which occur when the humidity rises and the temperature falls (resulting in precipitation) correlate with increased migraine attacks. A very interesting study in lab rats found that falling barometric pressure increases neuron discharge rates in the trigeminal nucleus caudalis (an area of the brainstem that plays a key role in migraine) [Messlinger, 2010].

Another very intriguing (albeit controversial) hypothesis implicates sferics, which are changes in electromagnetic fields resulting from natural atmospheric lightning discharges [Martin, 2013; Walach, 2010; Vaintl, 2001]. Interestingly, migraine incidence has been found to correlate with lightning activity – more migraine attacks occur on days with more lightning [Martin, 2013]. Remember that the brain essentially operates with electrical activity. Is it possible that lightning strikes in storm fronts alter electromagnetic fields to a point that a migraine brain's electrical activity is affected?

This sensitivity to weather changes saved a patient of mine. She had a horrible vestibular migraine attack during a storm and had to go to her daughter's home. A few hours after leaving her home, a tornado completely flattened it. If not for vestibular migraine, she may not be alive today. As they say, every dark cloud has a silver lining.

A great wind is coming, and that gives you either imagination or a headache

Catherine the Great, Empress of Russia (1729-1796)

Light

Bright and flashing lights are well-known migraine and vestibular migraine triggers. Artificial lights (e.g., fluorescent lights, electronic screens, lights from oncoming traffic) are more triggering than natural lights in most people. Natural light is full spectrum (contains all the light wavelengths in the colors of the rainbow) and dynamic (color temperature and light intensity varies). On the other hand, fluorescent and LED lighting emit higher levels of specific wavelengths of light.

The flicker of artificial lighting also plays a role in triggering migraine. In older fluorescent and LED lighting, the flicker was visible. Over time, advances have reduced flicker but even when imperceptible, flicker can cause headache and eyestrain [Veitch, 1995]. In some, flicker increases the excitability of the nervous system and worsens performance [Kuller, 1998]. The effects of flicker may be more pronounced in people with migraine, autism, epilepsy, and chronic fatigue syndrome.

Sunlight can also trigger migraine attacks. In the land of the midnight sun (near the Arctic in Norway), migraine attacks increase significantly from April until August, when the sun never sets. Many experience migraine attacks by being in bright sunlight, especially for too long. Some of my patients observe that abruptly stepping out into bright sunlight from the inside of a dark building triggers attacks.

Flashing, strobe, or flickering lights can also trigger vestibular migraine attacks. Flashing lights are common in TV shows, movies, and video games. Strobe effects can also occur when there is a light shining behind a ceiling fan, light coming through blinds, and when driving past a row of trees or picket fences with sunlight shining through.

The connection between flashing lights and epilepsy is well-recognized and may provide insight into how they trigger migraine and vertigo. A small number of epileptics (about 5%) suffer from photosensitive epilepsy, a condition where flashing lights provoke seizures. This phenomenon gained popular attention after a scene with flashing lights in a *Pokemon* episode caused seizures in hundreds of Japanese children in 1997. It is hypothesized that strobe lights cause the neurons in the visual cortex to fire in synchrony in those with vulnerable, hyperexcitable brains. When enough neurons fire in unison, the abnormal electrical activity spreads and causes a seizure.

Similarly, the visual cortices of people with vestibular migraine may be more vulnerable to the hyper-synchronous firing effect when exposed to strobe lights.

Flashing lights are also known triggers for vertigo and dizziness, not just migraine attacks. Flicker vertigo (or the Bucha effect) is a phenomenon where vertigo, dizziness, and nausea are triggered by strobe lights, flashing between 1 to 20 Hertz (flashes per second), which is the same frequency of human brain waves. Flicker vertigo was described by Dr. Bucha, who was called to investigate a series of unexplained helicopter crashes, and theorized the pilots experienced vertigo, disorientation, and nausea when the rotor blades strobed sunlight at a particular frequency.

The color of the flashing lights also plays a role in triggering migraine. Red flashing light is the most provocative for photosensitive epilepsy. In fact, that infamous *Pokemon* scene had red and blue flashing lights. My patients often report that flashing blue and red lights on fire trucks, ambulances, and police vehicles trigger their attacks.

Noise

Hyperacusis (sensitivity to sound) occurs during and in between vestibular migraine attacks. Hyperacusis may be due to dysfunctional trigeminocervical interactions with the inner ear or alterations in the cochlear nucleus in the brainstem. Loud sounds and noisy environments are not only unpleasant to vestibular migraine patients but may even be perceived as pain or trigger attacks.

Sirens are a particularly obnoxious trigger. Hyperacusis is most likely because of increased connections between the auditory centers of the brain, and the regions that perceive pain. Some of my patients observe repetitive or reverberating noises are especially provocative; this could be similar to the effect of flashing lights.

Air Pollution

Air pollutants include nitrogen dioxide, sulfur dioxide, carbon monoxide, ozone, dioxins, volatile organic compounds, and polycyclic aromatic hydrocarbons. How air pollution triggers migraine is not precisely known but there are several hypotheses.

The trigeminal endings in the nasal cavity may be irritated by the pollutants. Air pollution irritates and inflames the airway leading to higher levels of pro-inflammatory cytokines. These pollutants can also be absorbed through the lungs and travel through the circulatory system to the brain, triggering inflammatory reactions.

Multiple studies from different countries confirm that emergency department visits for migraine attacks increase on days with higher air pollution levels, particularly during hotter weather. Long-term air pollutants have also been linked to a higher frequency of migraine attacks.

Odors

Because many migraine patients are sensitive to smells, strong odors can often trigger a migraine attack. There are usually specific odors that trigger migraines. Perfumes are the most common offending odor, which is why many headache practices ban their staff from using perfumes or scented lotions. Pungent and unpleasant odors (e.g., paint, gasoline, bleach, cigarette smoke) are also common triggers.

The headache tree (*Umbellularia californica*) is a large tree native to California and the coastal forests of Oregon. It earned its name because the vapors released from its leaves can trigger migraine attacks. Italian scientists at the University of Florence reported the case of a gardener whose headache attacks occurred every time he pruned the tree. They found that vapors from the tree contained a chemical that triggered CGRP release in the trigeminal system [Benemei, 2010]. It is hypothesized that odors trigger migraine attacks by a similar pathway.

Mast cells are a subset of immune cells that are involved in allergic reactions. The surface of mast cells is covered with an antibody called IgE. When an allergen attaches to IgE, the reaction causes degranulation, which is the release of a cocktail of compounds (the most important of which is histamine) responsible for inflammation, swelling, pain, and increased blood flow. When mast cell degranulation occurs in the meninges, inflammation occurs in the local micro-environment, acidifying it, and sensitizing pain nerves, leading to the release of even more pro-inflammatory chemicals.

Histamine's influence on migraine is often under-recognized. Children with eczema and allergic disorders (diseases driven by histamine excess), suffer from more headaches. Injecting histamine through the veins can provoke headaches. Sleep deprivation, a common migraine trigger, is also known to increase histamine levels in spinal fluid. Furthermore, people with migraine have higher blood histamine levels, during and in between migraine attacks, and are much more sensitive to the effects of histamine. This may explain why anti-histaminergic medications like doxepin and cyproheptadine are effective in vestibular migraine prevention.

This relationship between migraine and histamine may also explain why people with vestibular migraine often suffer from seasonal allergies, rhinitis, and sinusitis. Furthermore, the link between histamine and migraine may be the reason for increased migraine attacks at certain times of the year (usually spring and fall). Some of my patients only experience vestibular migraine attacks during allergy season.

If you suffer from allergies and vestibular migraine, consulting an allergist can help. The optimal treatment of allergies goes beyond just taking an antihistamine. Nasal sprays, nasal rinses, mast cell stabilizers, leukotriene inhibitors, and immunotherapy (allergy shots) can all potentially help. An allergist can help tailor the best therapeutic plan for you.

Visual Stimuli

Busy and highly-patterned visual scenes are highly uncomfortable for people with migraine and vestibular migraine, and often trigger attacks. The French mathematician Jean-Baptiste Fourier theorized that visual scenes are composed of striped patterns of different sizes, orientations, and positions. In natural scenes, most of these stripes cancel each other out, which is why we do not typically see a series of straight lines in natural scenes. However, modern designs feature many regular, repetitive patterns and stripes, like windows, buildings, blinds, stairs, tiles, parking lots, sentences in books and documents, and grocery aisles.

Our brains did not evolve to deal with such unnatural patterns. They create visual discomfort and stress. This is why we feel relaxed when we look at natural scenes, not urban landscapes. In fact, such patterns alter the brain's electrical activity, creating gamma oscillations that increase the metabolic demand on the brain's visual-processing regions. When viewing natural scenes, the neurons in our visual cortex work asynchronously, which is less metabolically taxing. Visual scenes with lots of stripes (like urban landscapes) force the neurons to work synchronously, increasing the metabolic load. Recall that flashing lights can provoke migraine, vertigo, and seizures by forcing neurons to fire synchronously in large enough numbers. Similarly, excessive exposure to such visual stimuli can provoke seizures and vestibular migraine attacks. Large striped patterns with high contrast (i.e., alternating black and white stripes) are the most unpleasant stimuli, and vertical stripe patterns are more uncomfortable than horizontal lines. In addition to hyper-synchronous neuronal activity, the accumulation of toxic byproducts of increased metabolism may also contribute to migraine attacks.

Another form of visual stimulus that can aggravate vestibular migraine is called visually-induced motion sickness. Motion sickness typically arises from conflicting sensory information (discussed in Chapter 5). Visually-induced motion sickness occurs when visual input tells the brain that movement is occurring but the vestibular system tells the brain otherwise.

For example, if you are watching an action movie on a large screen TV while seated in your favorite recliner, your visual system interprets the rapid movements and shifting camera angles as actual movement and conveys this information to your brain. However, your vestibular system tells your brain that your head and body are stationary. People with migraine and vestibular migraine tend to be more sensitive to this conflicting information and develop nausea. This is why watching an IMAX or 3D movie, or watching a home video recording (where the camera jiggles around) is so unpleasant for those with migraine. Scrolling on electronic screens (especially big ones) and first-person shooter video games also induce a sensation of visual motion and provoke nausea. In those who are more susceptible, interacting with someone who is nodding or shaking their heads, or gesticulating excessively with their hands can provoke visually-induced motion sickness. Although the stimulus takes up the central visual scene in most, some are so sensitive that objects or people moving in their visual periphery make them dizzy.

Motion Sickness

Motion sensitivity and motion sickness are common in migraine and vestibular migraine (see Chapter 5). In fact, most patients have a childhood history of motion sickness. Motion sickness is related to low serotonin levels, just like migraine. Although it is usually unpleasant and nauseating, motion sickness can trigger a full-blown migraine attack if it is severe enough. If you have motion sickness, taking preventive measures before travel can help ward off a vestibular migraine attack (discussed in Chapter 17).

Menses

Menstruation is a well-recognized vestibular migraine trigger. Typically, vestibular migraines tend to increase in the few days leading up to menstruation and can persist for 2-3 days when the cycle is over. Fluctuations in estrogen levels, which cause changes in serotonin and CGRP levels, are the most likely reason for this. Some have suggested the ratio of progesterone to estrogen may also have a role as a migraine trigger. Chapter 18 covers the relationship between migraines and hormones.

Sleep

Irregular sleep patterns are a common vestibular migraine trigger. Depriving lab rats of REM sleep sensitizes the trigeminal system and causes the rat equivalent of a migraine attack when they are exposed to pungent odors [Cornelison, 2020]. Lack of sleep usually triggers the attack. While some experience vestibular migraine attacks the morning after a night of poor sleep, a study in migraine patients showed that most attacks tend to happen the following day.

Interestingly, sleeping in can also trigger migraine attacks. "Weekend migraines" or the "Saturday syndrome" occur in people with regular 9-to-5 jobs. These are migraines that begin on Saturday mornings, particularly after a hectic week. One explanation for these migraines is the change in sleep patterns. Sleeping in is a wonderful luxury, but may not be good for the hot migraine brain. If you don't usually nap, taking one can sometimes provoke a migraine attack. It is curious if naps really trigger migraine or if the premonitory phase of the migraine causes drowsiness and fatigue that compels one to nap.

Too Much Head Movement

Head motion-induced dizziness is problematic in vestibular migraine, as discussed in Chapter 5. Engaging in activities that require a lot of back-and-forth head movements is not only uncomfortable but can trigger vestibular migraine attacks in some people. House chores that involve a lot of back-and-forth head movements, like unloading the dishwasher, yard work, or transferring clothes to the dryer, can trigger an attack. At work, repeatedly looking back and forth between multiple computer screens, or from documents to computer screens, can be aggravating enough to trigger migraine attacks.

Dehydration

About a third of patients find that dehydration triggers migraine and vestibular migraine attacks. One theory is that serum osmolality changes affect metabolic activity in the migraine centers. Another theory is that an accumulation of cellular waste products and toxins that are not flushed away by adequate fluids trigger the migraine. Proving the importance of hydration in migraine, an emergency department study among people admitted for migraine attacks found that intravenous fluid hydration relieved migraine more effectively than injected pain medications.

Missing Meals

Missing or skipping meals can often trigger vestibular migraine attacks. While we don't yet understand how skipping meals can trigger a migraine, one possible explanation points to a neurotransmitter called orexin. Orexin-producing neurons project to many brain regions involved in migraine generation, including the locus coeruleus, periaqueductal gray, and trigeminal system.

Orexin also plays a role in obesity and this may explain why migraine is more severe in overweight individuals. Altered orexin levels are seen in the spinal fluid of migraine patients - lower levels are observed in episodic migraine, while higher levels are seen in chronic migraine. Skipping a meal may cause a drop in blood sugar levels, triggering the release of orexin in the hypothalamus, and resulting in a migraine attack.

Exercise

As we learned, exercise is very important for vestibular migraine patients. Low levels of physical activity can aggravate migraines, and in most, improved physical conditioning translates into better migraine control. Interestingly, a few reports detail how strenuous physical activity during the premonitory phase can ward off a migraine attack. However, it is also important to note that exercise may trigger migraines in some. The intolerance for excessive head movements (e.g., in dance classes, doing burpees), dehydration, heat, and hunger may be to blame. It is not clear why physical exertion triggers migraine attacks; some suggest that elevated lactate production (a byproduct of muscle anaerobic metabolism), altered orexin levels from the hypothalamus, increased nitric oxide levels (a vasodilator), or higher CGRP levels may be to blame.

Dietary Triggers

Migraine food triggers have been recognized for more than 200 years. These are discussed in detail in Chapter 14.

Chapter 12: Lifestyle Changes –Fortify your Brain

An ounce of prevention is worth a pound of cure
Benjamin Franklin (1706-1790)

Living well with vestibular migraine requires certain life changes to make your brain tougher and less vulnerable to vestibular migraine attacks and interictal symptoms. Recall how the hyperexcitable migraine brain suffers from inherent underlying bioenergetic, metabolic abnormalities that predispose it to dizziness, vertigo, nausea, photophobia, phonophobia, headache, brain fog, and all the symptoms that characterize vestibular migraine. Making the appropriate and necessary life changes can heal and correct these bioenergetic and metabolic imbalances, making the brain stronger and much less susceptible to vestibular migraine.

Think of your brain as a castle surrounded by walls. Migraine triggers are like burning arrows flying towards your castle. In people without migraine, these walls are high enough to stop most of these burning arrows and the defenders can easily extinguish the few that make it through. For those with migraine, the walls are lower and fewer defenders. Burning arrows easily breach the walls, overwhelm the defenders, and eventually, the castle is set alight (i.e., a migraine attack).

To reduce the number of migraine attacks, you have to build up the walls and defenders that protect your brain AND reduce the incoming burning arrows of migraine triggers. This can be achieved through lifestyle changes, nutraceuticals, exercise, and using the appropriate medication(s).

The two principles to guide these life changes: **routine** and **trigger reduction**. Routine is your best friend. Remember that the hot migraine brain dislikes change; anything outside its comfort zone can provoke a migraine attack. The migraine brain is like Goldilocks – not too much, not too little, but just nice.

Migraine triggers can be divided into unavoidable and avoidable triggers. Unavoidable ones are like weather changes or menstruation. Stress is an unavoidable trigger but your response to it can help you avoid a migraine attack. Many triggers, like certain foods, lack of sleep, or dehydration, can be avoided.

Reducing the number of vestibular migraine attacks is very important. The more migraine attacks a person suffers, the higher the risk of further attacks, chronic migraine, and PPPD. Migraine begets migraine. Dizziness begets dizziness. Vestibular migraine attacks rarely leave a person unscathed. After the acute attack dissipates, a person is left feeling disoriented, "off", or imbalanced for days or sometimes weeks afterward, like the embers from a large bonfire. Imagine having several attacks of vestibular migraine a week – before your brain can recover from one attack, it is hit with another and another. The embers are fanned into flames, which keep getting hotter, and the brain is sent into a worsening spiral of dizziness.

Sleep

Regular, proper sleep is essential for people with vestibular migraine. Here are a few pointers for restful sleep.

- Establish a regular healthy sleep routine. Sleep and wake up at a regular time every day, even on the weekends. Avoid both staying up late and sleeping in.
- Try not to nap during the day if you are not accustomed to it.
- Limit fluid intake at least an hour before bedtime to minimize the need to awaken during the night.
- Avoid caffeine in the evenings (within 5 hours of bedtime). Besides being bad for your migraine, caffeine also interferes with sleep quality.
- Avoid alcohol in the evenings. Even though you may feel sleepy and fall asleep after imbibing an alcoholic beverage or two in the evening, you actually get much less restful sleep with alcohol. Furthermore, alcohol is a diuretic and will awaken you at night to use the restroom.

- Consume a smaller evening meal. Eating a heavy, greasy meal too close to bedtime will interfere with your sleep quality. Also, try to avoid spicy foods in the evening; they can irritate the bladder or worse, the bowels.

- No electronic screens within two hours of bedtime. The blue light interferes with melatonin release in your brain and keeps you awake.

- If your pet wakes you up frequently, keep it out of the bedroom.

- No TV in the bedroom. Besides the blue light from the screen, watching TV activates your brain and keeps you awake.

- Don't use the bedroom for anything other than sleep and sex. If you work a lot in the bedroom, your brain may associate the bedroom with the stimulating mental activity involved in working.

- Turn the clock away. There is nothing worse for sleep than staring at the clock, and counting how many hours or minutes you have left before you have to wake up and get ready for the day.

- Get more light during the daytime. This will promote a healthy sleep-wake cycle.

- Regular exercise can help you sleep soundly. You should exercise at least 3 hours before bedtime. If you work out too close to bedtime, your body will not have sufficient time to wind down and relax.

- Optimize your sleep environment. Ensure the room is dark, quiet, and cool. Heavy curtains or eye masks can block out light. Keep the temperature between 65-72 degrees Fahrenheit. A good comfortable mattress and pillows are important and don't necessarily have to be expensive.

- Create a relaxing bedtime routine. A warm bath, slow music, meditation, reading, praying, sounds of nature (e.g., rain, waves), or autonomous sensory meridian response (ASMR) soundtracks can be very helpful. ASMR is an interesting auditory-tactile response, where a person experiences a tingling sensation on the scalp which moves down the neck and spine in response to specific auditory stimuli. There are a ton of YouTube videos promoting ASMR, and a huge variety of sounds that you can try out; from whispering or blowing, to bizarre noises (e.g., crunching plastic, dogs and rabbits eating). Meditation for sleep is discussed in Chapter 19.

- Some supplements that can help with sleep:
  - Melatonin and L-tryptophan (see Chapter 9)
  - Chamomile and passionflower tea contain apigenin, a compound that produces relaxation by promoting GABA production in the brain. Chamomile has the additional benefit of reducing depression and anxiety.

Meals

Regular meal time is important. Avoid skipping meals. If you do not have time for a lunch break at work, have some healthy snacks at hand. Instead of eating two or three large meals, consider eating four or five smaller meals. There are a lot of health benefits to intermittent fasting. Intermittent fasting involves not eating for most of the day, and only eating during a window. This window varies depending on the plan. Some people with migraine can do it without problems, but some can't.

Meal preparation at the beginning of the week may be useful for busy people. Warming up prepared food is much easier than cooking something from scratch. Furthermore, meal preparation can help avoid the temptation of fast food, or takeout meals, which are typically full of migraine food triggers. A diet plan will be discussed later.

Proper Hydration

- Drinking more water can actually reduce migraine attacks.
- Your body loses fluid throughout the day. Drink at least 64 oz of water (about 8 glasses) per day to replenish the lost fluid. On hot days, drink more water (at least 10 glasses), to compensate for additional fluid loss.
- If you are working out, ensure that you sip on water throughout your workout. It can be useful to drink more fluid before your workout to buffer against fluid loss.

- Limit alcohol and caffeine. They are diuretics and cause water loss.
- Adding natural water flavoring/enhancers can encourage you to drink more water and limit sugar intake.
- If you are on topiramate or zonisamide, adequate fluid intake is important to prevent kidney stones and heat stress from reduced sweating.
- Remember, by the time you feel dehydrated, it's too late, and you are already vulnerable to a migraine attack.
- A good way of reminding yourself to drink is using a time-marked water bottle, which provides a visual reminder of how much you need to drink by specific times of the day.

Lights & Screens

Measures for home and office lighting:

- Eliminate overhead fluorescent lights. Try to get accommodation for alternate lighting at work if possible.
- Do not place lights behind ceiling fans. This will create a strobe effect and make you dizzy.
- Try to use indirect soft lighting as much as possible.
- Green light tends to be the least provocative for migraine, and may enhance the mood. If possible, using green LED lights at home may help. Dr. Ramy Burstein, who described these interesting findings, developed the Allay Lamp that emits a pure green light.
- Avoid using blinds if possible. The striped pattern with light coming through the gaps often provokes dizziness. Curtains and drapes are better choices.

For electronic screens:

- Use anti-glare and blue light-blocking screens.
- Position screens to avoid the reflected glare from the sun.
- Lower the brightness of electronic screens as much as possible. If you can, use "dark mode" for these devices.

- Limit screen time, and take planned breaks. For example, try to take a 3-minute break from the computer screen every 30 minutes; look at a distant point to allow your eye muscles to relax. Make use of methods that increase efficiency and productivity (e.g., talk-to-text programs, premade templates, or predictive text applications).

- A Canadian study found that non-liquid crystal display (LCD) screens, which refresh at a much lower rate than LCD screens, improve screen tolerance in those with post-concussive syndrome [Mansur, 2018].

<u>Protective eye-wear</u>:

- Do not use sunglasses all the time. Sunglasses are fine for outdoor use, but do not use them indoors. Continuous use of sunglasses can lead to retinal dark adaptation, a physiologic response to darkness that increases light sensitivity.

- FL-41 tinted lenses are a much better choice. This rose-colored tint blocks the spectrum of light that is most triggering for people with migraine. You can ask your optometrist for the FL-41 coating on your prescription glasses. You can also purchase glasses sold by companies like Theraspecs, BluTech, and Axon Optics without a prescription. Look for big pairs that block out as much light as possible from the sides and top as well.

- Use polarized sunglasses when outdoors.

<u>To prevent visually-induced dizziness and motion sickness</u>:

- View your TV from at least 8 feet away.

- Bigger is not better. A huge TV or computer monitor causes a lot of visually-induced dizziness and motion sickness because it takes up more of your field of vision.

- Don't scroll fast. Look away if someone else is scrolling.

- Use electronic screens and TVs in a well-lit environment. This allows your visual system to use cues from stable surroundings to lessen the sensation of visual motion.

- Avoid flickering or flashing lights.

- Cover one eye if you get close to the TV or large monitor.

- When playing video games, the screen should be at least 1 foot away; a good rule of thumb is keeping a distance of at least 4 times the diagonal screen diameter (e.g., view a 5-inch screen from at least 20 inches away). Avoid playing video games for more than an hour a session.

Dry Eyes:

- Dry eyes can cause and exacerbate light sensitivity.
- Symptoms of dry eyes include excessive tearing, blurry vision, foreign body sensation (like there is an eyelash or dust in the eye), eye redness, and poor night vision. Using artificial tears can help alleviate the symptoms.
- Some medications (e.g., tricyclic antidepressants) may cause or worsen dry eyes.
- If light sensitivity is bad, consult an ophthalmologist to check for dry eyes. Sometimes treatments like cyclosporine (Restasis) may be needed. In severe cases, a minor surgical procedure to plug the tear ducts may be performed.

Noise

- Avoid using earplugs that muffle all sounds. Just like how dark sunglasses cause dark adaptation and worsen light sensitivity, frequent use of ear plugs that block out most noise can lead to worsening of hyperacusis. Choose earplugs that minimize excessive noise but still allow you to hear at comfortable levels. At the time of this writing, several products claim to do this, including Calmer by Flare Audio, Vibes, Experience by Loop, and Knops.
- Use soft thick rugs and upholstery that absorb sound waves.
- Soundproof windows can block a lot of noise from the outside.
- Gaps around doors and windows can let in a lot of unwanted noise. You can use caulk or weather stripping to seal off these gaps.
- If you need to quiet a particular room in the home so you can work or retreat temporarily, some companies can help you with using acoustic ceiling panels, wall tiles, floorings, and doors. Of course, this option will probably not be cheap.

Odors

For those with osmophobia, several measures can be taken to help minimize your exposure to odors that trigger your attacks.

- Avoid detergent aisles at the grocery store. If you need to purchase cleaning products, make a list, and make a beeline for what you need then get out of the aisle ASAP.
- Avoid the fragrance section of department stores.
- Use fragrance-free products (e.g., lotions, deodorants, laundry detergents, dish-washing detergents, dryer sheets, softeners, shampoos, etc.) wherever possible.
- If possible, politely request friends and family members avoid using fragrances, or scented lotions around you.
- Asking co-workers to avoid using such products is a bit touchier. It helps if you have a good relationship with them; tell them politely that you suffer from migraine and odors are a major trigger for you. It may help if you tell them that you are "allergic" to artificial fragrances and scents. If there is a specific co-worker who insists on marinating in perfume, you may need to relocate farther away. Sometimes a letter from your neurologist or migraine specialist may be needed to compel your superiors to accommodate such a request.

Tobacco

While the smell of cigarette smoke is a well-recognized migraine trigger, tobacco usage is also a trigger for migraines. Nicotine has been shown to stimulate the firing of pain nerves in the meninges. Furthermore, smoking can increase the risk of cardiovascular disease and stroke. Cutting out tobacco and nicotine usage, including vaping, is important in improving migraine control.

Grocery Shopping

A trip to the grocery store can be daunting for vestibular migraine patients. The local supermarket is basically like a minefield ready to set off an attack. However, there are some ways to make this experience less painful.

- Choose to shop at an off-peak time, when the number of shoppers is low and traffic is lighter. You're asking for trouble if you go between 5-7 pm when people leave work, or on Saturdays and Sundays.
- Make a list. Knowing what you need to purchase and going to get those items saves you the pain and time of browsing the aisles.
- If you infrequently take your rescue medications, you can consider using a rescue medication just before going shopping. Triptans can actually prevent visual stimuli from triggering a migraine. Be aware that some can make you drowsy; be sure someone is driving if you choose to take your rescue medication.
- Wear your FL-41 glasses. You can also wear a cap or hat to stop the light from above.
- Go with someone who can help you if you become too dizzy.
- Consider going to smaller neighborhood grocery stores instead of huge warehouse-style stores like Costco and Walmart.
- Recognize when your dizziness is getting worse and leave.
- Electronic grocery shopping services like Instacart can be invaluable. You can easily order your items online and have them delivered if you don't feel like you would be able to handle a grocery store.

Stress Management

As discussed previously, stress is a silent killer. It is impossible to avoid stress. However, we can control our response to stress, and as such reduce its impact on us, and diminish its potential to trigger a migraine attack. Many books have been written on stress management and a detailed discussion is way beyond the scope of this book. Here are some important points to help you deal with stress.

Become antifragile. Resilience can be understood as adapting in the face of adversity and stress, and bouncing back from such experiences. According to Professor Nassim Nicholas Taleb (who introduced the concept in his book "Antifragile"), antifragility goes beyond resilience; the resilient remain stable in the face of stress, but the antifragile get stronger, much like how Friedrich Nietzsche put it: what does not kill you, makes you stronger. Antifragility ensures that you don't just "bounce back" from stress or adversity, but instead, flourish and thrive. The antifragile embrace challenges because it allows them to grow.

Time management. Stay ahead of stress by prioritizing tasks and organizing our days. Don't let the demands of daily tasks overwhelm and drown you.

Let it out. Bottling up your stress makes it worse and more toxic. Find a confidant that you can be completely honest with. Talking about what stresses you and your emotions neutralizes their potency. This is called affect labeling (discussed in Chapter 19). If you prefer not to discuss private thoughts with a familiar person, see a professional counselor or psychologist. If you are not comfortable sharing, try journaling.

Set aside time for you. You need to take care of yourself. It is so easy to be busy caring for others, and forget to care for yourself. Setting aside even a small amount of time to focus on yourself, and do what relaxes you can be very helpful in managing your stress levels.

Learn to say no. Create boundaries, and set limits. Find the courage to say no, and politely decline situations that you know will stress you out. If you already have a lot on your plate, say "no" when someone asks you to do more. Saying no to bosses and colleagues can be difficult; instead of rejecting a request, a better approach may be to say, "Will it be ok to do X after I have completed A, B, C, and D? Would you like me to prioritize X and postpone A, B, C, or D?". Family and social commitments can also be challenging to decline but you have to find the time to care for yourself and not allow yourself to be pulled in multiple directions.

Support Network. A strong support network can be immensely helpful in managing stress levels. This is discussed in Chapter 20.

Diet. A healthy diet can do wonders for one's stress and mood. Stress often makes us crave highly processed, sugary foods. These foods momentarily make us feel good but as the blood sugar levels drop, so does our mood. More about diet is discussed in Chapter 14.

Exercise. Exercise is one of the best ways to improve stress levels, and elevate the mood. Setting aside time to exercise is essential for health. This is discussed more in Chapter 10.

Mindfulness. Prayer, & Meditation. Chapter 19 discusses how mindfulness, prayer, and meditation can help with stress related to vestibular migraine.

Home Safety: Fall Prevention

Vertigo, dizziness, and imbalance increase your risk for falls. To protect yourself from falls, make some simple modifications to your home environment.

- Be sure that there are no cracks or buckled floors.
- Avoid thresholds at door entrances.
- Ensure that floors (especially in the bathroom and kitchen) are non-slippery.
- Keep floors free of clutter.
- Avoid loose rugs with warped edges.
- Install grab bars in the restroom.
- Ensure that carpets and runners on stairs are fastened.
- Have a firm chair with good back and neck support so that you have somewhere to rest when you are dizzy.
- Install night lights. Complete darkness can be very disconcerting for people with dizziness. You don't want to fall when going to the restroom at night.

- Beware of lurking dogs and cats. Tripping over pets, particularly on stairs, can be dangerous.

Weight Control

Migraine is comorbid with obesity, particularly in women under the age of 50. Obesity is linked to a higher risk of migraine, chronic migraine, and transformation from episodic to chronic daily headaches.

One potential reason is increased inflammation. Adipose (fat) tissue is not an inert tissue that just stores excess calories. Adipose tissue is actually a neuro-endocrine organ that releases a variety of chemical compounds, including adiponectin, and cytokines. These chemicals activate pro-inflammatory pathways, and as we discussed before, this inflammatory state not only aggravates migraines, but increases the risk for many other pathologies, including cardiovascular disease.

If you are overweight, losing weight may help improve your migraines. Topiramate is a medication that can both control vestibular migraine and help curb appetite to aid weight loss. A sensible diet, and an exercise program will also help with weight control. If you have a lot of trouble controlling your weight, consulting with a specialist can be helpful. Glucagon-like peptide-1receptor agonists like semaglutide (Ozempic, Rybelsus, or Wegovy) or tirzapatide (Monjauro or Zepbound) have gained popularity as weight loss drugs. At the time I am writing this, I have not encountered any vestibular migraine problems in patients using these medications.

Traveling

Traveling presents some challenges for people with vestibular migraine but with the right preparation, may be fairly painless.

- Sleep properly the night before.

- Dress comfortably. No tight clothes or shoes.
- Plan ahead of time. Don't rush. The stress of rushing to the airport, getting through TSA lines, and squeezing like sardines on the plane can trigger a migraine attack.
- Be sure to carry your rescue and preventive medications in your hand luggage. If airlines can lose people's pets, don't count on them delivering your medication safely.
- Prepare for motion sickness (see Chapter 17)
- Don't skip meals. Pack some migraine-friendly snacks that can release sustained levels of energy.
- Avoid airport food. Besides being overpriced and revolting, fast food is loaded with migraine-triggering additives.
- Try to stick to your migraine diet.
- Hydrate. Remind yourself to drink enough fluids.
- Use your blue light-blocking glasses.
- Use noise-canceling headphones and prepare a list of your favorite relaxing tunes.

Holidays

The holidays can be tough on vestibular migraine. The stress of travel and holiday preparation, the food triggers, the lack of sleep, the rush to shop, the crowds, and the bright lights can often cause a lot of vestibular migraine attacks. However, it is important not to isolate yourself from friends and family. Loneliness is highly detrimental to your mental, emotional, and even physical health. With planning and preparation, you can enjoy the holidays and minimize the chances of a vestibular migraine attack.

- Plan ahead as much as possible. No last-minute rushes. Shop for gifts as early as possible and avoid the hordes of last-minute shoppers. If possible, shop online. If you plan to cook, prepare ingredients as far ahead as possible and consider freezing them.
- Maintain your sleep routine.

- Maintain your migraine diet routine. Holiday meals can be loaded with migraine food triggers.
- Hydrate, hydrate, hydrate.
- Try to get some exercise.
- Set aside time for meditation.
- If possible, request that people don't use perfumes or scented lotions.
- Be careful with alcohol, caffeine, and excessive salt and sugar.
- Make it a pot-luck. Assign each person a dish to lessen your workload. This will also give you time to bond and reconnect with your loved ones.
- It's ok to buy prepared, ready-to-serve food. Buying a sweet potato pie from Costco and peppermint bark from Sam's Club is ok. You don't have to make every single thing from scratch. You're not Martha Stewart.
- Have your rescue medication on hand.
- Don't forget to pack your preventive medication.
- Listen to your body. Take a short break from the festivities to relax if you need it.
- Plan an end time. Instead of letting celebrations last all night, ensure that they end at a reasonable time to allow enough rest.
- Plan recovery time. Plan to allow at least a full day of rest and recuperate before you return to work.

Miscellaneous Tips

1. Scalp and head muscle tightness and pain can aggravate migraines and headaches.

- Avoid tight hats, caps, and headbands.

- Avoid tight braids, hair extensions, weaves, and ponytails. Some weaves are so tight they actually pull the corner of the eyes towards the ears. I know patients whose headaches improved dramatically after they stopped getting tight weaves and braids.

- Avoid tight headphones.

2. Weather changes can't be prevented but you can use apps that provide barometric pressure readings. When the pressure drops and a storm approaches, take your rescue medication or acetazolamide to head off a migraine attack.

3. Weather apps and local meteorological news reports provide information about air pollution levels. Try to stay indoors more when the level of pollutants is high.

4. Prepare a migraine first-aid kit that you can bring around with you to work, school, or travel. This will help immensely during a migraine attack. Your kit should contain:

- A small bottle of water.

- Your rescue medication. It is best to have two doses unless it is a medication that is taken once a day only.

- Anti-nausea treatment.

- Earplugs and sunglasses

Chapter 13: The Gut-Brain Axis

All disease begins in the gut.

Hippocrates (460-370 BC)

The gut-brain axis refers to the complex, two-way relationship between the digestive tract and the brain. Medicine and science have known that the brain controls the gut, but we have only begun to recognize the influence of the gut on brain function. Several pathways connect the gut and brain: the hypothalamic-pituitary-adrenal (HPA) axis, the autonomic nervous system, and the gut microbiome. Many lines of evidence point to the importance of the gut-brain axis in migraine. There is a higher prevalence of gastrointestinal disorders in people with migraine. Migraine can also manifest with various gastrointestinal symptoms. One's diet affects migraine control as well.

The Vagus Nerve

The role of the vagus nerve in migraine cannot be disputed. The beneficial effect of vagus nerve stimulation on vestibular migraine confirms the importance of the vagus nerve in migraine pathophysiology. Indirectly, the vagus nerve is also important to vestibular migraine because it is central to the gut-brain axis.

Recall that the autonomic nervous system is divided into the sympathetic and parasympathetic systems. A more recently discovered component of the autonomic nervous system is the enteric nervous system (ENS). The ENS arises from primordial vagus nerve cells. The ENS consists of almost half a billion neurons, the largest collection of nerve cells outside the brain and unsurprisingly, the gut is called the second brain. The ENS regulates and controls all gut functions, including immune response, nutrient absorption, local circulation, motility, and movement of fluid, electrolytes, and metabolites.

The vagus nerve is the largest cranial nerve, exiting the brainstem and skull to travel through the neck into the chest and abdomen. Its Latin name, which means "wandering", refers to its long path from the brain to the organs of the body. The vagus nerve controls the function of the internal organs (digestive, respiratory, cardiac, urinary), and reflexes like coughing, sneezing, gagging, swallowing, and vomiting. As the major highway for the parasympathetic nervous system, it connects the ENS to the brain, allowing information to flow in both directions. The vagus nerve is central to the communication between the brain and the gut.

The main brainstem nucleus of the vagus nerve (nucleus tractus solitarius; NTS) is connected to the amygdala and influences levels of neurotransmitters like dopamine, norepinephrine, and serotonin. Following vagotomy (an outdated surgical procedure to treat gastric ulcers by severing part of the vagus nerve), the incidence of psychiatric disorders increased. The vagus nerve is closely connected to the immune system and the HPA axis; it is a crucial counterweight of the inflammatory reflex. Circulating pro-inflammatory cytokines act on the vagal brainstem nuclei, triggering an increase in vagal activity to inhibit inflammation. In addition, the vagus nerve is the conduit for the gut microbiota's influence on the brain (discussed later); in animal experiments, severing the vagus nerve abolishes the benefits of the gut microbes.

The Gut Microbiome

The gut microbiome is the fantastically diverse community of viruses, fungi, and bacteria that dwell in our digestive tracts. There are trillions of microbes inhabiting our guts, 10 times more than the total number of cells in our bodies, carrying 800 times more unique genes than the human genome. Many species have not even been identified but large collaborative research projects like the Human Microbiome Project, British Gut Project, American Gut Project, and MetaHIT are underway to catalog the wonderfully complex ecosystems inside us.

This microscopic community begins at birth when we acquire the initial inhabitants from our mothers through the vaginal canal, breastfeeding, and skin contact. It stabilizes by 2-3 years of age as we are weaned and fed solid food. This also corresponds to a critical phase of development. During this period, the brain undergoes an astounding transformation; it grows by more than 50% in the first 3 months of life, and reaches 90% of adult size by age 5. The importance of the gut microbiome on brain development is unquestionable. Lab mice grown in sterile environments, or treated with antibiotics to kill off bacteria, suffer from neurological deficits and exaggerated HPA axis responses. Microbe-free lab mice display anxious and depressive behaviors, and impaired fear extinction [Chu, 2019]. In migraine rat models, wiping out their gut bacteria worsened pain responses but restoring their gut microbiota reversed it [Crawford, 2022]. Lab rats with more frequent and severe migraine pain experienced a change in their gut microbial composition [Wen, 2019].

Each person's gut microbiome is unique. Even two healthy people don't have exactly the same microbial composition. However, the composition can be altered, for better or for worse, by various influences over our lives. The biggest influence on the gut microbiome is one's diet; up to 50% of the variation in gut microbiota can be attributed to the diet. Other influences on the gut microbiota include exercise, stress levels, toxins (e.g., bisphenol A, heavy metals), and antibiotic use.

The HPA axis is one avenue for the brain, immune system, and gut microbiome to communicate. The HPA axis is the main stress response system. Stress greatly influences the gut microbiome. Just two hours of stress is enough to change the gut microbial composition [Galley, 2014]. Stressful events in infant animals alter the gut microbiota and raise the levels of inflammatory markers for life. Interestingly, surgically removing the adrenal glands abolishes such changes, emphasizing the central role of the HPA axis in how stress affects the gut microbiome. Similar stress-triggered changes also occur in humans' gut microbiota. The stress of neonatal ICU hospitalization changes infants' gut microbial composition [D'Agata, 2020]. Stressful childhood experiences lead to lifelong alterations in the gut microbiome. In one study, childhood trauma and stresses changed the gut microbial population and caused anxiety, gastrointestinal symptoms, and altered prefrontal cortex responses to fearful expressions [Callaghan, 2020].

Moreover, because our microbiome is inherited from our mothers, the effects of stress can be passed from mother to offspring. Maternal stress and higher cortisol levels during pregnancy alter the mother's gut microbiome. Such changes are passed on to her baby resulting in a hyper-reactive HPA axis in the infant and long-term changes to the stress response [Cryan, 2019]. It is not difficult to see how inheriting a dysfunctional gut microbiome could account for generational trauma. The good news is that maternal and early life stress need not condemn one to a future of dysbiosis. Probiotic supplements can prevent fear and anxious behaviors in animal pups and their offspring [Callaghan, 2016]. Probiotics reversed depression-like behaviors in adult lab rats that were traumatized as infants [Desbonnet, 2010].

The digestive tract contains the highest concentration of immune cells in the body. The gut immune system interacts intimately with the microbiota, and this relationship affects immune responses in other parts of the body. The main objective of the gut immune system is to prevent microbes from invading the body by maintaining the integrity of the gut mucosa and releasing chemicals (e.g., antibodies) that directly attack or recruit other immune cells to attack these microbes. The microbiota evolved methods to modulate the immune system, keeping the inflammatory response at bay to allow them to survive, but not suppressing it so much that pathogenic microbes can flourish. Thus, a harmonious, symbiotic relationship between the host's immune system and gut microbiome ensures the host survives and thrives. Maladaptive changes in the gut microbiota can trigger inflammatory responses, which then spill over into the rest of the body. Conversely, immunological dysregulation (e.g., autoimmune disease, COVID-19) can negatively affect the gut microbiome and gastrointestinal physiology.

The gut microbiome produces a rich stew of biochemical molecules with diverse health benefits. Short-chain fatty acids (SCFAs) are produced when gut microbes digest and ferment fiber. Three major SCFAs are butyric acid, propionic acid, and acetic acid. These molecules enhance gut health by supporting energy homeostasis, maintaining the integrity of its lining (preventing toxins from leaking into the circulation), reducing inflammation, and stimulating mucus production (which traps and eliminates wastes and toxins). SCFAs help protect the brain against the effects of stress, enhance neurogenesis, strengthen the blood-brain barrier, decrease neuroinflammation, support healthy microglia (the brain's resident immune cell) function, and modulate the levels of many neurotransmitters (like GABA, dopamine, glutamate). [Silva, 2020]. Fascinatingly, the levels of SCFAs in the brain are much higher than those found in the blood, indicating that they must be getting to the brain by another route, most likely the vagus nerve since SCFAs in the gut can alter activity in the brainstem nuclei of the vagus nerve. In terms of real-world effects, SCFAs control appetite, food cravings, depression, and anxiety, while improving sleep, learning, memory, and sociability.

The gut microbes produce a myriad of vitamins that are essential to human health, particularly neurological function. These include thiamine (B1), folate (B9), riboflavin (B2), biotin (B7), niacin (B3), pantothenic acid (B5), pyridoxine (B6), and cobalamin (B12). These vitamins support the health of the host organism and the gut microbiome. In addition, gut microbes produce neurotransmitters that are critical to neurological function. GABA can be obtained from fermented foods containing Lactobacillus and is also produced by the gut microbiome. After absorption by the intestinal mucosa, only a small amount of GABA enters the brain from the circulation. Dietary GABA raises brain GABA levels by activating the vagus nerve. Approximately 95% of the body's serotonin is produced by the gut, from the action of microbes on tryptophan, and a small amount is produced in the brain. Within the gut, serotonin can act on both the ENS and vagus neurons.

Dysbiosis refers to maladaptive (negative) changes in the composition and ecology of the gut microbiome. Dysbiosis is associated with many illnesses, including many neurological conditions, including migraine, long COVID, MS, depression, anxiety, autism, and neurodegenerative disorders like Alzheimer's and Parkinson's disease. For example, the gut microbiome in Parkinson's disease produces lower amounts of SCFAs and dopamine [Rutsch, 2020]. People with depression have different gut microbiota from non-depressed people and those successfully treated with antidepressants [Akkasheh, 2016]. Transplanting gut microbes from MS patients into lab mice can trigger the disease [Berer, 2017]. In fact, several non-communicable conditions, like obesity, depression, and anxiety, can be "transferred" to lab animals when they are transplanted with the microbiota from humans with these conditions.

Some evidence suggests that the gut flora of people with migraine is different from those without migraine [Gonzalez, 2016]. One study showed that women with migraine have a less diverse gut microbiome compared to women without migraine [Chen, 2019]. Migraine patients have higher levels of gut bacteria that metabolize nitrates, nitrites, and nitric oxide [Gonzalez, 2016]. The exact changes that result in disease are unclear at this time but the general themes underlying dysbiosis include reduced microbial diversity, proliferation of pathogenic microbes, and loss of symbiotic flora. Science is merely on the cusp of discovering how dysbiosis causes neurological diseases; while we know that it is present in these conditions, we do not yet know precisely how or why it occurs.

Louis Pasteur (1822-1895), the renowned French scientist and father of microbiology, discovered that fermentation by lactic acid bacteria produced lactate which inhibited the growth of microbes that cause food spoilage. The concept of beneficial microbes at that time was nothing short of revolutionary. In the early 20th century, Elie Metchnikoff was intrigued by the long lifespan of Bulgarian villagers living in the Caucasus mountains. He observed they regularly drank a fermented milk drink (later found to contain *Lactobacillus bulgaricus)* and developed the idea that cultivating beneficial bacteria in the gut was the key to good health. Thus, the concept (and business) of probiotics was born.

Prebiotics are substances consumed and digested by the host microbiome to sustain a healthy population and provide the microbes with the material needed to produce the aforementioned beneficial biochemical substances. Dietary fiber can be divided into soluble, and insoluble fiber. Soluble fiber consists of inulin, fructooligosaccharides (FOS), galactooligosaccharides (GOS), pectins, beta-glucans, and resistant starches. Insoluble fiber consists of cellulose, hemicellulose, and others; it bulks the feces to facilitate elimination and is good for constipation. Soluble fiber is the main food source for the gut microbes. Consuming prebiotics promotes the growth of healthy gut microbes and increases the production of SCFAs, which are byproducts of fiber digestion by these microbes.

Probiotics refer to supplements that contain the live bacteria that a person wants to colonize the digestive tract. Probiotic supplementation can alter various aspects of neurological function, including neuroplasticity, neurotransmission, and inflammation. Evidence is emerging that probiotics produce real-world benefits for various neurological and psychiatric conditions. *Psychobiotics* are probiotics that can improve anxiety, depression, and other psychiatric symptoms, by influencing neurotransmitter levels.

Both animal and human studies support the benefits of pre-and probiotics. Recolonizing microbe-free lab mice with the appropriate gut bacteria reduces anxiety and depression, and restores normal fear extinction [Chu, 2019]. Pre-and probiotic supplementation in humans helps with depression, anxiety, and the impact of stress on the brain and body. Furthermore, supplementation has also shown promise in treating conditions that are often co-morbid with migraine, like irritable bowel syndrome, and fibromyalgia. One study in migraine mice models showed that probiotics reversed pain responses caused by wiping out their gut bacteria with antibiotics [Tang, 2020]. In humans, one study [Martami, 2019] showed that an 8-week course of probiotics reduced migraine severity, frequency, and rescue medication use. Another study [De Roos, 2017] showed no improvement with probiotics. The mixed results are most likely due to differences in the probiotic formulation.

Pre- and pro-biotics can also improve brain fog. In experiments, administering pro- and prebiotics to animals with dysbiosis restores memory and cognitive function. One showed that gut microbiome composition influences attention, processing speed, and cognitive flexibility; and modulates activity in the thalamus, hypothalamus, and amygdala [Fernandez-Real, 2015]. In toddlers, different gut microbial populations may affect learning abilities [Carlson, 2018]. In adults, probiotic supplementation improves memory, mood, stress response, anxiety, social behavior, decision-making, and learning [Cryan, 2015].

A growing body of evidence suggests that changes in the gut microbiome can reduce the impact of stress on the HPA axis and the brain. Probiotic supplements blunt the stress-provoked spike in glucocorticoid levels. Many of these studies (usually using *Bifidobacterium* and *Lactobacillus* strains, the bacteria often associated with fermented dairy products) show promising benefits for stress, and its impact on depression and anxiety [Cryan, 2019]. Probiotics are protective against the impact of stress on memory and prefrontal cortex function [Papalini, 2019]. The effects of pre- and probiotics on the brain are mediated through the vagus nerve; in animal studies, severing the vagus nerve abolishes such benefits [Bravo, 2011]. Growing evidence in human studies shows that probiotic supplementation can reduce cortisol levels, depression, and anxiety. Furthermore, long-term probiotic use may alter GABA gene expression in the hippocampus, amygdala, and prefrontal cortex, enhancing the activity of the prefrontal cortex while reducing overactivity in the limbic system [Bravo, 2011].

While there are no studies that investigate the role of the gut-brain axis, gut microbiome, and pre/probiotic supplementation in vestibular migraine, there is a growing body of evidence that point in that direction. The gut-brain axis is an exciting new frontier to explore in vestibular migraine treatment and research.

Chapter 14: Diet & Vestibular Migraine

Let food by thy medicine, and medicine be thy food.
Hippocrates (c. 450 – c. 380 BC)

The relationship between diet and migraine attacks has been recognized for over 200 years. Specific foods are very well-known (and avoidable) migraine triggers. Some are less well-recognized, but may nonetheless provoke migraine attacks in vulnerable people. So, are people with migraine allergic to specific foods? Is an allergy the reason these foods trigger migraine attacks in vulnerable people? Food allergy studies show that migraine attacks improve when food allergens are eliminated [Alpay, 2010; Arroyave Hernandez, 2007]. Bear in mind that these studies confirm the allergy by detecting actual antibodies against food allergens.

Certainly, consuming a food that you are allergic to provokes an inflammatory response, and we already know that inflammation plays an important role in vestibular migraine. However, the relationship between food triggers and migraine goes beyond a straightforward allergic relationship. There are specific molecules and chemicals in food that can trigger migraine attacks without causing an allergic reaction. We will discuss these in this chapter.

As you read this chapter, think about designing your diet plan for vestibular migraine based on a double-pronged strategy: *AVOID* and *EMBRACE*. Avoid foods that trigger your migraine attacks. Some, like caffeine, red wine, and nitrites, are widely acknowledged as typical triggers, and should be avoided. However, some food triggers (e.g., avocadoes, soy) only affect certain people. These are trickier to detect. Since everyone has unique and specific food triggers, keep a journal to track and identify your triggers. This approach will help you discover if you have more peculiar triggers. It is also a good idea to avoid unhealthy foods. Migraine brains need healthy environments to function optimally; avoid foods that are not conducive to good health, like highly processed, sugary, pro-inflammatory, and salty foods. Embrace foods that heal your brain, like those with anti-inflammatory and antioxidant properties, those that optimize the brain's bioenergetic processes, and those that promote gut health.

Caffeine

The relationship between caffeine and migraine is complicated. When used sparingly, caffeine is an effective rescue agent. However, consuming too much caffeine regularly can exacerbate migraines significantly and cause medication overuse headache. While some people with migraine cannot tolerate any amount of caffeine, most can consume *some* caffeine. The caffeine limit for migraine patients is 200 mg per day, which is the equivalent of 1-2 cups (8-16 oz) of coffee per day; more than this will worsen migraines.

Caffeine works by blocking the adenosine receptor. Adenosine receptors are widely found throughout the brain. One of adenosine's functions is to promote sleepiness; caffeine perks us up by blocking this effect. However, with chronic caffeine consumption, the brain reacts by producing even more adenosine receptors and adenosine. Over time, we need more caffeine to feel that "jolt" of alertness. This higher level of adenosine activity lowers the headache threshold. Blocking adenosine stops a migraine and headache when caffeine is used *infrequently*. Chronic, frequent use of caffeine leads to a state of increased adenosine activity, which worsens migraines, and causes medication overuse headache.

To be safe, I advise my patients to limit their intake to one cup per day. It is important to emphasize that caffeine does not just mean coffee - tea, chocolate, energy drinks, energy snacks, and many sodas contain caffeine (sometimes huge amounts). Remember that decaffeinated does not mean caffeine-free – decaffeinated coffee only has to be 97% caffeine-free according to USDA rules. As such, remember that there are still small amounts of caffeine. This can affect those who are sensitive to caffeine. If you consume large amounts of decaffeinated beverages, your total caffeine intake will rise.

Lina suffered from vertigo almost 4-5 days out of each week. After consulting with me, I diagnosed her with vestibular migraine. I inquired about caffeine intake to which she said no, but when I asked about tea, sodas, or energy drinks, she told me she drank 1-2 gallons of sweet tea every day. Being a proper Southern lady, she clutched her pearls when I told her she had to cut down her sweet tea consumption by a lot. She finally eliminated her sweet tea intake completely and her vertigo attacks stopped without even needing medications.

Caffeine can aggravate anxiety in those who suffer from or a predisposed to anxiety disorder. Amounts of caffeine (1-3 cups) usually consumed by most people can worsen anxiety in these people. If you have anxiety and panic disorder, simply eliminating caffeine can help control your symptoms.

Chocolate

Chocolate has long been blamed as a migraine trigger. An important question to ask is whether the migraine prodrome causes chocolate cravings or whether chocolate really triggers a migraine attack. Could it be that the serotonin-deficient migraine brain craves a serotonin-rich food like chocolate? Cacao is an amazing superfood with antioxidant and mood-improving properties. It would be a shame to just give up cacao and unsweetened cocoa if they weren't the potent migraine triggers they've been made out to be.

A brief understanding of chocolate may help us determine its role as a migraine trigger. Cacao beans are harvested and then undergo fermentation, drying, roasting, crushing, and grinding to prepare them to be made into chocolate. It can be made into a paste called chocolate liquor, which is then further processed by mixing in more cocoa butter and sugar (and sometimes vanilla and lecithin). Cocoa powder is produced from chocolate liquor by separating it from cocoa butter. Chocolate products list the percentage of cacao (amount of cocoa powder plus cocoa butter); the darker the chocolate, the higher the cacao content. However, with more awareness regarding health foods, cacao is usually now used to refer to raw, minimally-processed beans, and cocoa refers to the processed product used for chocolate. Cacao nibs are pieces of beans that have been roasted, cracked, and deshelled.

Even though studies of cocoa products in migraine have not produced a clear link, many swear it is a trigger. Several compounds in chocolate may trigger migraine, including nitrates, caffeine, tyramine, and phenylalanine. Many commercially-sold chocolate contain tons of sugar and additives which could also trigger migraine attacks. Cacao contains caffeine as well, but the lack of fermentation and processing may mean that it contains far less of the other compounds that can trigger migraine.

Alcohol

The connection between wine, particularly red wine, and migraine has been recognized for millennia. Aulus Cornelius Celsus, the ancient Roman encyclopedist known for his medical work *De Medicina*, wrote about how wine triggered headaches. Consumption of alcohol during periods of stress can also increase migraine frequency – the likely combination of stress and alcohol consumption. Directly related to the consumption of alcohol, there appear to be two windows for migraine attacks to occur: one within hours and the other about a day later.

In the first scenario, alcohol consumption triggers a migraine attack within hours. This may be because alcohol provokes the release of histamine release from mast cells as well as CGRP. Some people experience migraine attacks with all forms of alcohol. However, in most, only certain beverages trigger attacks, the most common culprit being red wine. Consuming 300 ml (10 ounces) of red wine can trigger a headache within 30 minutes to 3 hours but drinking vodka with a similar amount of alcohol does not trigger such a headache, suggesting that other substances in red wine, and not alcohol per se, are responsible for migraine attacks. These include histamine, sulfites, phenylethylamine, prostaglandins, tyramine, phenolic flavonoids, and tannins.

Red wine contains 20 to 200 times more histamine than white wine. Sparkling wines and champagne contain more histamine than white wine as well. Furthermore, alcohol inhibits an enzyme called diamine oxidase, which breaks down histamine. Flavonoids and tannins may also be to blame for provoking migraine attacks; these compounds are responsible for the color of red wine and darker liquors (e.g., bourbon, brandy). Unsurprisingly, darker liquors tend to be more triggering than light-colored ones (e.g., vodka, gin). Beer does not seem to be a migraine trigger; however, unpasteurized, and tap beer contain higher amounts of tyramine that can provoke migraine attacks.

The second scenario occurs during the hangover. As the alcohol levels drop, the hangover starts, usually the day after alcohol is consumed. Increased adenosine levels are one reason for hangover headaches. People with migraine develop hangover headaches with lower levels of alcohol compared to people without migraine. Furthermore, hangover headaches tend to be more severe in people with migraine, compared to people who do not, and can often trigger actual migraine attacks.

Tyramine

Tyramine is the by-product of tyrosine (an amino acid) breakdown. It is a known migraine trigger but it remains a mystery as to how it triggers attacks. An interesting study [Moffett, 1972] showed that tyramine-containing capsules caused actual electrical changes in the brain (as measured by an EEG) in a significant number of people who experience headaches after eating foods with tyramine.

One hypothesis is that tyramine behaves as a "false neurotransmitter" that displaces norepinephrine from receptors, resulting in higher blood norepinephrine levels that constrict blood vessels. Repeated exposure to tyramine may lead to lower brain norepinephrine levels by increasing the levels of a metabolite called octopamine that displaces norepinephrine in nerve terminals. Tyramine content in food rises when it is aged, cured, or ripened at room temperature. Fresh and frozen food in general have low tyramine levels. Examples of tyramine-rich foods:

Meats	Liver, meat with tenderizers, bacon, hot dogs, sausages, pepperoni, corned beef, jerky, bologna, pastrami, smoked fish/meat, dried fish, pâté
Fruits	Oranges, lemons, limes, grapefruits, coconuts, raspberries, figs, dates, pineapple, overripe bananas, nutmeg, red plums, papayas, avocados
Vegetables	Raw onions, tomatoes, eggplants, snow peas, olives
Legumes	Fava beans, broad beans, lima beans, edamame
Cheese	Stilton, cheddar, blue, feta, parmesan, Swiss, Muenster, gorgonzola, Camembert, Roquefort
Nuts	Brazil nuts, peanuts, pecans, pistachios, walnuts, nut butters
Baked goods	Sourdough, fresh home-made yeast bread (allow 24 hours before consuming)
Fermented vegetables	Kimchi, sauerkraut, miso, tempeh, pickles, natto
Fermented dairy products	Yogurt, buttermilk, sour cream, kefir
Fermented drinks	Kombucha, *Tepache de Piña* (a traditional Mexican fermented pineapple beverage), beet kvass, apple cider
Alcoholic beverages	Red wine, sparkling wine, champagne, tap beer, unpasteurized beer, ale, chianti, vermouth, sherry
Condiments	Soy sauce, balsamic vinegar, red vinegar, fish sauce, teriyaki sauce, shrimp paste/sauce, mustard, *colatura di alici* (fermented anchovy sauce), *murri/almori* (fermented barley), A1 sauce, Worcestershire sauce, Marmite/Vegemite/Vitam-R/Cenovis, Bovril

Histamine

The role of histamine in migraine was discussed in Chapter 11. Histamine can also be found in certain foods. Just like tyramine, histamine is found in foods that have been degraded by microbes; as a rule of thumb, the fresher the food, the lower the levels of histamine and tyramine. As such, fermented foods contain high levels of histamine. Some foods like citrus cause the body to release more histamine. The good news is that most foods that raise histamine levels are also tyramine-rich foods. Therefore, a low-tyramine diet is also low in histamine.

There are only two exceptions to watch out for. Firstly, beware of improperly stored fish like tuna, mackerel, bonito, skip-jack, sardine, yellowtail, herring, and mahi-mahi which contain high amounts of histidine. If the fish are not frozen below 4 degrees Celsius after being caught, bacteria begin to flourish and convert histidine into histamine. Histamine poisoning (called *scombroid ichthyotoxicosis*) is similar to severe allergic reactions, characterized by facial and neck flushing, headache, diarrhea, and rash. Cooking does not destroy histamine. Proper storage on fishing vessels, food safety inspections, and quality control protocols have made this a rare occurrence. Secondly, be careful with champagne, which has very high levels of histamine.

Soy Products

Soy products include tofu, edamame, miso, soymilk, and soy yogurt, as well as many vegan food items (chik'n nuggets, meatless grounds, vege patties, etc). Soy has been reported to trigger migraines in susceptible individuals. Phytoestrogens (plant estrogens) in soy could potentially cause fluctuations in estrogen levels which can aggravate migraine. Some soy products (particularly fermented ones) also contain high amounts of tyramine. The link between soy and migraine is not very strong; if soy is your predominant source of protein and you don't notice it triggering your migraine attacks, you can keep soy in your diet.

Gluten

Celiac disease is a condition where the gut is allergic to gluten, a protein found in wheat and some grains. People with celiac disease develop gastrointestinal symptoms (e.g., diarrhea, bloating) and actual inflammatory changes in their intestines in response to gluten.

Non-celiac gluten sensitivity refers to a condition where people experience symptoms related to gluten consumption in the absence of true celiac disease. However, it is challenging to conclusively diagnose gluten sensitivity. The best way to figure out if you are sensitive to gluten is to eliminate gluten from your diet to see if the symptoms improve. If the symptoms improve, a recurrence of symptoms with the reintroduction of gluten will confirm your sensitivity.

There is a higher incidence of migraine in people with celiac disease and gluten sensitivity. In these people, gluten is pro-inflammatory and can trigger migraine. However, the role of gluten as a migraine trigger in people without these conditions is much less clear. It is certainly reasonable to pursue a gluten-free diet, to see if migraines improve. A worsening of migraines with gluten reintroduction confirms you are sensitive to it.

Dairy

The link between dairy and migraine is unclear. Some people find that dairy triggers migraine attacks, but many do not. Like gluten, if you are lactose intolerant or allergic to milk, dairy products can certainly trigger migraine attacks. That being said, diagnosing a food allergy is difficult. It is reasonable to try eliminating dairy and re-challenging your body to see if dairy really triggers your attacks.

Sugar affects the brain like a drug. When given a choice, lab rats choose sugar over cocaine [Lenoir, 2007]. Diets high in sugary foods (e.g., sodas, baked goods) are associated with a higher risk of anxiety and depression. Furthermore, high-sugar diets impair neurogenesis (formation of new neurons) and increase neuronal death [Jacques, 2019]. Sugar is not a migraine trigger, per se. However, high-sugar diets are detrimental to brain health. Consuming sugary foods can also spike blood sugar levels and trigger migraine attacks.

Salt intake is more often linked to Meniere's disease and not migraine. However, some patients find that consuming excessively salty foods triggers migraine attacks. Eating a salty meal causes vasoconstriction and hypoxia (lack of oxygen) in the hypothalamus [Roy, 2021]. Chronic high salt intake reduces blood flow to the brain and leads to the accumulation of toxic proteins associated with dementia [Faraco, 2019]. Furthermore, a high-salt diet is clearly linked to negative cardiovascular effects.

Now, of course, cravings for sugary or salty foods may be a migraine prodrome. In view of the detrimental health impact of high sugar and salt diets, it is best to limit one's intake. It is imprudent to add another physiological stressor for the sensitive migraine brain.

Food Additives

Monosodium Glutamate (MSG)

Is MSG good or bad? Glutamate is a natural amino acid found in many foods and is responsible for the *umami* (or savory "mouth flavor") taste. MSG alone does not have much flavor. It enhances the savory flavors and aromas. MSG is the flavor enhancer originally derived from seaweed. Today, most MSG is synthesized from bacteria.

MSG and glutamate are found in a large variety of foods. They occur naturally or can be added to processed foods. Examples of food that you wouldn't suspect contained MSG include ripe tomatoes, autolyzed yeast, nutritional yeast, broths/stocks (chicken, beef, vegetable), malt extract, and bouillon. Many tyramine-rich condiments and foods also contain high levels of glutamate, which is why we find them oh-so-tasty.

Other names for synthetic MSG include sodium 2-aminopentanedioate; sodium glutamate; glutamic acid, monosodium salt, monohydrate; L-glutamic acid, monosodium salt, monohydrate; L-monosodium glutamate monohydrate; monosodium L-glutamate monohydrate; sodium glutamate monohydrate; UNII-W81N5U6R6U; flavor enhancer E621. Monopotassium glutamate (E622) and monoammonium glutamate (E624) are flavor enhancers that do not contain sodium but have the glutamate molecule.

So, what's the deal with MSG? Opponents claim it is a toxin that causes a host of health problems, including diabetes, hypertension, neurological problems, and heart disease. Supporters blame anti-Asian bigotry as the reason behind the demonization of MSG and claim that it is completely safe to use. Like most questions about whether a particular food is good or bad, the answer is nuanced.

Glutamate is a naturally-occurring chemical and plays an important role in taste. We are drawn to foods with naturally high glutamate content because of the taste, like ripe tomatoes. Naturally occurring glutamate is used across multiple cultures, from seaweed extract in East Asian cuisine, to fermented anchovy sauce (*garum*) used by ancient Greeks and Romans, to fermented barley (*almori*) in Middle Eastern foods. MSG found in natural condiments such as these, and in Asian home cooking typically have lower glutamate levels compared to processed foods like chips, canned food, and snacks which often contain large amounts of added synthetic MSG to entice you to keep eating.

The FDA labels MSG as "generally recognized as safe" (GRAS). The European Food Safety Authority (EFSA) recommends no more than 30 mg per kilogram of body weight daily. According to the EFSA, this limit is not associated with any detrimental health effects but reduces exposure to heavy metals like arsenic and lead, which may contaminate manufactured MSG.

For people without migraine, moderate MSG consumption is harmless although several studies indicate that MSG increases the risk of obesity (perhaps because it enhances food enjoyment). Just like sugar and salt, MSG is probably not harmful if used in moderation but has negative consequences if used excessively. Healthy men given a single high dose of MSG experienced increases in headaches and blood pressure [Baad-Hansen, 2010]. Healthy adults given a large amount of MSG experience headaches and dizziness [Shimada, 2013].

For people with migraine, the MSG/glutamate may trigger attacks when consumed in larger than usual amounts. For example, if you have canned soup and chips when you usually don't, the MSG load may trigger an attack. Recall how the migraine brain is already in a hyperexcitable state. Since glutamate is an excitatory neurotransmitter, increased glutamate levels aggravate this hyperexcitable state further, triggering a migraine attack. Furthermore, MSG increases the sensitivity of the scalp, jaw, and facial muscles to pain [Shimada, 2013]. Limit your exposure to MSG/glutamate the way you should reduce your exposure to tyramine, blue light, noise, and caffeine. Cut out as much of it from your diet as possible by limiting your consumption of processed foods. Sticking to fresh, home-prepared meals keeps MSG intake to a minimum.

Nitrates & Nitrites

Nitrates and nitrites can also occur naturally in vegetables (like spinach, celery, and beetroot). Nitrites and nitrates are also added to meat to preserve it, add a salty flavor, and keep it looking pink or red (without nitrites, meat turns into an unappetizing brown color). Nitrates are inert but can be converted by bacteria into nitrites, which in turn, are transformed into nitric oxide or nitrosamines.

Nitric oxide has important functions in the body. It relaxes the walls of blood vessels, which helps with blood pressure and circulation. However, too much nitric oxide causes vasodilation that can trigger migraine attacks.

People with migraine are more sensitive to nitrates because their guts have more nitrate-reducing bacteria. These bacteria create more nitrite, leading to higher levels of nitric oxide that trigger migraine attacks. When sodium nitrite in processed meats is exposed to heat, it reacts with amino acids to form nitrosamines, which are harmful and carcinogenic. Nitrates and nitrites in vegetables do not form nitrosamines due to the lack of amino acids and the presence of antioxidants.

Check the label of foods for sodium nitrate/nitrite, and potassium nitrate/nitrite. Beware of labels that claim that no nitrates or nitrites are added – some manufacturers add celery juice/powder or celeriac, which is a natural source of nitrates and nitrites. For people with migraine, nitrites and nitrates can trigger migraine, regardless of their source.

Sulfites

Sulfites can be found naturally in foods but are also used as additives. Like nitrites and nitrates, sulfites are added to foods to preserve their freshness and prevent browning. Look for additives that contain the words sulfite, bisulfite, metabisulfite, thiosulfate, or dithionate. Sulfur dioxide and sulfurous acid are also sulfite additives. Foods that contain sulfites include dried fruit (except dark raisins and prunes); non-frozen bottled lemon and lime juice; wine; grape juices; pickled cocktail onions; sauerkraut; vinegar and wine vinegar; maraschino cherries;

commercially peeled, mashed, or dried potatoes; and tomato paste, puree, and ketchup.

Artificial Coloring

There are nine approved food dyes in the US. Yellow #5 (Tartrazine, E102), Yellow #6 (Sunset Yellow, E110), Blue #1 (Brilliant Blue FD, E133), Blue #2 (Indigotine, E132), Green #3 (Fast Green FCF, E143), Red #40 (Allura Red AC, E129), and Red # 3 (Erythrosine, E 127) are used in multiple products. Citrus Red #2 (C.I. Solvent Red 80, E121) is only approved to color orange peels. Orange B (C.I. Acid Orange 137) is only approved for hot dog and sausage casings (potentially carcinogenic).

There are reports of food dyes (particularly Yellow #5 and Red #40) triggering migraine attacks, although there are no studies to confirm this link. Of note, it is very difficult to study the effects of these dyes on migraine since they can be found in many products, and their names are often buried in the list of unpronounceable chemical names listed in the ingredients. By eliminating as many processed foods from your diet as possible, you can minimize your exposure to these artificial coloring agents.

Artificial Sweeteners

Artificial sweeteners are often blamed for migraine attacks. There are several commercially available artificial sweeteners, and a brief understanding of their metabolism may help us understand their role in triggering vestibular migraines.

Acesulfame potassium (Ace K) is absorbed from the gut and distributed through all tissues. It is excreted in the urine whole, without being metabolized at all. It can be transferred across the placenta and into breast milk.

Aspartame (Equal) is an artificial sweetener used widely in many beverages and foods. It is the ester of aspartic acid and phenylalanine. High levels of phenylalanine and aspartic acid can potentially trigger migraines. Furthermore, its metabolites, including methanol, formaldehyde, and formic acid may be neurotoxic. Aspartame is the artificial sweetener that is often blamed for triggering migraines [Koehler, 1988; Newman, 2001; Van den Eeden, 1994].

Saccharin (Sweet n Low) is absorbed into the systemic circulation and disseminates through all tissues. It can also pass the placental barrier and be excreted in breast milk. Like acesulfame, it is not metabolized and is excreted whole in the urine.

Sucralose (Splenda) is not absorbed or metabolized and passes right into the feces. There is only one case report of sucralose triggering migraine in the medical literature [Bigal, 2006].

Stevia leaf extract was used as a sweetener by indigenous South American people and was introduced to Japan in the 1970s. It was eventually allowed into the US as a dietary supplement in 1991. Most of the stevia leaf extract passes through the gut and is excreted in the feces.

Monk fruit (*Siraitia grosvenorii*) extract has gained popularity as a natural low-calorie sweetener. The compounds that create sweetness are called mogrosides. Mogrosides are metabolized in the large intestine by bacteria that cleave off the glucose molecules. Only small amounts are absorbed into the circulation and most are excreted in the feces.

Aspartame seems to be the artificial sweetener usually implicated as a vestibular migraine trigger. Acesulfame and saccharin are absorbed into the circulation and could also theoretically trigger migraines, although there are no studies that report this. As a general rule, sweeteners that are not absorbed into the circulation, like sucralose, stevia, and monk fruit, are much less likely to trigger migraines since they remain in the intestine and are excreted in the feces.

The following table summarizes food additives to watch out for:

Additives	Ingredients to watch out for
Monosodium glutamate (MSG)	Seaweed extract (kombu), kelp, carob, autolyzed yeast, nutritional yeast, brewer's yeast, yeast food, broths/stocks (chicken, beef, vegetable), bouillon (chicken, beef, vegetable), Ajinomoto, Ve-Tsin, maltodextrin, oligodextrin, barley malt, malt extract, malted barley, "natural flavor", carrageenan, yeast food, textured protein, "seasonings", hydrolyzed soy, sodium/calcium caseinate, whey protein.
Nitrites & Nitrates	Look out for sodium nitrate/nitrite, potassium nitrate/nitrite, and celery juice/powder. Foods to avoid: bacon, hot dogs, sausages, pepperoni, corned beef, jerky, bologna, pastrami
Sulfites	Look for words with -sulfite, -bisulfite, -metabisulfite, -thiosulfate, -dithionate, sulfur dioxide, and sulfurous acid. Foods to avoid: dried fruit (except dark raisins and prunes); non-frozen bottled lemon & lime juice; wine; grape juice; pickled cocktail onions; sauerkraut; vinegar & wine vinegar; maraschino cherries; commercially peeled, mashed, or dried potatoes; tomato paste, puree and ketchup
Sweeteners	High fructose corn syrup, acesulfame potassium (Ace K), aspartame (Equal), saccharin (Sweet n Low)
Artificial Coloring	Yellow #5 (Tartrazine, E102), Yellow #6 (Sunset Yellow, E110), Blue #1 (Brilliant Blue FD, E133), Blue #2 (Indigotine, E132), Green #3 (Fast Green FCF, E143), Red #40 (Allura Red AC, E129), Citrus Red #2 (C.I. Solvent Red 80, E121), Red # 3 (Erythrosine, E 127), Orange B (C.I. Acid Orange 137)

The Ketogenic Diet

The ketogenic ("keto") diet is high in fat and protein but very low in carbohydrates. It aims to put the body in ketosis, a metabolic state mimicking starvation where it uses ketone bodies instead of glucose as its primary fuel. The keto diet has been used for a long time to control refractory epilepsy. The first report of the keto diet in migraine appeared in 1928 [Schnabel, 1928].

Several small studies have shown that the ketogenic diet can help control migraine headaches [Bongiovanni, 2021; Di Lorenzo, 2015; Di Lorenzo, 2019; Lovati, 2022]. No one really knows how the keto diet helps neurological disorders. Some hypotheses include weight loss, controlling brain hyperexcitability, improving mitochondrial energy metabolism, and inhibiting inflammation. There may be an increase in migraine activity in the first few weeks of the diet as the brain adjusts and switches its fuel source. In general, improvement may be seen in the first month but it can take up to 3 months for the benefits to be seen.

It can be used in the short term to control migraine but it is not healthy or sustainable in the long run. It is difficult to constantly prepare meals and measure the amounts of fat and carbs. The keto diet tends to be very low in fruits, whole grains, and vegetables which results in a lack of important vitamins (e.g., folate, thiamine, vitamin C, B2, B6), minerals (e.g., calcium, magnesium), antioxidants, and fiber. It may cause constipation, fatigue, headaches, and increased blood lipids. In the long term, the keto diet is linked to a higher risk of gout, nephrolithiasis (kidney stones), osteoporosis, anemia, cardiomyopathy, and optic nerve damage.

The Mediterranean Diet

A typical modern Western diet (high in sugar, salt, unhealthy fats, and highly processed foods) is linked to many medical (e.g., diabetes, hypertension) and neurological diseases. Lab mice fed this diet experience a dramatic change in their gut microbial composition within 24 hours [Cryan, 2019].

A growing body of scientific data proves that the Mediterranean diet is, by far, the best diet for neurological health. As of 2018, the Mediterranean diet has been studied in almost 13 million people [Dinu, 2018]. It decreases the risk of certain cancers (prostate, breast, and colorectal), promotes a healthy body weight, reduces obesity, enhances cardiovascular health, diminishes the risk of neurodegenerative diseases (e.g., Alzheimer's, Parkinson's) and controls autoimmune disease activity. The Mediterranean diet also dramatically improves the composition of the gut microbiota, increasing the diversity and numbers of healthy microbes, and suppressing negative ones. Of special interest in vestibular migraine, this diet has been proven to improve neuroplasticity, anxiety, and depression.

The scientifically proven benefits of the Mediterranean diet can be attributed to several overarching principles. It contains high levels of antioxidants, anti-inflammatory agents, bioactive polyphenols, fiber, and healthy fats. The Mediterranean diet also contains lower levels of refined carbohydrates (like sugar, and white flour), and unhealthy fats (saturated animal fats, and trans fats). The diet emphasizes a high intake of vegetables, legumes, fresh fruit, non-refined (whole grain) cereals, nuts, and olive oil, particularly extra virgin olive oil (EVOO). Poultry, fish, and dairy products are consumed in moderation, while red meat and sugar intake are kept low.

The Mediterranean diet is more sustainable and healthier. It is a lifestyle and not a diet fad. For those with migraine, you can easily adopt a migraine-friendly Mediterranean diet that adheres to the abovementioned principles without migraine food triggers.

Migraine Superfoods

There are migraine superfoods that you should embrace. These contain nutrients that help control migraine, antioxidants that decrease inflammation (a huge part of migraine pathophysiology), and many other health benefits.

- *Green leafy vegetables* (especially kale, collard greens, microgreens, cabbage, Brussels sprouts, broccoli, turnip greens, Swiss chard, arugula, bokchoy) are a great source of fiber, riboflavin (vitamin B2), magnesium, folate, vitamin C, and antioxidants.

- *Asparagus* is a great source of fiber, folate, vitamin C, vitamin E, and antioxidants.
- *Seeds* (e.g., sesame, pumpkin, sunflower, chia, flaxseeds) are a great source of magnesium, coenzyme-Q10, folate, and Omega-3 fatty acids.
- *Garbanzo beans, lentils, black beans, and pinto beans* are a great source of plant-based protein, fiber, folate, magnesium, and vitamin B6.
- *Mushrooms* (e.g., button, cremini, shiitake, portobello) are a low-calorie, and delicious source of vitamin B2, folate, vitamin B6, vitamin C, and antioxidants.
- *Whole grains* are a good source of fiber, riboflavin (B2), and magnesium.
- *Eggs* are nutritious and provide vitamins B2, B6, B12, D and E. You can purchase Omega-3 enriched eggs to increase your dietary intake of omega-3 fatty acids.
- *Fish* (particularly fatty fish) is a great source of omega-3 fatty acids, coenzyme-Q10, magnesium, and vitamin D.
- *Fresh fruits* (particularly blueberries, blackberries, acai berries, goji berries, and pomegranate) are a great source of vitamin C, and antioxidants.
- *Tart (Montmorency, sour, or dwarf) cherries* contain high levels of vitamin C, antioxidants, and melatonin.
- *Ginger and turmeric* are great for migraine control and have potent anti-inflammatory and antioxidant properties. Ginger has added anti-nausea benefits as well. Add them to dishes for flavor (don't forget to add some black pepper to improve absorption of curcumin).
- *Garlic* adds a lot of flavor to food and is loaded with antioxidants, vitamin C, and B6.

Designing Your Diet

All the information on food triggers can be overwhelming. How do you create your very own diet plan? Must you avoid every single food trigger? Must you avoid all these triggers your whole life? How do you know which food(s) provoke your migraine attacks? This is a simple approach to help you.

Start with the Detoxification Phase, which lasts for 3-4 months, during which you will eliminate every food trigger. At the end of the Detoxification Phase, you may gradually introduce food items, one at a time, to test your tolerance for them. If a particular food does not trigger a migraine attack, it is safe for you to continue consuming it. If a specific food item provokes a migraine attack, avoid it.

Detoxification Phase

- Cut out all caffeine. This includes coffee, tea, energy drinks, and sodas. Decaffeinated coffee or teas also contain small amounts of caffeine and should be avoided.
- Cut out foods with MSG/glutamate.
- Cut out foods with nitrites and nitrates.
- Cut out all alcohol.
- Cut out all chocolate.
- Cut out foods with sulfites and sulfates.
- Cut out all tyramine-rich foods.
- Cut out soy products.
- Cut out all added salt. In other words, avoid adding extra salt to your food. Use seasonings for flavor.
- Avoid sugar and simple (refined) carbs.
  - Avoid syrups, especially high-fructose corn syrup.
  - Avoid foods that contain a lot of sugar, like ice cream, cakes, pastries, cookies, jelly, spreads, and jam.
  - Avoid refined carbs like white bread, white rice, and white flour, which spike blood sugar levels, and are devoid of most nutrients.
  - Stick to complex carbs like whole wheat, oats, and brown rice; because of the higher fiber content, these carbs are digested slowly, providing a gradual rise in blood sugar and keeping you feeling fuller for longer.

241

The higher fiber content is also great for your gut bacteria.

- Cut out aspartame (Equal), acesulfame, and saccharine.
- Drink *at least* 8 glasses (64 oz) of water every day.
- Gluten and dairy are not migraine triggers in most. If you like, you can eliminate them from your diet as well during the Detoxification Phase.

As much as possible, try to eat fresh food. Cut out canned and processed foods. Preparing your meals is a bit more tedious but allows you to control what ingredients are used. Eat more of the migraine superfoods. The following table summarizes some of the food items that you can consume during the Detoxification Phase.

Grain-based foods	Oats, whole wheat, brown or black rice, corn Pasta (look for vegetable pasta, or whole wheat) Noodles Cereal and granola (no nuts, dried fruit) Flour (all-purpose, self-rising, bread, whole wheat)
Vegetables	Fresh or frozen vegetables (except those listed above)
Fruits	Fresh fruits (except those listed above)
Seeds	Chia seeds, flaxseed, sunflower seeds, pumpkin seeds
Meat	Fresh or frozen chicken, turkey, pork, lamb, beef
Fish	Look for fatty fish (mackerel, salmon, tuna, trout, cod, halibut)
Seafood	Fresh or frozen shrimp, squid, crab, lobster, shellfish
Dairy	Fresh milk, dry (powdered) milk, ricotta, American cheese, cream cheese, cottage cheese, butter, cream
Plant-based milk	Oat milk, rice milk, hemp milk
Baked products	Store-bought bread (except sourdough) Home-baked bread at least one day old
Eggs	Fresh eggs. Omega-3 eggs are best.
Spices & Seasonings	Garlic, cooked onion, green onion, rosemary, thyme, oregano, turmeric, ginger, black pepper, cilantro, coriander, cumin, curry powder, fennel, bay leaves, basil, paprika, mint, peppermint, spearmint, clear vinegar, cinnamon, vanilla
Sweeteners	Honey, sucralose (Splenda), Stevia, monk fruit

The Detoxification Phase diet may sound tasteless and terrible but it really isn't. By cutting out processed foods and a lot of junk from your diet, you will actually feel better while simultaneously controlling your vestibular migraines. This phase should not just be about avoiding trigger foods. You should embrace the migraine superfoods.

Alicia Wolf's cookbook *The Dizzy Cook* is an excellent reference about all the food items you should avoid and those that are safe, while also providing an extensive list of recipes for migraine-friendly dishes. Our book, *The Mediterranean Migraine Diet*, provides many recipes for a migraine-friendly Mediterranean diet.

The Re-Challenge Phase

After the Detoxification Phase, you can choose to maintain the food restrictions or begin reintroducing foods to your diet. This is the Re-Challenge Phase, where you reintroduce various foods to test if they are migraine triggers. If a food does not trigger a vestibular migraine attack within 24 hours of consumption, it's most likely not a trigger for you.

You should slowly add food items back to your diet. *Slowly.* Stay away from the big, well-known triggers like MSG, caffeine, alcohol, fermented foods, aged/cured foods, aspartame, saccharine, nitrates/nitrites, sulfites, and ultra-processed foods. Continue to limit sugar and added salt.

Start by adding fruits and vegetables that were disallowed during the detoxification phase. Add one item at a time. This will allow you to identify a migraine trigger easily. If you start by eating a bunch of different items, it would be impossible to pinpoint the trigger. For example, you can start with avocados. If that triggers a migraine attack, no more avocadoes for you. If it does not, go ahead and add oranges, and so on.

You can then try adding soy products back into your diet if you like. Start with soymilk or tofu. Beware of highly processed soy products like vegetarian meat substitutes since these contain a lot of other additives that could trigger migraine attacks. If you eliminated gluten and/or dairy products from your diet you can also slowly reintroduce them (one by one, of course) if you'd like.

You may also try adding certain nuts back into your diet. Start with almonds since they are a rich source of magnesium, fiber, and healthy fats. You can then decide if you would like to add pecans, walnuts, or pistachios. It may be best to continue avoiding Brazil nuts and peanuts until your migraine symptoms have been well-controlled.

Six months from the time your symptoms are well-controlled and stable, you may start adding some alcohol if you like. Vodka is the safest to start with. Stay away from dark beers, dark liquors, champagne, sparkling wine, and red wine. If you really want to drink wine, try using a product called "The Wand" by Pure Wine (www.drinkpurewine.com), which can remove sulfites and histamines. Chocolate and cocoa products can be reintroduced cautiously as well. Look for higher-quality chocolate products that are not loaded with sugar and artificial flavors.

You may also *gradually* allow **some** caffeine back into your diet if you want. You can start with decaf and then introduce "half-caf". However, I would advise no more than 1 cup of coffee (8oz) or tea per day. More than one cup a day will aggravate migraines. Non-caffeinated herbal teas can be a very good substitute for caffeinated beverages. Ginger teas can help with nausea and migraine control. Peppermint or spearmint can help with nausea. Chamomile and passionflower are good for relaxation.

Fermented foods are fantastic for gut health. You can try reintroducing some (e.g., yogurt, kimchi, kefir) in small amounts slowly to see if these trigger your vestibular migraine attacks. Continue to limit those that contain high amounts of glutamate/MSG.

The migraine diet has health benefits beyond controlling migraine attacks. For your well-being and health, avoid foods with added nitrites/nitrates, sulfites, artificial coloring, aspartame, acesulfame, and saccharin. Limit your consumption of simple carbohydrates, sugar, salt, and MSG. Remember, read food labels. Avoid products that have too many incomprehensible chemical compounds listed as ingredients. As much as possible, consume whole, fresh foods and avoid highly-processed, artificial products.

A Word of Caution: Orthorexia

Orthorexia is an eating disorder characterized by a preoccupation with what one believes is healthy eating. Note that the person is overly concerned with what they *believe* is "pure" or "clean". Those with orthorexia spend unusually large amounts of time thinking about and avoiding "unhealthy" foods. If they consume (inadvertently or otherwise) something considered "unhealthy", they experience significant psychological distress.

Now, one's diet definitely has an impact but one's diet cannot solve everything. Orthorexia is the result of the prevalent cultural belief that any health goal can be achieved with the correct and pure diet. People with chronic health conditions like vestibular migraine are often stressed and discomfited by the lack of control over their diseases. Many turn to the illusion of diet control to gain power over their illnesses. When confronted by the uncertainty and unpredictability of their illness, the mind tries to cope by controlling what it can i.e., food.

Since there are migraine food triggers, many fall for the simple but false idea that a clean diet is *the* solution to their illness. When one's symptoms do not improve, the next logical step is to "clean up" one's diet further. Perhaps one did not eliminate *enough* migraine triggers. As time goes by, the person's food horizons shrink as more and more foods are eliminated. This is where things get dangerous. The underlying psychopathology of this process is discussed in Chapter 19. In unpredictable illnesses like vestibular migraine, the amygdala enters a state of hyperactivation and a vicious state of growing anxiety about an ever-increasing list of potential threats.

More and more foods become suspect. As the fires of central sensitization are kindled, the brain becomes rigid, intolerant of change, and hypervigilant of anything that causes it to feel different. Innocuous foods become "migraine triggers" and in some extreme cases, the person feels worse or triggered after eating *anything*. This is a very unhealthy and unsustainable situation as you can imagine.

Don't let your mind become obsessed and fixated on food triggers. The migraine diet is one tool in your arsenal, not the only one. I tell my patients that the diet *can* help but it is not the ultimate, one-and-only solution. It is not the only treatment option for vestibular migraine. There are a host of many other treatment options at your disposal, including supplements, medications, exercise, and lifestyle changes.

T

Therapeutic Options

Overview of all available preventive and rescue treatments for vestibular migraine

Chapter 15: Preventive Treatments

Medicine is the science of uncertainty and an art of probability

Sir William Osler (1849-1919)

If non-pharmacologic treatments and lifestyle changes do not sufficiently control vestibular migraine, you should consider starting preventive treatment. The goal of preventive therapy is to improve your quality of life by reducing the number, severity, and duration of migraine attacks, as well as relieve interictal symptoms. By controlling your migraine attacks, you decrease the need to use rescue medication(s), which helps not only reduce your medication costs, but also prevents medication-overuse headache, side effects, and progression to chronic migraine.

As with nutraceuticals, there are many migraine preventives to choose from. There is not much data to show one or two particular treatments are the absolute best for migraine. All of them can potentially help (or else we would not prescribe them!). Since everyone's genetic makeup is different, what works for one person may not necessarily work for another. Different people just metabolize medications differently. Similarly, side effects cannot be predicted. What causes side effects for one person may not cause any for another. For example, not every patient develops brain fog from topiramate, and only a small number of patients have trouble weaning off venlafaxine.

It is important to understand these uncertainties when selecting a migraine preventive. In the same vein, do not give up on a good physician just because a medication prescribed did not work or caused an unexpected side effect. It is quite impossible to predict response or side effects (beware those who guarantee treatment success – these are often con artists!).

Before weighing out your choices, there are two important considerations. Firstly, make sure you do not have any contraindications to the medications. For example, if you have severe asthma, you should avoid beta-blockers. Health conditions that can preclude the use of certain medications are covered in this chapter. Secondly, you also need to consider if you are planning to get pregnant in the near future. The FDA categories of A, B, C, D, X, and N is no longer in use. Currently, the FDA uses the Pregnancy and Lactation Labeling Rule (PLLR), which requires a risk summary based on human, animal, and pharmacological data. This is supposed to provide women and physicians with more information to make a decision but is more cumbersome, in my opinion.

How to Choose Your Migraine Preventive(s)

Get the most bang for your buck

If one medication can treat migraine and other conditions you may have, choose that first. For example, if you have insomnia and vestibular migraine, amitriptyline can help both. If you have hypertension, essential tremor, and vestibular migraine, propranolol can potentially help all three conditions.

Start low, go slow

I always start with the lowest possible dose, and gradually increase it over time, stopping at a dosage that my patient tells me works well for them. This helps minimize the risks of side effects and allows us to use the minimum effective dose. I do not have a "target dosage" for most medications unless there is a set dosage like with the CGRP monoclonal antibodies.

Patience is a virtue

I understand that vertigo and dizziness are horrible, and everyone wants to immediately control them. Trust me, I wish there was a vestibular migraine preventive that immediately relieved my patients' symptoms. However, supplements, lifestyle modification, and preventive medications typically take 2-3 months to show benefit. Some people experience benefits earlier, and others take a bit longer. Do not give up too early unless you experience an intolerable side effect. You need to give treatment(s) a chance to work.

Remember to take your meds

The treatment can only work if you use it. Make sure you take the medication or use the treatment as prescribed. Try to establish a routine to ensure that you take your medication. For example, place the medication bottle in the kitchen area, and take it with breakfast and/or dinner as prescribed.

How does one measure success?

A preventive drug can be considered successful if (1) it reduces migraine attack frequency or days by at least 50% within 3 months, or; (2) it significantly decreases the duration and/or severity of the attacks, or; (3) it reduces rescue medication usage, or; (4) if it improves your ability to work or participate in activities. Of course, the ultimate goal is to reduce the attacks as much as possible, and even eliminate them completely. However, keep these measures of success in mind – if a medication helps reduce migraine frequency by at least half, it means that it is working and you should not give up on it. The dosage can be either increased further (provided you do not experience side effects), or another medication can be added (if you cannot tolerate higher doses). To objectively measure if a medication is working or not, keep a diary of your migraine attacks.

Mix n' Match

The goal of treatment is, of course, monotherapy, meaning optimal treatment with one single medication. Sometimes that is not possible – either because side effects occur at higher doses, or because a person derives modest benefit regardless of dose escalation. In this situation, a second medication is usually added to the first. In rare cases, a third medication may need to be added to optimize migraine control. While not "ideal", the goal of treatment is to achieve adequate control of migraine, and bring a person's quality of life as close as possible to normal.

Beware the nocebo effect

Expectations affect outcomes. We are quite familiar with the placebo (Latin "I shall please") effect; the term was first used in medicine in the 18th century. The placebo refers to a beneficial, desirable, or pleasant outcome from a treatment. Its opposite, the nocebo (Latin "I shall harm") effect, was described in 1961 by Walter Kennedy. The nocebo effect occurs when a person's negative expectations regarding a treatment cause the person to suffer more negative effects than it would otherwise cause.

The nocebo effect is psychological but produces real biological impacts. If you expect to experience a side effect, you will. This phenomenon has been studied extensively. There are brain changes that occur when a person expects a negative outcome from a treatment. An inert sugar pill causes "side effects" in those who believe that they will experience side effects even though there is no biological reason for it. This is why some placebo-treated patients report clinical trials experience "side effects"; they believe that the sugar pill is the real medication and expect to suffer side effects. In migraine trials, over 40% of participants experience the nocebo effect [Mitsikostas, 2011; Zhang, 2022]. People with longer illnesses are at higher risk of nocebo effects most likely because they have been conditioned by their previous experiences with medications. Furthermore, a person is at higher risk of the nocebo effect if they know someone who experienced or reported a side effect [Faasse, 2015].

Marketing and branding also have an effect on treatment response. People who receive a placebo with a fancy, brand-name label report greater "benefits" and fewer "side effects" compared to those who are given a placebo with a bland, generic label [Faasse, 2016]. In an interesting study [Faasse, 2013], college students were given a branded placebo (Betaprol) for blood pressure and anxiety in one test. When the same students were given placebos labeled "Generic" or with a different brand (Novaprol) in the second test, they reported the placebo wasn't as effective and caused more side effects.

A phenomenon called voodoo death is an extreme manifestation of negative expectations; healthy people who believe strongly that they are cursed actually die soon after - they literally will themselves to death. Similarly, if you believe that a medication won't work, guess what happens... it won't work. Studies have shown that people who believe their pain will not get better, don't get any relief even when given potent opioids.

It is very important to be aware of the nocebo effect. If you allow yourself to be afraid and paranoid about side effects, you will experience them. You will suffer the very thing you fear. Keep an open mind and be realistic when you start any new medication. Reading about a medication is good and being informed is great; however, don't freak yourself out reading all the potential side effects listed online. Social media is especially fraught; some may describe legitimate side effects but most are just being dramatic to get more attention.

In general, the risk of side effects with medications is low. At low doses, the likelihood is *extremely* low. Will you let this low risk keep you from getting better? Is it logical to continue suffering with your illness because of a small possibility of side effects? Why let the unfounded fear of side effects stand in the way of your healing? There's a small chance of being killed while driving but does that keep you from leaving the house? Being negative and pessimistic deprives you of the potential benefits of available medications. Even if you feel "weird" when you start a new medication, stick with it; such minor side effects usually resolve within a couple of weeks.

If at first, you don't succeed, maybe try again

Just because a treatment did not work once, that does not mean it should not be tried again at a different dosage. If a very low dose of a particular medication did not work, perhaps the dosage should have been increased, instead of abandoning it. Similarly, if you had side effects from a particular medication, perhaps the starting dose was too high or the dose was increased too rapidly. It could be worth trying it at a lower dose and increasing it more slowly to allow your body time to adapt to it.

Wean off

Finally, unless you are taking a very low dose of a particular medication or develop a serious adverse effect, do not stop it abruptly. Stopping a medication abruptly can be detrimental if you have been on it for a considerable duration; for example, stopping an antidepressant suddenly can cause a withdrawal syndrome that makes you extremely dizzy, and stopping an anticonvulsant medication abruptly may cause seizures especially if you're on a higher dose. If you want to discontinue any medication, always contact the prescribing physician for advice on how to taper off.

Newer does not mean better

Thank goodness for all the advances in migraine therapies! However, it is important to realize that newer does not necessarily mean better. The new drugs are not really more effective than older medications, even though they may be safer, and better tolerated. For example, the efficacy of ubrogepant and lasmiditan is similar to the triptans. In addition, the injectable

CGRP monoclonal antibodies have comparable efficacy to older migraine preventives, but can take up to 6 months for their benefits to be realized.

The Issue of Tolerance

Tolerance is defined as a loss of benefit from a previously effective treatment, i.e., the drug "losing" its effect or "wearing out". For example, if you initially find valproate to control your migraine well but after 6 months, the migraines worsen. Tolerance to migraine preventives is, unfortunately, not well studied, but estimated to affect between 1 to 8% of people with migraine [Rizzoli, 2011].

The mechanism of tolerance is not very well understood at this time. Pharmacokinetic tolerance occurs when the body becomes more efficient at breaking down, and expelling of a medication; higher doses are needed to overcome this effect. Pharmacodynamic tolerance occurs when the cells alter their response to a particular drug. This is similar to what happens with caffeine, which blocks the adenosine receptor. The body responds by making more receptors, and producing more adenosine resulting in a need for higher doses of caffeine to get the same jolt.

If tolerance occurs, a drug holiday could be considered – stop the medication for some time, and then resume taking it. Another option is to switch to a different medication. Don't completely abandon the medication that you have developed tolerance to; it could be something you can reconsider in the future if other treatments fail.

Tricyclic Antidepressants (TCAs)

In the 1950s, TCAs were used to treat depression, but have since been replaced by safer and more tolerable antidepressants. TCAs have found new life as a treatment for various neurological disorders, particularly those that cause pain (e.g., neuropathic pain, fibromyalgia). Most TCAs act by increasing serotonin and norepinephrine levels, similar to selective norepinephrine reuptake inhibitors (SNRIs).

Robust evidence supports TCA efficacy for migraine prevention. Furthermore, TCAs are also useful in treating tension-type headache, and as such, benefit patients with more than one type of headache.

Side effects include dry mouth, constipation, difficulty urinating, drowsiness, blurry vision, increased appetite, vivid dreams, and weight gain. Serious side effects include irregular heart rate, palpitations, hallucinations, and angle-closure glaucoma. It should be avoided in people with cardiac arrhythmias unless cleared by a cardiologist. Caution showed be exercised in people with epilepsy.

The two commonly used TCAs in migraine are *amitriptyline* (Elavil), and *nortriptyline* (Pamelor). In migraine prevention studies, amitriptyline is slightly more effective than nortriptyline. However, amitriptyline also tends to cause more side effects, particularly sedation and cognitive impairment in older adults.

Since amitriptyline causes drowsiness, it is taken at bedtime and is useful for insomnia. Nortriptyline tends to be much less sedating compared to amitriptyline, and is useful for those wishing to avoid drowsiness; it can be taken during the day. In my experience, weight gain tends to occur more with amitriptyline compared to nortriptyline.

Desipramine (Norpramin) and *protriptyline* (Vivactil) are less commonly used. They cause less sedation and weight gain compared to amitriptyline. They are reasonable choices if a person benefits from amitriptyline or nortriptyline but have intolerable side effects.

Doxepin is a TCA with strong anti-histamine activity, and as such, can be used in those with concomitant allergies.

However, it is very sedating, and is usually used for insomnia, rather than for migraine prevention.

Beta-Blockers

Beta-blockers and TCAs are the most studied migraine preventives, with solid scientific data to back their efficacy in migraine prevention. Beta-blockers can also treat tremors, anxiety, hypertension, postural orthostatic tachycardia syndrome, and some types of cardiac diseases. Some people use beta-blockers for performance anxiety (e.g., stage fright).

Side effects include fatigue, bradycardia (low heart rate), hypotension (low blood pressure), erectile dysfunction, weight gain, and vivid dreams. The weight gain usually occurs at the beginning of treatment, then plateaus. Physically active people and athletes should be aware that beta-blockers reduce endurance and exercise tolerance, because it blunts the physiologic rise in heart rate in response to the demands of physical exertion. Beta-blockers should be avoided in people with asthma and chronic obstructive pulmonary disease (COPD) due to the risk of bronchospasm (narrowing of the airways), and in those with bradycardia (resting heart rate less than 60 beats per minute).

Caution should be exercised in those with Raynaud's disease, diabetes mellitus, myasthenia gravis, congestive heart failure, and heart block; discuss beta-blocker use with your physician(s) before use. The data suggesting that beta-blockers worsen depression is very weak; they can be safely used in people with depression.

Propranolol (Inderal) is FDA-approved for migraine prevention. Propranolol is the best-studied beta-blocker in migraine, with benefits usually taking between 8 to 12 weeks to notice (but may be seen as early as 4 weeks). *Metoprolol* (Lopressor) is another well-studied beta-blocker used in migraine prevention. A few studies indicate that *bisoprolol, nadolol,* and *atenolol* may help prevent migraine.

Oral timolol is FDA-approved for migraine prevention but the evidence for it is less robust compared to propranolol and metoprolol. Timolol eye drops are available in 0.25 and 0.5% strength, and are prescribed for glaucoma, but have also been found to be effective for migraine rescue and prevention. I find it useful for migraine rescue and prevention as well; I use timolol eye drops for pregnant women, women planning to get pregnant, and those who find it difficult to tolerate oral medications.

The drops cause a brief burning sensation and are very well-tolerated. If you do not like the burning sensation, you can put the drops under your tongue.

Calcium Channel Blockers

Verapamil (Calan or Verelan) is used to treat hypertension, and certain cardiac arrhythmias. It is also moderately useful for migraine prevention. Side effects include constipation, weight gain, and peripheral edema (leg swelling).

In people with cardiac arrhythmias, a cardiologist must be consulted before calcium channel blockers are started. Gum enlargement is also known to occur. The high incidence of side effects makes verapamil a difficult medication to use for migraine prevention.

Other calcium channel blockers used in vestibular migraine prevention, but not available for prescription in the US include *flunarizine* and *cinnarizine*. These are particularly interesting because they also have anti-histaminergic and anti-dopaminergic properties. A potentially serious complication of these medications is Parkinson's-type movement disorders. Only a modest benefit has been reported with *nifedipine* in migraine prevention.

Anticonvulsants

Anticonvulsants are also called anti-epileptic drugs. Recall how migraine and epilepsy share common pathophysiologic features i.e., abnormally excitable brain regions. Anticonvulsants work by reducing this hyperexcitability, and can be very effective migraine preventives. In addition, they can be useful in people who also have bipolar disorder, neuropathic pain, or fibromyalgia.

As a general rule, all anticonvulsants may cause some dizziness, blurry vision, tiredness, and disequilibrium when first started. This is a common occurrence, and it is important to hang in there. Don't give up too early. Allow your body some time to get used to the medication, and these side effects will disappear. For migraines, the starting dosages are usually very low and unlikely to cause side effects. There is a very low (less than 0.5%) risk of suicidal thoughts with anticonvulsants. If you develop thoughts of hurting yourself after starting any anticonvulsant, stop taking it immediately and contact your physician.

Topiramate

Topiramate (Topamax) is an effective and widely-prescribed migraine preventive, and has shown efficacy in vestibular migraine as well. Benefits can be seen as early as 4 weeks, but usually take about 2 months. Higher doses usually work better, but cause more side effects.

Possible side effects include tingling (usually in the lips and fingers), taste changes (metallic taste), reduced appetite, and weight loss. Topiramate's appetite-suppressing effect makes it useful for weight control; it is combined with phentermine and marketed as an anti-obesity drug called Qsymia. The most bothersome side effect is cognitive slowing, causing slowness and difficulty thinking and the reason it's sometimes called "Dope-amax". In my experience, about 10% of my patients who take it experience this side effect.

If topiramate helps your migraine but causes pesky side effects, try switching to extended-release topiramate (brand names Qudexy and Trokendi), which is often better tolerated. The extended-release topiramate formulations are more expensive, and not uncommonly, insurance companies refuse to pay for them.

There is a small risk of kidney stones and reduced sweating (which can cause heat exhaustion); drink at least 64 oz of water (8 glasses) per day can prevent these adverse effects. It is eliminated through the kidneys and in people with renal disease, the dose must be adjusted accordingly. In some cases, topiramate cannot be used if a person has renal disease. If you have renal disease and are taking or planning to take topiramate, consult a nephrologist. Annual ophthalmic or optometric examination is important because of a very rare risk of angle closure glaucoma. It should be avoided in pregnancy or in women planning to get pregnant due to the risk of cleft palate and lip in the baby.

Zonisamide

Zonisamide (Zonegran) is an anticonvulsant that has similar properties to topiramate. However, it is effective in people with migraine who cannot tolerate, or who do not respond to topiramate. The side effects, and precautions are similar to that of topiramate. Zonisamide is a reasonable choice for people who do not improve with topiramate, or experience intolerable side effects from it.

Lamotrigine

Lamotrigine (Lamictal) is a migraine preventive and mood stabilizer. It is safe to use in the long term, and is very well-tolerated in general. Because of its mood-stabilizing properties, lamotrigine is useful in people with both migraine and mood disorders. Lamotrigine is metabolized in the liver and may affect the levels of certain anticonvulsants (valproate, carbamazepine, oxcarbazepine, phenytoin), antibiotics (trimethoprim, rifampin, pyrimethamine), and oral contraceptives.

While lamotrigine has few side effects, there are two very rare but serious adverse effects. The first is a very serious skin reaction called Stevens-Johnson syndrome and toxic epidermal necrolysis. While about 10% of people who start lamotrigine may get a benign rash, less than 0.1% experience serious skin reactions. These dermatological reactions typically occur within the first 2-8 weeks of starting treatment. To minimize the risk, lamotrigine must be started at a very low dose and increased slowly. Lamotrigine should also be avoided in people on valproate because it elevates lamotrigine levels and thus increases the risk of serious adverse effects. If you develop a rash when you start lamotrigine, stop it immediately and go to an emergency department for evaluation.

The second potential serious adverse effect is called hemophagocytic lymphohistiocytosis (HLH). HLH is an extremely rare disorder caused by the uncontrolled proliferation of immune cells that release a high amount of inflammatory chemicals. It is characterized by rash, fever, swollen lymph nodes, and spleen and liver enlargement. At the time I am writing this, less than 10 people have confirmed HLH caused by lamotrigine. If you develop a fever within 2-8 weeks of starting lamotrigine, stop it immediately and go to an emergency department.

To reduce any confusion about rashes and fever related to lamotrigine, do not start lamotrigine within 2 weeks of vaccinations or any illness that causes a fever. Do not start lamotrigine with another new medication. If you just started lamotrigine, wait 2-8 weeks before getting vaccinated.

Gabapentin

Gabapentin (Neurontin) has been shown to be modestly useful for migraine prevention. Gabapentin can also be used in neuropathic pain, and fibromyalgia. Side effects include weight gain, drowsiness, confusion, imbalance, and dizziness. It has to be started at a low dose and slowly increased to minimize these side effects. Its sedating effects, and the long time needed to achieve the target dose, make gabapentin somewhat difficult to use in vestibular migraine prevention. Gabapentin is excreted by the kidneys, and therefore needs to be adjusted or avoided in people who have renal disease. There is evidence that gabapentin and lamotrigine have synergistic actions.

Pregabalin (Lyrica) was developed as a successor to gabapentin. It is considered a Schedule V controlled substance (low potential for abuse). Pregabalin works similarly to gabapentin and has comparable side effects, although the dosage can be increased faster compared to gabapentin. Pregabalin has been shown to help with migraine prevention in small studies.

Divalproex Sodium or Sodium Valproate

While divalproex/valproate (Depakote) is an effective migraine preventive, it has a lot of side effects and requires serial monitoring lab studies. Side effects include weight gain, hair loss, liver problems, low platelets, tremors, and elevated ammonia levels. It should not be used in people with severe liver disease and pancreatitis. It can also cause serious birth defects (called spina bifida and neural tube defects); women of childbearing age who take divalproex/valproate must use contraception. Due to the high incidence of side effects and safety profile, I do not use it much for migraine prevention.

Levetiracetam

In several studies, levetiracetam (Keppra) showed benefit as a migraine preventive, typically at 2 months, and with continued use for 6 months. It is not widely used as a migraine preventive but can be a reasonable option if other treatments are not effective. It is generally a well-tolerated and very safe medication. In adults, the most common side effect (about 10-15%) is an irritable mood. It is excreted by the kidneys, and its dosage should be adjusted in people with renal disease. There are some rare reports of serious skin reactions like Stevens-Johnson syndrome and toxic epidermal necrolysis with levetiracetam (see the section on *Lamotrigine*). Low levels can be found in breast milk, but no harmful effects on babies have been reported. Some evidence indicates that levetiracetam may decrease breast milk production. Its use in pregnancy and during lactation should be discussed with an obstetrician.

Lacosamide

Lacosamide (Vimpat) is a newer anticonvulsant that can be administered in intravenous form to treat acute migraine attacks. Lacosamide can also be taken daily as a migraine preventive. In animals, it blocks CGRP release from the trigeminal nucleus. Lacosamide can be used to treat neuralgias as well. It is important to get an EKG before, and after starting lacosamide due to a rare risk of cardiac arrhythmias. There is a small risk of mood disturbances (e.g., depression, panic, anxiety, irritability), mania, and insomnia. Lacosamide is classified as a controlled (Schedule V) drug due to the very low incidence of euphoria. It causes birth defects in animal studies, and should be avoided by women planning to get pregnant, or who are pregnant. Lacosamide has not been well-studied in breastfeeding mothers; although small amounts can be secreted into breast milk, there have been no known reports of harm at this time.

Acetazolamide

Acetazolamide (Diamox) is a diuretic used to treat a variety of neurological conditions including altitude sickness, glaucoma, epilepsy, and intracranial hypertension.

It can be useful for migraine, and treating migraine aura status (prolonged migraine aura), but the side effects are often problematic. These include tingling and numbness, nausea, drowsiness, tinnitus, metallic taste, and diarrhea. More serious side effects include kidney stones, and electrolyte abnormalities (low potassium and sodium levels). Rare but serious side effects include Stevens-Johnson syndrome (see the section on *Lamotrigine*), and blood cell count abnormalities. It should be avoided in people with renal disease, and sulfa allergies. Acetazolamide can be used to prevent menstrually-related migraine.

Acetazolamide acts by blocking an enzyme called carbonic anhydrase, which is responsible for keeping the blood alkaline (by retaining bicarbonate). Topiramate and zonisamide have weak carbonic anhydrase-blocking properties, and are much better tolerated compared to acetazolamide.

Selective Norepinephrine Reuptake Inhibitors (SNRIs)

SNRIs are more helpful for migraine control compared to selective serotonin reuptake inhibitors (SSRIs). This may be because both norepinephrine and serotonin levels are affected in migraine, not just serotonin. SNRIs are better tolerated compared to TCAs, and are a good option for people who have migraine and depression or anxiety. SNRIs are also effective for PPPD, a common co-morbid condition in people with vestibular migraine.

Side effects include sexual dysfunction, fatigue, sweating, dry mouth, and nausea. All antidepressants have a very small risk of causing suicidal thoughts. A very rare side effect of SNRIs is increased blood pressure. SNRIs and SSRIs may trigger mania if used in people with bipolar disorder.

Venlafaxine (Effexor) has the best evidence for migraine prevention among SNRIs. Benefits are usually observed at 8 weeks. It is available in an extended-release capsule and immediate-release tablets. The extended-release capsule is dosed once a day, and immediate-release tablets are dosed up to three times a day.

Venlafaxine may cause insomnia if taken in the evening. Nausea and gastrointestinal upset are a bit more common in venlafaxine compared to other SNRIs. I advise my patients to take venlafaxine with food in the morning to mitigate this side effect. A rare side effect I've observed is constipation, which may be severe.

However, this side effect of venlafaxine makes it useful in people who have the diarrhea-type of irritable bowel syndrome (IBS). The majority of people do not experience any weight changes; infrequently, weight gain or loss may occur. Some experience withdrawal symptoms (irritability, sleep disturbances, mood changes, dizziness, brain zaps) when trying to wean off venlafaxine; most have no trouble with a slow taper but if there is a concern about withdrawal, a much slower taper can be considered.

Desvenlafaxine (Pristiq) is the metabolite of venlafaxine. It is very similar to venlafaxine, and generally may cause fewer side effects. Insomnia seems to be more common with desvenlafaxine, compared to other SNRIs. In general, desvenlafaxine dosage can be increased faster than venlafaxine but it is formulated as extended-release tablets, and as such, cannot be broken.

Duloxetine (Cymbalta) is an SNRI that can be useful in migraine prevention, although evidence for it is much less robust compared to venlafaxine. Duloxetine is particularly useful for chronic pain conditions as well, like fibromyalgia, or neuropathic pain, and as such, would be a good choice in people with MDDS and chronic pain. It appears to have fewer side effects and a lower risk of withdrawal compared to venlafaxine. Duloxetine is formulated as extended-release capsules.

Milnacipran (Savella) is FDA-approved for fibromyalgia, not depression. The reason for this approval was to avoid the stigma attached to using antidepressants in fibromyalgia. One study showed it helped prevent migraines, and can be used in people who have both fibromyalgia and migraine. It may cause significant sexual dysfunction. One unusual side effect in men is testicular pain and painful urination. At the time of this writing, milnacipran remains a branded medication, and as such, may be expensive depending on one's insurance coverage.

There is not much evidence to support the use of SSRIs for migraine prevention. *Fluoxetine* (Prozac) may be a useful migraine preventive, but the studies have been small. Mirtazapine (Remeron) helps with tension-type headaches, and because it is sedating, can help with insomnia.

There is little evidence to support the efficacy of *escitalopram* (Lexapro), *fluvoxamine* (Luvox), or *sertraline* (Zoloft) in migraine. It is important to treat mood disorders in people with migraine. Depression anxiety, panic, and PTSD are much more common in people with migraine, especially those with vertigo and dizziness. If an SSRI or SNRI helps with the mood but not vertigo and dizziness, I would advise staying on it, and starting another medication for migraine prevention.

Serotonin syndrome is a very rare condition caused by very high levels of serotonin, usually due to overdosing on SSRIs. It is characterized by elevated heart rate, increased body temperature, tremors, sweating, confusion, hallucinations, and agitation; if severe, it can be life-threatening. In 2006, the FDA warned about using SSRI/SNRIs and triptans together due to the theoretical risk of serotonin syndrome. Some physicians and pharmacists refuse to prescribe triptans to people who are taking SNRIs/SSRIs. However, studies since then have disproven this.

Cyproheptadine

Cyproheptadine (Periactin) is often used to treat migraine or migraine equivalents in children, and can also be used to treat allergies and itching, as well as to stimulate the appetite. It can also be used for migraine prevention in adults. It would be reasonable to use cyproheptadine in adults with vestibular migraine if they also have significant seasonal allergies, insomnia, or if they are underweight. The main side effects are drowsiness and weight gain. I use cyproheptadine in my patients who have had side effects with many other medications, or those who have allergies; in my experience, it is very well-tolerated and quite effective.

Angiotensin Blockers

Angiotensin-converting enzyme (ACE) inhibitors (e.g., *lisinopril, enalapril*) have been shown to help reduce migraine attacks. ACE inhibitors are also used to lower blood pressure, and could be a useful option if a person has both vestibular migraine and hypertension. A dry cough can be a particularly pesky side effect. More serious side effects include abnormally high blood potassium levels, kidney impairment, and angioedema (swelling under the skin and mucous membranes).

Angiotensin II receptor antagonists (ARBs) like *candesartan* (Atacand) and telmisartan (Micardis) can be used for people who develop a dry cough with ADE inhibitors. I generally recommend that people who use ACE inhibitors or ARBs have a primary care provider who can help monitor kidney function, electrolyte levels, and blood pressure.

Buspirone

Buspirone (Buspar) is an anti-anxiety medication that is quite well-tolerated. It is not particularly effective for anxiety, when compared to other medications like SSRIs or SNRIs., and is therefore considered a second-line medication for anxiety. One study showed that buspirone helped with migraine prevention, independent of its effects on anxiety [Lee, 2005]. While its effect on migraine is likely modest at best, it could be considered in people with vestibular migraine and anxiety.

Muscle Relaxants

Muscle relaxants have been shown to help with migraine prevention and rescue, and could be useful in people with concomitant muscle spasms and pain. The main drawback of muscle relaxants is drowsiness which can be somewhat mitigated by using it at bedtime and very slowly building up the dosage.

Tizanidine (Zanaflex) is the best-studied muscle relaxant for migraine headache prevention followed by *baclofen* (Lioresal). Other muscle relaxants that can also be used are *cyclobenzaprine* (Flexeril), *methocarbamol* (Robaxin), and *chlorzoxazone* (Parafon Forte). For migraine prevention, muscle relaxants are usually dosed three times a day. For rescue, muscle relaxants can be used as needed for migraine attacks and do not carry the risk of medication overuse headache.

Memantine

Memantine (Namenda) is a medication used to moderately slow the cognitive decline in dementia. It can also treat some forms of nystagmus. A few small studies have supported the potential benefit of memantine as a migraine preventive. The role of memantine in reducing brain fog in migraine has not been studied.

Dizziness is the most common side effect, and can often limit how high the dose can be increased. Other side effects include drowsiness and constipation. I have generally reserved memantine use for people with vestibular migraine, who also have dementia, or in people in whom other medications have not helped.

Montelukast

Montelukast (Singulair) is used for the treatment of allergies and asthma. The results in migraine prevention studies are mixed. Doses used in these studies (10 to 20 mg daily) are safe. While the evidence to support its use is not strong, it is not unreasonable to try montelukast, particularly if a person also has asthma and allergies. It is a generally very safe and well-tolerated medication; however, it is important to note that the FDA issued a black box warning regarding the possibility of suicidality with montelukast.

CGRP Monoclonal Antibodies

CGRP monoclonal antibodies were the first medications designed specifically for the treatment of migraines. There are currently four CGRP monoclonal antibodies available: *erenumab* (Aimovig), *fremanezumab* (Ajovy), *galcanezumab* (Emgality), and *eptinezumab* (Vyepti).

Erenumab, fremanezumab, and galcanezumab are administered subcutaneously (under the skin). Erenumab and galcanezumab are given once a month. Fremanezumab can be given once a month or every three months. Eptinezumab is given intravenously every three months.

Erenumab can be given in doses of 70 or 140 mg once a month; there does not seem to be a difference in terms of efficacy or side effects, although the 140 mg dose seems to reduce the use of rescue medications slightly more. Fremanezumab can be given as a 225 mg dose once a month, or 675 mg (three 225 mg shots) every 3 months. The efficacy between the monthly and quarterly administrations is similar. Galcanezumab is given as a 240 mg loading dose followed by 120 mg monthly doses.

Erenumab, fremanezumab, and galcanezumab must be kept refrigerated (not frozen). When you are ready to inject it, take it out from the refrigerator and leave it out for 30 minutes to warm to room temperature. Do not put it in warm water to try to speed up the process. Allowing these medications to warm to room temperature makes the injection less painful.

Eptinezumab is administered intravenously (100 or 300 mg) once every three months, as an outpatient infusion. These infusions are performed under the supervision of healthcare professionals.

The efficacy of the CGRP monoclonal antibodies is comparable to the other migraine preventives. However, some people have remarkable responses and became completely free of migraine ("super responders"). It is important to be patient and not give up too early; benefits are first observed at 3 months but may take 6-12 months to fully realize. I usually recommend using these medications for 6-12 months before making any decision about stopping them. Because it's given intravenously, eptinezumab reaches peak plasma concentration within 48 hours, and as such, may show benefit much earlier compared to subcutaneously-administered CGRP monoclonal antibodies. As such, eptinezumab may be more useful when rapid control of vestibular migraine is desirable.

The CGRP monoclonal antibodies appear to be well-tolerated. Known side effects include injection site reactions (e.g., redness, itching, pain), and constipation. The number of upper respiratory tract infections also appears slightly increased in people using CGRP antibodies, although the reason for this is unclear. The risk of constipation is higher with erenumab. Hypertension may occur infrequently; this typically occurs within a week of initiating treatment. Otherwise, there does not seem to be a higher risk of cardiovascular disease in those treated with CGRP monoclonal antibodies. One unusual side effect that is being reported by patients is increased hair shedding, and in some, hair thinning; this appears to be the result of CGRP blockade and has been described with gepants as well.

However, it would be better to avoid using these medications with recent (less than 6 months) stroke, subarachnoid hemorrhage, or myocardial infarction. Because older studies showed that CGRP blockade worsened outcomes following subarachnoid hemorrhage, these medications should be used judiciously in those with known brain aneurysms.

It is unclear interactions occur between these medications and monoclonal antibodies used for other diseases like multiple sclerosis, psoriasis, and rheumatoid arthritis. CGRP is important in the development of placental blood vessels and should be avoided in pregnancy or in women planning to get pregnant in the near future. If you have been on one of these medications, hold off on trying to get pregnant for at least 5 months after discontinuation.

Gepants

Gepants are oral CGRP blockers. The potential side effects are similar to the CGRP monoclonal antibodies, and include constipation, nausea, dizziness, gastrointestinal upset, and increased hair shedding/thinning. The benefit of gepants is that more frequent dosing overcomes the withdrawal effect some experience a week before injecting the CGRP monoclonal antibodies. Furthermore, a shorter half-life means that gepants are cleared more quickly from the body, which is helpful in the event of unexpected side effects, or if one wants to get pregnant. It is also easier to travel with oral tablets, instead of monoclonal antibodies that need to be kept cold. There are two gepants are currently available for migraine prevention.

Atogepant (Qulipta) is a once-daily tablet available in 10, 30, and 60 mg doses. While effective, the incidence of nausea and gastrointestinal upset is quite high. Unfortunately, many of my patients have been unable to tolerate atogepant.

Rimegepant (Nurtec) can be used for both migraine rescue (see next chapter), and prevention. It comes in a single dose of 75 mg. The dose for migraine prevention is 75 mg every other day. Rimegepant is very well-tolerated, and in my experience, has the lowest incidence of side effects.

Onabotulinumtoxin A (Botox)

Botox is FDA-approved for the treatment of chronic migraine. The story of Botox and migraine is one of medical serendipity. People with migraine who got Botox for cosmetic reasons noticed that both migraines and wrinkles disappeared. Botulinum toxin is produced by a bacterium (*Clostridium botulinum*) that lives in anaerobic (oxygen-poor) environments. It can enter the body through food (especially contaminated home-canned foods or preserved meats), or wounds. The toxin causes paralysis of skeletal muscles by blocking the release of acetylcholine at the neuromuscular junction. Commercial forms include onabotulinumtoxin A (Botox), abobotulinumtoxin A (Dysport or Azzalure), incobotulinumtoxin A (Xeomin or Bocouture), rimabotulinumtoxin B (Myobloc), and prabotulinumtoxin A (Jeuveau).

While Botox is FDA-approved for chronic migraine treatment, there is evidence that Dysport and Xeomin can control migraine as well. How botulinum toxin works on migraine is not fully understood. Besides relaxing muscles, Botox may block the release of chemicals involved in propagating pain and in peripheral sensitization.

The protocol used for Botox is based on the Placebo-controlled phase III Research Evaluating Migraine Prophylaxis Therapy (PREEMPT) study and involves the injection of specific muscles in the face, scalp, and neck muscles. There can be some variation in the administration protocol. For example, if a person develops shoulder or neck weakness, these sites should be avoided for future injections. Botox is typically administered every 12 weeks. Even though some patients suffer a recurrence of migraine 2-4 weeks before the next injection, it can be extraordinarily difficult to get insurance approval for earlier injections. Nerve blocks performed around week 8 can help control headaches until Botox can be administered at week 12. It can take 6 months before the full benefits of Botox on migraine are realized. Some people do very well when on Botox and CGRP monoclonal antibodies, but insurance approval for both can be difficult.

Botox is generally quite safe. Side effects are mainly injection-related (pain and swelling), and cosmetic. Some may get "devil's eyebrows" where the outer portion of the brows are elevated. The cosmetic effects can be mitigated by adjusting the injection sites and doses. There is a small risk of excessive muscle weakness causing droopy eyelids. Difficulty swallowing may occur but is rare if injected at the sites targeted in migraine treatment. It can cause flu-like symptoms that last for a few days after administration. Insurance approval may be cumbersome; a person must carry the diagnosis of chronic migraine, and most insurance companies require failing several migraine preventives first.

In patients with concomitant chronic migraine and vestibular migraine, I have observed mixed results. In some, Botox controlled their headaches really well but not vertigo, and in others, it controlled both headache and vertigo. The small number of vestibular migraine patients on Botox makes it tough to evaluate treatment responses. If a person has significant headaches and vestibular migraine, it is reasonable to use Botox.

Nerve Blocks

Nerve blocks are local injections of numbing agents (lidocaine or bupivacaine) administered along the pathway of specific nerves to numb them to relieve chronic headache. They have been shown to reduce migraine severity and frequency, and can be administered in pregnant women. The nerve blocks most likely do not help with vertigo and dizziness but can relieve headaches.

The occipital nerves are often treated with nerve blocks, but other nerves in the face and scalp (e.g., auriculotemporal, supraorbital, supratrochlear) can also be treated. They have been shown to reduce migraine severity and frequency, and can be administered in pregnant women. These injections are very safe, and only involve some local pain, and very minor bleeding in the vast majority.

The sphenopalatine ganglion (SPG) is a cluster of nerves associated with the trigeminal nerve. The SPG is located inside the nasal cavity. SPG blocks can be effective at controlling migraine and other headache disorders. The procedure involves placing a catheter into the nostrils and administering lidocaine or bupivacaine with the patient lying down with the head hanging off the edge of the bed. It is a safe procedure, and may cause some numbness of the throat, minor bleeding from the nose, lightheadedness, or a bitter taste.

Neuromodulation

Neuromodulation can be understood as the alteration of nerve activity through the targeted delivery of an electrical or magnetic stimulus. Neuromodulation is not a new concept. In ancient Rome, people with intractable headaches had a black torpedo or electric ray placed on their heads. The imperial Roman physician, Scribonius Largus, was a huge fan of this treatment. He wrote, "To immediately remove and permanently cure a headache, however long-lasting and intolerable, a live black torpedo is put on the place which is in pain, until the pain ceases and the part grows numb."

Electric rays are no longer prescribed (they could make a medical comeback like maggots and leeches...), but the concept of neuromodulation is becoming more popular. Neuromodulation provides drug-free, well-tolerated treatment options for people who cannot tolerate or prefer not to use medications.

Non-Invasive Vagus Nerve Stimulation

The vagus nerve is the longest cranial nerve, starting in the brainstem and extending throughout the body, innervating organs in the chest and abdomen. The vagus nerve controls parasympathetic nerve function, the part of the autonomic nervous system controlling processes that take place when the body is in a state of relaxation (i.e. "rest and digest" or "feed and breed"). Deep breathing, yoga, and exercise induce a state of relaxation and reduce stress by stimulating the vagus nerve. Electrical stimulation of the vagus nerve can stop seizures, improve depression, and control headaches. The vagus nerve is intimately connected with the trigeminal and vestibular nerves in the brainstem; these connections can explain how vagus nerve stimulation helps vestibular migraine.

The Gammacore device is an FDA-cleared non-invasive vagus nerve stimulation device for cluster headache and migraine. It is a rectangular device that is placed on the neck, where two electrodes make contact with the skin overlying the course of the vagus nerve. The Gammacore device delivers a 2-minute electrical stimulation of the vagus nerve; the intensity of the stimulation can be adjusted by the user and should be increased until a gentle pulling sensation of the angle of the mouth occurs. It can help with both migraine prevention and rescue. It is safe, and very well-tolerated. I published the first study showing that Gammacore treatment was effective at eliminating vertigo and headache in vestibular migraine attacks. A pilot study from Europe showed that using it regularly helped reduce PPPD. It is an exciting and potentially very useful therapy for vestibular migraine.

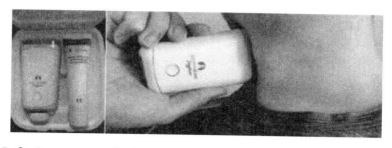

Left: Gammacore device and conducting gel in the charging case. Right: Placement on the neck, along the course of the vagus nerve.

External Trigeminal Nerve Stimulation

The Cefaly device is an FDA-cleared external trigeminal nerve stimulating device for migraine headache treatment. It is a triangular device that attaches to an electrode pad that is placed on the forehead between the brows, about 1-2 inches above the bridge of the nose. The device stimulates the ophthalmic branch of the trigeminal nerve, which in turn induces electrical changes in regions of the brain responsible for migraine and vestibular migraine.

The Cefaly Dual has two settings: *acute* and *prevent*. The acute setting lasts for one hour, and is used for migraine rescue. The prevent setting lasts for 20 minutes, and is usually used once a day. The main side effect is forehead and scalp tingling. Personally, I find it weird but not too uncomfortable. However, it can be intolerable for those with sensitive scalps. The device has a preset stimulation protocol that starts at the lowest intensity and gradually rises to the maximum intensity at about 14 minutes; at any time, if you find the sensations too unpleasant, you can hit a button that stops the intensity from rising further.

I published the first study that showed that the Cefaly device helps relieve vertigo and headache in vestibular migraine. For vestibular migraine, I recommend using the *prevent* setting twice a day, once in the morning and once in the evening. Use the *acute* setting when you have a vestibular migraine attack. I have also found that the Cefaly device reduces dizziness provoked by visual stimuli, making it a useful therapy for people with vestibular migraine, and PPPD. Use the *prevent* setting twice a day, and before entering environments that make you dizzy. As of October 13, 2020, a prescription is not needed to purchase the Cefaly device. You can order it directly from the manufacturer's website.

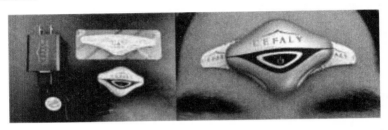

Left: the Cefaly device, electrode pad, and charging cable.
Right: placement of the electrode and the Cefaly device.

Other neuromodulation therapies

Relivion MG is a device that delivers stimulation to both the trigeminal and occipital nerves. It is FDA-cleared for migraine headache rescue, but unfortunately, at the time of this writing, is not widely available for prescription, as the manufacturer is only working with a small number of physicians. Based on my experience with the Cefaly Dual, it is likely that Relivion could work for vestibular migraine as well. It also seems somewhat more difficult to use as the sponges have to be wet and fit snugly on the front and back of the head.

Nerivio is a device that delivers electrical stimulation to the upper arm for migraine headache rescue. The armband is controlled by an app on the patient's phone. It uses a mechanism called conditioned pain modulation, where the brain's perception of pain is altered by a stimulus from a different part of the body. Theoretically, the device delivers an uncomfortable stimulation to the arm which stops the migraine attack, by distracting and refocusing the brain's attention on the new source of discomfort. One patient informed me that Nerivio relieved both her headache and vertigo during vestibular migraine attacks. I do not have much experience with the device in other patients, at this time.

Transcranial magnetic stimulation is a technique of stimulating specific brain regions using an external magnetic coil. It is usually used for depression, but has shown some benefit in migraine. Repetitive transcranial magnetic stimulation (rTMS) treatments are administered by licensed practitioners at their clinic locations, unlike the Gammacore and Cefaly devices.

Single-pulse transcranial magnetic stimulation (sTMS) can also help with migraine; a portable device (called sTMS mini) manufactured by eNeura was FDA-cleared for acute and preventive treatment of migraine. However, it was very expensive and not covered by insurance. As such, I have not had experience with this device in vestibular migraine. The manufacturer filed for bankruptcy in late 2020 and was taken over by a different company. The new device is called SAVI Dual, and although cheaper, remains costly with limited insurance coverage at the time of this writing.

Transcranial direct current stimulation utilizes very low currents delivered to specific brain locations depending on the goals of treatment. It can be effective in migraine, and has been shown to help with tinnitus, anxiety, and cognitive impairment. Its use remains experimental at this time, and not easily accessible. There are some homemade devices sold online but these may not stimulate the correct brain regions, and are ineffective at best, or unsafe, at worst. It should be delivered by a practitioner who is familiar with the treatment, and who has the proper equipment that can accurately stimulate the targeted brain locations.

Both transcranial magnetic and direct current stimulation should be avoided in people with epilepsy due to the possible risk of triggering seizures.

Chapter 16: Rescue Treatments

That no one dies of migraine seems, to someone deep into an attack,
an ambiguous blessing.
Joan Didion

A vestibular migraine attack is a fire that starts small and grows. The more attacks occur, the higher the risk of chronic migraine and constant dizziness; if the brain does not have enough time to recover between vestibular migraine attacks, the less likely a person is to return to a normal baseline and hence, suffer from more dizziness which then lowers the threshold for even more vestibular migraine attacks.

If many fires are sparked without being properly extinguished, the castle continues to smolder, increasing the risk for even more fires. Rescue treatments are the fire crews that extinguish these attacks to prevent the vicious feed-forward cycle of more frequent vestibular migraine attacks.

Remember that rescue treatments should be taken as early as possible when the fire is small. Once the fire turns into an inferno, rescue treatments are ineffective. In migraine headache, the point of no return is when central sensitization occurs. Central sensitization is the hyperexcitable state of pain where literally everything hurts (even lightly touching the scalp), a phenomenon called allodynia. At this point, it is extremely difficult to break the migraine attack. Learn how to recognize when your migraine attack is starting, and use your rescue treatment as soon as it begins. Nip it in the bud!

How to Use Your Rescue Treatment(s)

There are three broad strategies used to select rescue treatments:

The *escalation across attacks approach* is the most conservative. First, use a safer and/or cheaper medication. If that fails, when you have another attack, use the next medication which may be either more expensive or cause more side effects. For example, if ibuprofen is ineffective, take rizatriptan for the next attack, and if that does not work, take ubrogepant for the subsequent attack. This approach is slow and a person can continue to suffer vestibular migraine attacks while searching for the right rescue therapy.

The *stratified approach* allows a person to choose which medication to use based on the severity of the attack. For instance, for mild attacks, use acetaminophen or timolol eye drops. For moderate ones, an oral triptan may suffice. For severe attacks, intranasal sumatriptan, diazepam, and/or a promethazine suppository may be employed. This is a useful approach if a person can quickly discern the nature of the attack. For instance, I know when a migraine headache is starting (compared to a minor tension-type headache) because my mouth gets dry. It is not helpful if attacks start at a low level and progress because a person cannot quickly predict how severe the attack will be.

The most effective approach is called *escalation within attacks*. Start with the medication with the least side effects and/or lowest cost. If that works, great. If not, use a medication that may cause more side effects (or is more costly), but is more effective, and so on. For example, start off with rizatriptan (a generic and very well-tolerated rescue medication). If rizatriptan does not work within two hours, rimegepant (a newer medication that costs more but is very well-tolerated) can be employed. Alternatively, clonazepam (older, effective, and cheaper but tends to be sedating) may be administered. Two hours later, if rimegepant does not help, inject subcutaneous sumatriptan (highly effective but costly with more side effects). Over time, you will learn which medication works best, and can simplify the steps in this approach.

Regardless of which approach you find works best, the most fundamental rescue treatment principle is: *hit hard and early*. That's right. Don't dawdle. A big mistake many make is hesitating and second-guessing themselves. Learn how to identify what symptoms precede a migraine attack. As soon as you recognize the signs, hit your rescue treatments. With the triptans, we have known that by the time central sensitization occurs, rescue treatments are much less effective. The ubrogepant pre-headache study showed that using it in the prodrome phase was 2.1 times more likely to stop a migraine attack in its tracks [Dodick, 2023]. Over time, you will learn what treatments are the most effective. Once you know what works best, use them as early as possible.

How to Choose Your Rescue Treatment(s)

Do you have a headache with vertigo?

If a headache is a significant component of your vestibular migraine attack, consider using an analgesic rescue treatment. If you don't have headaches with vertigo, analgesics may not be helpful.

How bad is nausea?

If you have severe nausea or vomiting, tablets may not be of much use. It would be better to use orally-disintegrating tablets, subcutaneous injections, nasal sprays or rectal suppositories to deliver the rescue medication.

How long does a typical attack last?

While the duration of the attacks varies, use the typical duration of your attacks as a guide. For attacks that last less than a day, shorter-acting agents (e.g., rizatriptan, ibuprofen, ubrogepant, diazepam) can be used. For attacks that last more than 24 hours, longer-acting medications (e.g., rimegepant, clonazepam, naproxen) should be used.

Try two-in-one treatments

Some treatments can be used as both preventive and rescue. For example, Gammacore, Cefaly work as both migraine preventive and rescue agents. Supplements like ginger and magnesium can also be used in both capacities.

How do you measure success?

There are several ways to measure if a rescue agent works well. A migraine rescue treatment can be considered successful if:

• it decreases the duration of the attack significantly (for example, if it cuts your attack from two days to half a day), or;

• if it reduces the severity of the attack (e.g., from 10/10 to 5/10), or;

• if it can help you get back to your life as soon as possible, AND;

• causes minimal side effects.

For example, an effective rescue treatment diminishes the severity and duration of a migraine attack and allows you to return to your usual activities within 1-2 hours (compared to suffering for half a day if you did not use it). It is also important that the rescue treatment causes minimal side effects; for example, a rescue agent that gets rid of your headache but makes you incredibly drowsy for an entire day isn't very helpful.

Ease of use

A rescue medication should be easily accessible and administered. Ideally, it should be something that you can have with you at all times and easily use when a migraine attack occurs. For example, a tablet that dissolves under the tongue, or nasal spray is ideal. Intravenous medications (e.g., DHE) are very effective but have to be administered under the supervision of healthcare professionals and as such, are not easily accessible.

Find the best combo

Sometimes a single medication works beautifully, but at times you may need to combine two or even three medications from different classes for best results. For example, a person may find that diazepam and sumatriptan together work well, but another prefers ketorolac, rimegepant, and promethazine.

Beware of medication overuse headache (MOH)

Also called rebound headache, MOH is a condition caused by excessive use of analgesic medications. In this condition, drugs that are supposed to relieve headaches paradoxically cause and aggravate the headache. This is a state where the brain becomes "addicted" to these analgesics and needs higher and more frequent doses just to feel no pain. Opioids, caffeine (e.g., Excedrin) and barbiturates (e.g., Fioricet and Fiorinal) carry the greatest risk of MOH. It can also occur with acetaminophen, NSAIDs (except naproxen), triptans, and dihydroergotamine. If you use acetaminophen, NSAIDs, or triptans more than three days a week for more than three months, you are at high risk for developing MOH.

The only treatment for this condition is to stop all analgesic medications cold turkey. The headache will be severe for two to ten days, while your brain detoxifies and withdraws from the analgesics. Starting a preventive medication during the detoxification period can help speed up recovery. Oddly enough, MOH only occurs when a person frequently takes analgesics for a headache. It does not occur if a person takes analgesics for a different condition (e.g., arthritis, back pain). Preventing MOH is far better than curing this miserable condition.

Triptans

Triptans relieve migraine (a state of serotonin deficiency) by activating serotonin receptors, specifically 5-HT1B (which constricts dilated blood vessels) and 5-HT1D (which stops CGRP release from pain-sensitive nerves).

Triptans relieve headaches within two hours in half to three-quarters of patients. However, about a quarter of migraine patients do not respond to triptans, and only about one-third are completely free of a headache at 2 hours.

Triptans are most effective when used early in a migraine attack (i.e., within two hours). I always advise my patients to administer a triptan within an hour of a migraine attack for best results. You can usually repeat a dose two hours later if you still have migraine attack symptoms. Triptans should not be used more than twice in 24 hours. I also advise against using triptans for more than two days (i.e., a total of 4 doses) in a week, due to the risk of MOH.

"Triptan sensations" describe a rare but well-recognized constellation of side effects, including flushing, chest pressure, neck tightness, tingling in the limbs, a feeling of heaviness, and jaw tightness. Some describe drowsiness or feeling hung over after using triptans, although this may actually be a postdrome migraine symptom. Caution is advised in people with vascular disease (e.g., coronary artery disease, peripheral artery disease, stroke, ischemic bowel disease) and uncontrolled hypertension.

There are seven triptans. They can be divided into two groups based on the onset of action – fast-acting (within an hour) and slow-acting (between 1-2 hours). Five (sumatriptan, rizatriptan, eletriptan, almotriptan, zolmitriptan) are fast-acting, while two (naratriptan and frovatriptan) are slow-acting.

Sumatriptan (Imitrex) was the first triptan developed. It can be administered as an oral tablet, subcutaneous injection, or intranasal spray. Sumatriptan suppositories are available in the EU but not in the US. A battery-powered transdermal patch sumatriptan preparation (Zecuity) was approved in 2013 but withdrawn from the market due to skin irritation and burns. Sumatriptan is effective but may cause more side effects compared to the other triptans. The most effective triptan therapy is subcutaneous sumatriptan injections but it also causes the most side effects. The injection is available as an auto-injector, or as a vial that you will draw up in a syringe to inject.

Among the oral triptans, *rizatriptan* (Maxalt) and *eletriptan* (Relpax) have the highest rate of two-hour pain freedom. Rizatriptan is the most well-tolerated triptan, with good efficacy and time of onset. *Zolmitriptan* (Zomig) is also effective for rescue. Eletriptan and rizatriptan have the best rate of 24-hour headache freedom. Zolmitriptan has both oral and nasal spray preparations. *Frovatriptan* (Frova) is a slow- but long-acting tripta, with a half-life of 24-30 hours. Frovatriptan is useful for people who have longer migraine attacks (although the slower onset of action may require concomitant use of an NSAID), and can also be used for the prevention of menstrual migraines. *Naratriptan* (Amerge) has a longer half-life compared to other triptans (6 hours), and also can be used for the prevention of menstrual migraine. *Almotriptan* (Axert) does not particularly stand out compared to the other triptans but can be tried if a person fails the other triptans.

Oral triptans usually take between 30-60 minutes to start working and are therefore, not very helpful for migraine attacks that last less than 30 minutes. Nasal spray triptans (sumatriptan and zolmitriptan) have a rapid onset of action (about 15 minutes), and excellent efficacy. Which triptan to choose? For oral tablets, I typically start with rizatriptan or sumatriptan. For those who need a rapidly-acting rescue, I use either intranasal or subcutaneous sumatriptan, or intranasal zolmitriptan. For people who have vestibular migraine attacks lasting days, and for the prevention of menstrual migraine, I prefer to use naratriptan or frovatriptan.

It is important to note that failure to respond to one triptan does not predict failure to all triptans; switching to a different triptan may help identify one that works. Combining a triptan with an analgesic (either acetaminophen or NSAID) increases the efficacy. You can take separate medications together, or take combination drugs. For example, Treximet is a combination of sumatriptan 85 mg and naproxen 500 mg which is more effective than taking sumatriptan alone. A meloxicam-rizatriptan combination has shown efficacy in Phase 3 clinical trials and may be available for prescription soon.

Ditans

The ditans are a new class of migraine rescue treatments that only block 5-HT1F serotonin receptors, which gives them the migraine rescue benefits of the triptans without the vascular risks since 5-HT1B receptors are found on blood vessels. This class of rescue medication can be safely used in people with coronary artery disease, peripheral vascular disease, or ischemic stroke risks.

Lasmiditan (Reyvow) is the first of this class. It is taken at migraine onset; only one dose daily is needed. Lasmiditan can be used in people with vascular diseases that prevent triptan use, or those who experience intolerable side effects with triptans. Treatment failure with triptans does not predict response to lasmiditan.

Almost 20% of those who take lasmiditan experience dizziness. It can affect driving ability; the effect peaks at 90 minutes, but you should not drive or operate machinery for 8 hours after taking it. Drowsiness may occur in some people. Because a small number of study subjects "liked" how lasmiditan made them feel, the Drug Enforcement Agency classifies lasmiditan as a Schedule V drug. While no human pregnancy data is available, it can harm animal fetuses, and as such should be avoided during pregnancy. There is a potential for MOH and lasmiditan should be used no more than two days per week.

Dihydroergotamine (DHE)

If the ditans are cruise missiles that target only a specific receptor in the brain, DHE is a conventional bomb that hits multiple receptors. DHE is an ergot extract that activates 5-HT1B and 5-HT1D receptors, like triptans, but DHE also activates other serotonin receptors, and dopamine receptors, as well as blocks the release of prostaglandins.

DHE can be used for refractory migraine with very good results. It is typically administered as an intravenous, subcutaneous, or intramuscular injection. Intravenous DHE has to be administered in a hospital or infusion center. Subcutaneous and intramuscular DHE can be injected in a clinic, or at home. DHE can also be given as an intranasal spray (Migranal or Trudhesa).

DHE is highly effective but often causes nausea and vomiting. Pre-treatment with anti-nausea medications is needed before injecting DHE. Some people experience diarrhea, abdominal cramps, leg cramps, and a transient worsening of the headache. It does not cause sedation, and can be mixed with lidocaine to minimize injection site burning. Intranasal DHE sprays can cause nasal congestion; using a decongestant spray (e.g., oxymetazoline) afterward may help. DHE should be avoided in pregnancy, vascular disease, and uncontrolled hypertension. DHE cannot be used within 24 hours of using a triptan.

Analgesics

Acetaminophen

Acetaminophen (Tylenol) or paracetamol (Panadol) is a common analgesic and antipyretic (fever-reducing) medication. The precise mechanism by which acetaminophen helps migraine is unknown. It is typically useful for mild to moderate migraine headaches. A typical dose is 1000 mg taken at the onset of migraine; it can be repeated 2 hours later if needed.

Unlike NSAIDs, acetaminophen does not cause gastric ulcers or bleeding or affect the blood's ability to clot. It is safe to use pre- and post-operatively for pain control. While acetaminophen is safe and well-tolerated, do not exceed 4000 mg in 24 hours. Dosages higher than this can cause liver damage. Since many over-the-counter products also contain acetaminophen, it is important to monitor your total intake to ensure you do not exceed this daily limit. It is safe to use in pregnancy. Expired acetaminophen breaks down into compounds that are toxic to the liver. People with liver disease or liver transplants should consult their specialists before using it.

Acetaminophen can cause MOH, and should not be used more than three days in any given week. Preparations that contain caffeine (e.g., Excedrin), opioids (e.g., Lortab, Tylenol #3), and butalbital (e.g., Fioricet) have a much higher risk of MOH.

Non-Steroidal Anti-Inflammatory Drugs (NSAIDs)

NSAIDs are effective for acute migraine treatment. They inhibit the synthesis of prostaglandins from arachidonic acid, resulting in anti-inflammatory, analgesic, and antipyretic effects. The anti-inflammatory effects combat the neurogenic inflammatory processes that drive migraines.

Ibuprofen is quick-acting (within 1 hour), with a short half-life of 2 hours. Liquid capsules are faster absorbed than oral tablets. A typical dose is 400- 600 mg taken at the onset of a migraine attack. Due to the short half-life, the dose may need to be repeated.

Diclofenac has a very fast onset of action, and a short half-life (less than two hours). The tablet formulations reach maximum plasma concentrations in under an hour. The powdered formulation for oral solution (Cambia) reaches peak plasma levels in under 15 minutes. The typical dose is 50 mg at the onset of migraine. Due to the short half-life, a repeat dose is sometimes needed. Cambia is very expensive compared to generic tablets; it is reasonable to try the tablets before using Cambia.

Aspirin has a longer half-life (6 hours) compared to ibuprofen and diclofenac; the effervescent formulation is faster acting than regular tablets, with similar efficacy to sumatriptan. Aspirin may cause or aggravate tinnitus.

Naproxen (Aleve) is a slower- but longer-acting NSAID with a half-life of 14 hours. As such, the need to repeat a dose is lower and the risk of MOH is almost nil. It is useful for migraine attacks that last more than half a day. In addition, the cardiovascular risk profile of naproxen is the lowest compared to other NSAIDs.

Meloxicam (Mobic) is a long-acting NSAID that is typically taken once a day for conditions like arthritis. Taking it with foods that contain fat (e.g., peanut butter) improves its bioavailability. Because it is longer-acting, it can be used if migraine attacks last more than half a day.

Celecoxib (Celebrex) was intended to cause fewer gastrointestinal side effects. Unfortunately, it has been linked to an increased risk of cardiovascular events and stroke. It has a half-life of about 8-12 hours, and may need to be taken twice a day. An oral solution of celecoxib (Elyxyb) is available for migraine rescue.

Ketorolac (Toradol) is rapidly absorbed and has a half-life of about 5 hours. It can be given in tablet, injection, or rectal suppository form; the latter two are advantageous for people who have significant nausea and vomiting during a migraine attack. Ketorolac must not be used for more than 5 consecutive days due to potential kidney toxicity.

Excedrin is a brand name for a combination of acetaminophen, aspirin and caffeine. There are similar generics. The presence of caffeine in Excedrin and similar products increases the risk of MOH significantly. Such products should be used very judiciously.

NSAIDs can reduce the blood's ability to clot and should not be taken concurrently with blood thinners (e.g., warfarin) and anti-platelet agents (e.g., clopidogrel). Due to the risk of bleeding, NSAIDs should be avoided for at least one week before any planned surgical procedure. These drugs should be avoided in people with gastric bypass surgery, kidney disease, peptic ulcer, gastroesophageal reflux disease, and inflammatory bowel disease. NSAIDs (particularly meloxicam and celecoxib) may increase the risk of cardiovascular events (like heart attacks) and strokes if used regularly.

All NSAIDs, except naproxen and meloxicam, can cause MOH, and should not be used more than three days in any given week. NSAIDs should be avoided in women who are pregnant. In early pregnancy, NSAIDs may increase the risk of miscarriage and fetal malformations. After 30 weeks of gestation, NSAIDs may decrease amniotic fluid production and can cause premature closure of the fetal ductus arteriosus (an important blood vessel connecting the pulmonary artery to the aorta allowing blood to bypass a fetus' lungs).

Opioids & Butalbital

Opioids are substances derived from or chemically similar to opium. These include morphine, hydrocodone, oxycodone, hydromorphone (Dilaudid), fentanyl, meperidine (Demerol), tramadol, butorphanol (Stadol), and codeine.

Opioids are detrimental for people with migraine. They reduce the efficacy of other medications and dramatically increase the risk of chronic migraine and MOH. Long term use causes opioid-induced hyperalgesia, a condition not dissimilar to MOH, where opioids induce and increase pain sensitivity. Furthermore, opioids can even trigger migraine attacks. Unfortunately, many emergency departments use opioids for migraine as a quick pain fix. Aside from the negative impact of opioids on migraine, opioids can cause seizures, nausea, vomiting, and addiction. The terrible burden of opioid addiction on our society is well-recognized.

Butalbital is a barbiturate that is often combined with other medications like acetaminophen, caffeine, aspirin, and even opioids like codeine. These combinations are sold under several brand names, including Esgic, Axocet, Butapap, Fioricet, and Fiorinal. Butalbital-containing medications carry a very high risk of MOH. Butalbital can cause intoxication and drowsiness similar to that produced by alcohol; respiratory depression and death occur at toxic levels. Furthermore, butalbital can cause addiction and dependence. People who have taken butalbital-containing medications regularly at high doses can suffer severe withdrawal when it is stopped and often have to be admitted to psychiatric facilities for detoxification. It is still available in the US but is banned in the EU.

Opioids and butalbital-containing medications are sometimes used in pregnant women since many of the other medications are less safe. This does not mean that they are very safe; they just carry fewer possible risks to the fetus. It is important to be very judicious when using these medications during pregnancy, since they can enter the fetal circulation. In non-pregnant women, the use of opioids and butalbital carries too many risks and dangers. I only prescribe butalbital in exceptional circumstances and never prescribe opioids in vestibular migraine.

Gepants

The gepants are small-molecule medications that block CGRP. The first generation gepant (telcagepant) was discontinued during development due to liver toxicity. However, over time, the chemical structures have been modified and current gepants are very safe. Due to the important role of CGRP in new blood vessel formation, they should be avoided in pregnancy or if pregnancy is planned, and within 6 months of a myocardial infarction or stroke. Caution is advised in people with Raynaud's phenomenon and intracranial aneurysms. The gepants do not carry any risk of MOH. Unlike triptans, they can be taken at any time during a migraine attack. However, they are more effective when taken early in the course of a migraine attack.

Ubrogepant (Ubrelvy) was the first gepant approved for migraine rescue. It can be taken at migraine onset, and repeated two hours later if needed. The maximum daily dose is 200 mg. Ubrogepant should be avoided if a person is taking certain anti-fungal medications (ketoconazole, itraconazole) and clarithromycin (an antibiotic) which block a liver enzyme called CYP3A4. Concurrent use can lead to very high ubrogepant levels. If you have to take a course of anti-fungal drugs or clarithromycin, complete that treatment and wait 48 hours before taking ubrogepant. Since CBD oil, phenytoin, rifampin, barbiturates, and verapamil lower ubrogepant levels, you may need a higher dose (100 mg) if you are on these medications.

Rimegepant (Nurtec ODT) was the second gepant approved for migraine rescue, and is an orally dissolving tablet. It is a particularly exciting treatment due to its rapid onset (within 15 minutes) and long half-life. Rimegepant can provide migraine relief for up to 48 hours, and is therefore, a useful medication to use for patients with long or frequent migraine attacks. It is available only as a 75 mg dose to be taken once a day. Rimegepant is also metabolized by the CYP3A4 liver enzyme. Like ubrogepant, it should not be taken with the antifungals and antibiotics listed above. Medications that lower ubrogepant levels may also lower rimegepant levels; however, unlike ubrogepant which has 50 mg and 100 mg dosing options, rimegepant is only available as a 75 mg tablet.

Zavegepant (Zavzpret) is a nasal spray gepant that is administered once at the onset of a migraine attack. The benefits may be seen as early as 15 minutes. The main side effect is an unpleasant aftertaste that can last for up to 30 minutes after administration. Some people experienced nausea or nasal passage discomfort afterward.

An interesting study found that two people who were on CGRP monoclonal antibodies obtained even better migraine control when they used rimegepant. This suggests that using gepants and CGRP monoclonal antibodies together may provide more benefit than using each separately.

Benzodiazepines

Benzodiazepines are effective treatments for vertigo, dizziness, anxiety, insomnia, and muscle spasms. However, sedation and the risk of dependence limit their use. There are several options for vestibular migraine, and the choice of treatment generally depends on the duration of the attacks.

Benzodiazepines cause drowsiness and should of course, not be taken with alcohol, or opioids. They can cause cognitive impairment in elderly patients. In very rare cases, a paradoxical response occurs; instead of sedation, a person becomes anxious, agitated, and irritable. Benzodiazepines should be avoided in people with a history of alcohol abuse. Those with liver disease must use lower doses. Benzodiazepines should be avoided during pregnancy.

Diazepam (Valium) reaches peak plasma concentration 30-90 minutes after oral administration and has a half-life of 30-56 hours. However, the peak effects of diazepam last for about 3-4 hours because diazepam is widely distributed throughout the body. The metabolites are active and can remain in the system for

2-7 days. In other words, even though diazepam's effects usually should last for 3-4 hours, the drug and its active metabolites can remain in your system for a much longer period. Those who are more sensitive to diazepam and its metabolites may experience drowsiness for a longer period than expected.

Lorazepam (Ativan) reaches peak plasma levels about two hours after oral administration and has a half-life of about 10-20 hours. Its duration of action lasts between 8 to 12 hours. Compared to diazepam, lorazepam has a shorter half-life, but a longer duration of action. Lorazepam generally has a more predictable action (compared to diazepam), because it does not distribute widely in the body, and its metabolites are inactive.

Clonazepam (Klonopin) has a half-life of about 18-60 hours, reaches peak plasma concentration 1-2 hours after oral administration, and a duration of action of 6-12 hours.

Alprazolam (Xanax) is of little use in vestibular migraine due to the very short duration of action (about 30 minutes), and the high risk of addiction.

For vestibular migraine attacks that last about a few hours to half a day, I generally prefer to use diazepam. For longer attacks, lorazepam or clonazepam can be used. Due to the longer half-life of clonazepam, it can be used for people who have longer vestibular migraine attacks or for those suffering from a cluster of vestibular migraine attacks. Lorazepam's shorter half-life makes it more useful for those with attacks that last between half to a day, or for those who want to avoid feeling drowsy the next day.

Anti-Nausea Medications

Anti-nausea medications are useful for vestibular migraine and migraine attacks since nausea is such a common accompanying symptom. They are seldom used in isolation but are often combined with other migraine rescue medications. They also can be used in people suffering from persistent nausea.

Anti-Dopamine Medications

Anti-nausea medications that also block dopamine action provide additional benefits for migraine rescue. However, an unwanted and serious side effect of anti-dopaminergic medications is movement disorders. The risk is highest with metoclopramide and prochlorperazine.

Acute use (for migraine rescue) can cause dystonia (painful muscle contractions), and akathisia (an unbearable sensation of inner restlessness and uneasiness often described as "crawling out of one's skin"). Administering diphenhydramine (Benadryl) with these medications often prevents these acute movement disorders but it causes drowsiness.

Chronic, regular use of anti-dopaminergic medications (for persistent nausea) can lead to irreversible movement disorders like Parkinsonism and tardive dyskinesia (a disorder characterized by persistent involuntary movements of the body or face, resembling a rabbit chewing). It is important not to use these medications for more than 5 consecutive days to avoid these long-term adverse effects.

Prochlorperazine (Compazine) can be administered as an oral tablet, rectal suppository, or injected intravenously or intramuscularly. Of all the anti-nausea medications, it has the best migraine rescue effects.

Metoclopramide (Reglan) can also be administered as an oral tablet, or injected intravenously or intramuscularly. It is slightly less effective than prochlorperazine.

Promethazine (Phenergan) is available by mouth (tablet or syrup), rectal suppository, topical gel, or intramuscular injection. Intravenous use is generally avoided. Promethazine has the lowest risk of movement disorders compared to prochlorperazine and metoclopramide but is sedating.

Trimethobenzamide (Tigan) carries a lower risk of Parkinsonism but may cause acute movement disorders like dystonia.

Domperidone (Motilium) is not available for prescription in the US. It can be used for acute migraine rescue and nausea, and in fact, is recommended by the Canadian Headache Society. There is a small risk of fatal cardiac arrhythmia, especially at higher doses but is otherwise quite safe.

Anti-Histaminergic Medications

Antihistaminergic drugs are used for motion sickness and nausea, and are believed to target the histamine receptors in the brainstem. These medications are rarely used in isolation for migraine rescue; they are usually combined with other medications.

The main side effect is drowsiness. Other side effects include dry mouth, constipation, urinary difficulty, and visual blurriness. They can also worsen cognitive function, particularly in the elderly, and should be used judiciously in this population.

Diphenhydramine (Benadryl) is an antihistamine that can be used during migraine attacks. It can also be administered with anti-dopaminergic medications to mitigate the risk of movement disorders.

Doxylamine is an antihistamine that has been sold as a sleep aid (Unisom). It is combined with vitamin B6 as an extended-release tablet (Diclegis, Diclectin, or Bonjesta) for nausea and vomiting in pregnant women.

Dimenhydrinate (Dramamine) is an over-the-counter antihistamine for nausea and motion sickness. It is basically weak diphenhydramine. In my experience, it is not very useful in migraine rescue.

Meclizine (Bonine/Antivert) is an over-the-counter medication often used for the treatment of vertigo, dizziness, nausea, and motion sickness. While it can help motion sickness, it is not very effective for vertigo, dizziness, and nausea; very few of my patients actually derive benefit from meclizine.

Other Anti-Nausea Medications

Ondansetron (Zofran) can be a helpful anti-nausea agent that does not cause drowsiness, or movement disorders. It can be given by mouth (regular tablet, orally dissolving tablet, thin film), rectal suppository, or injected intravenously or intramuscularly. It is well-tolerated. There is a possibility of ondansetron causing headaches or constipation. The FDA has warned about ondansetron causing a rare but potentially fatal arrhythmia; make sure your cardiologist is aware that you are taking ondansetron if you have any underlying heart problems.

Scopolamine or Hyoscine is an anticholinergic medication that is often used for motion sickness and nausea (especially postoperative nausea and vomiting). It can be given orally or as a transdermal patch. One patch is designed to release scopolamine over 3 days. Wash your hands thoroughly after touching the patch; if you don't, and inadvertently touch your eye, your pupil will dilate and remain dilated for hours. Side effects include confusion, memory problems, dry mouth, dry eyes, and blurry vision. It should be avoided in those with prostate enlargement and glaucoma. As tempting as it is to replace a patch every 3 days, do NOT do so. Never use transdermal scopolamine for more than 72 hours!

Aprepitant (Emend) is a new anti-nausea medication. It has been used to control DHE-associated nausea and vomiting. It costs a lot and does not seem to have any additional benefit compared to other drugs.

Corticosteroids

Corticosteroids may help as a migraine rescue treatment by stopping neurogenic inflammation. In previous chapters, we discussed how the chronically stressed body is less able to produce a spike of cortisol in response to acute stress. Prescribing a short course of corticosteroids may help the body deal with such stress, and break a prolonged migraine attack.

The use of corticosteroids for migraine rescue is controversial and inconclusive. Some practitioners believe in it, while others don't. I find they can be useful in people who are experiencing a cluster of vestibular migraine attacks and reduce the usage of rescue medications (thus preventing MOH and reducing costs). Corticosteroids are not without side effects and can often cause gastrointestinal upset, increased appetite, insomnia, tremulousness, irritability, and heartburn. Typically, short-term corticosteroid treatments are safe. Problems arise when they are used for more than two weeks. Caution should be exercised in diabetics because corticosteroids can increase blood sugar levels. One very rare side effect of corticosteroid use is avascular necrosis (bone death due to loss of blood supply).

I usually prescribe a steroid taper, where a person starts at a higher dose, and decreases it over a few days. This is similar to the Medrol Dosepak often prescribed for allergies.

Timolol Eye Drops

Timolol eye drops can be used for migraine prevention and rescue. The rapid absorption of timolol through the blood vessels in the eye makes timolol eye drops a quick-acting rescue agent. Instill one drop in each eye at the onset of a vestibular migraine attack. If you do not experience sufficient relief 30 minutes later, use a different rescue medication.

Non-Pharmacologic Migraine Rescue

Drug-free measures can certainly help during a migraine attack, and can be used in conjunction with rescue medications.

Reduce stimulation. Find a dark quiet room and turn off your phone. Too much light and noise aggravate the migraine.

Use cold. Apply ice-cold compresses to the head and back of the neck. Cooling towels are very affordable and create a cooling effect by evaporating water. The Headache Hat is a large wrap containing ice packs that can be wrapped around the head and neck. The Cryo Helmet is a helmet-like device that can be filled with ice packs and worn on the head.

Drink fluids. Dehydration often triggers a migraine attack, and adequate hydration can help mitigate the attack. Furthermore, if you are vomiting, you need to replenish the lost fluid.

Sleep it off. As discussed before, sleep can help terminate an attack. One of the rescue therapies is to take your migraine rescue treatment(s) and melatonin, get your bedroom as dark and cool as possible and sleep.

Menthol-containing topicals. Typical locations include the back of the neck at the base of the skull and temples. Peppermint oil is a natural source of menthol. Other menthol-containing topical applications include Mentholatum, Vicks, and Icy Hot. A couple of my patients dab Bengay on their foreheads during a migraine attack; however, this may burn too much for most people.

Supplements. Try magnesium and ginger root. Try smelling essential oils (specifically rose or lavender). However, if you have sensitivity to smells, these oils may aggravate your symptoms.

Neuromodulation. Non-invasive vagus nerve and external trigeminal nerve stimulation can be used. From my research, both are effective for vestibular migraine attacks. Nerivio Migra utilizes a smartphone-controlled stimulator worn on the upper arm; it delivers electrical pulses generating a conditional pain modulation that inhibits a migraine headache. There is no data about its use in vestibular migraine yet.

True love has a habit of coming back...
and so do migraines.

Shiva Tomar

I

Interictal Symptoms & Co-Morbid Disorders Treatment

Chapter 17: Symptomatic Management

It cannot be done all at once. To overpower vertigo – the keeper of the abyss – one must tame it, cautiously.
Phillipe Petit

The military strategy of divide and conquer can also help you conquer the multitude of symptoms that arise from migraine and vestibular migraine. Together, all these symptoms form a seemingly invincible and terrifying army. However, by breaking these problems down into individual components and attacking each one separately, you will find that you can manage vestibular migraine much more successfully.

This chapter will detail strategies and options for treating disorders and symptoms that often coexist with vestibular migraine and migraine. These are separated into specific problems, with recommendations on how to deal with them. The recommendations here are up to date at the time of writing, but because medical science advances at a breathtaking pace, more treatments or strategies may become available by the time you read this.

Brain Fog & Fatigue

There is considerable overlap between brain fog and fatigue in migraine, and I suspect they share many pathophysiologic similarities. The first step in dealing with these symptoms is to look for other disorders that may also cause these symptoms. Physical deconditioning is a very common cause of fatigue, which is why exercise is so important in MDDS. Sleep disorders, particularly those that rob a person of restful sleep, can cause fatigue and brain fog. A variety of other medical problems may cause fatigue and brain fog including hypothyroidism, vitamin D deficiency, vitamin B12 deficiency, low testosterone levels, anemia, and postural orthostatic tachycardia syndrome (POTS). Long COVID) is emerging as a major cause of fatigue and brain fog.

There are no specific treatments for migraine-related brain fog or fatigue, unfortunately. The good news is that controlling migraine with the appropriate preventive therapy often leads to improvement in these symptoms. Fatigue and brain fog are most likely due to bioenergetic dysfunction and neurogenic inflammation.

Vitamin B2, CoQ10, and magnesium can help improve the brain's energy metabolism. Some of my patients find that magnesium L-threonate seems to help brain fog better than other magnesium preparations. Anti-inflammatory supplements like turmeric, Ginkgo, Pycnogenol, and omega 3-fatty acids may also be useful.

Getting proper sleep is essential. Poor sleep quality causes fatigue, and excessive daytime sleepiness that worsens brain fog. This is usually my first target for brain fog – if you are not sleeping well, you will not be thinking well. On the other hand, exercise improves brain functions, reduces inflammation, promotes better sleep, and stimulates the release of neurochemicals that enhance cognitive function. The importance of regular exercise cannot be emphasized enough.

Often missed, many medications may cause drowsiness, and cognitive impairment. Meclizine, dimenhydrinate, promethazine, benzodiazepines, topiramate, opioids, gabapentin, blood pressure-lowering medications, and amitriptyline can cause fatigue and brain fog. It sometimes can be tough – a medication may control your migraine well but cause brain fog and fatigue. If this is the case, work closely with your neurologist to switch to a different medication.

Transdermal scopolamine deserves special mention because some physicians prescribe it for nausea, vertigo and dizziness. Scopolamine may cause significant cognitive problems and its use should be limited to post-operative nausea and motion sickness control. One patch is designed to last for 3 days. As tempting as it is to replace a patch every 3 days, do NOT do so. I saw a patient who had such horrible cognitive complaints her family thought she was developing dementia; after stopping transdermal scopolamine (which she had been using continuously for 5 months!), her cognition returned to normal.

While waiting for the fog to lift, there are some strategies that you can use to help cope. Routine is important, and can help eliminate the need to expend precious mental energy on decisions. If you can automate certain decisions, do so. Consider a capsule wardrobe; wear the same set of clothes during the week. You can also consider a more limited diet; plan to prepare and eat a set number of meals. Business leaders often use this technique to save their brain power for things that matter most. Apple CEO Steve Jobs always wore a black turtleneck, jeans, and white New Balance sneakers. Prioritize daily tasks; perform the most important tasks at the time of the day you feel your cognition is best. Learn to say no; save your mental energy for important tasks, and turn down tasks that are not essential. Try to take a break during the day; sometimes even a short nap or rest can do wonders. Organize your home, and day; keep a list of tasks to perform so you can keep track.

Light Sensitivity

See Chapter 11

Mood Disorders

Anxiety and depression are common comorbid disorders in vestibular migraine. If you have significant anxiety or depression, you should consider consulting a psychiatrist. The following are some measures to consider in the treatment of anxiety and depression.

Non-Pharmacological Options: Regular exercise is the best mood enhancer. Exercise triggers the release of serotonin, dopamine, norepinephrine, and endorphins that help the mood. A good, healthy diet is also key to helping one's mood. While alcohol is often used to dull the symptoms of anxiety and depression, long-term use worsens these mood disorders. Caffeine and sugary foods worsen anxiety and should be avoided. Ultra-processed foods are bad for brain health and mood. Mindfulness meditation is also a very useful therapy for mood disorders.

Supplements: Several supplements may also help improve the symptoms of anxiety and depression. Vitamin D3, B2, B12, B6, and folic acid have been shown to improve the mood and also enhance the effects of antidepressant treatments. Rosavin is an extract of Siberian rose (Rhodiola rosea) that has anti-depressant and anxiolytic properties; take 400 to 500 mg (standardized to 3% rosavin and 1% salidroside) about half an hour before breakfast. Chamomile tea can help improve depression, anxiety, and insomnia.

Psychological Therapies: CBT can be helpful in people with anxiety and depression by targeting unhelpful patterns of thinking, and behaviors, and provides better ways of coping. Psychodynamic therapy is an in-depth talk therapy that focuses on a person's interactions and relationship with their world. Interpersonal therapy focuses on a person's relationship with others, and is centered on the idea that interpersonal relationships are the root of psychological disorders. Psychotherapy is a way of improving a person's well-being by addressing behaviors, beliefs, emotions, and thoughts that negatively impact the person's life.

Motion Sickness

An ounce of prevention is worth a pound of cure. Before your trip, get enough sleep and do not consume a heavy meal, caffeine, alcohol, or foods high in histamine (e.g., cheese, cured meats) right before a trip. Basically, avoid migraine food triggers! Stay hydrated.

If flying, get seats above the wings. Turbulence is minimal in this area. If riding in a car, sit in the front seat. Face forward and look outwards. In a train, choose a window seat that faces the direction the train is moving in. If you are not able to look at the horizon, try wearing glasses with a fluid level that provides an artificial horizon. If on a cruise, get a room with a window. Focus on the horizon as much as possible, especially at the beginning of the trip. Avoid spending too much time in the windowless parts of the ship.

During your trip, try these strategies:

• Eliminate visual input by wearing sleep eye masks (not when you're driving of course!)

• Open the window to let air blow on your face. If you're in a plane or vehicle where this is not possible, use a portable electric fan.

• Controlled slow deep breathing and mindfulness breathing exercises can suppress motion sickness.

• Get that road trip playlist ready! Pleasant music reduces motion sickness [Keshavarz, 2014].

• Buckle yourself in a seat with a solid back and headrest [Chang, 2013; Keshavarz, 2017]

Non-pharmacological measures:

• L-tryptophan is needed for serotonin synthesis, and may help prevent motion sickness. Take 500-1000 mg of L-tryptophan about an hour or two before riding in a vehicle.

• Ginger is an effective anti-nausea agent. Take ginger before a trip. Consume some during a trip if needed.

• High dose (1000 mg) vitamin C can prevent motion sickness when taken before a trip [Jarisch, 2014].

• Some essential oils can help relieve motion sickness [Keshavarz, 2015]. Peppermint oil is especially useful, but others that may help include rose, eucalyptus, and lavender oil. You can try applying a small amount on the forehead and, if you like, just above the upper lip.

• Cannabidiol can control nausea associated with motion sickness. CBD is not legal in all states and because it is illegal according to federal law, transporting products across state lines could get you in trouble. Users should be aware that marijuana may impair their judgment and ability to operate a vehicle.

• Acupressure at the P6 point (see Chapter 9). Pressing on this point with the thumb for 2-3 minutes has been reported to help with nausea. Alternately, Sea Band is an acupressure device that can be worn at this acupressure point; studies into the device have not shown any positive results, but some of my patients swear by it. It is quite affordable and safe, and I see no harm in trying it.

• My experience with the Cefaly device shows that it helps some of my patients prevent motion sickness. They typically use it before riding in a car.

• The Gammacore device could also potentially help. In two patients with benign paroxysmal positional vertigo (BPPV), stimulation with Gammacore relieved nausea from the examination and prevented nausea during BPPV treatment [Beh, 2020].

Medications for motion sickness include meclizine (Antivert), dimenhydrinate (Dramamine), diphenhydramine (Benadryl), baclofen, promethazine (Phenergan), scopolamine, and benzodiazepines. All these medications can cause drowsiness – do not drive after using them. Although effective for nausea, ondansetron (Zofran) has not been shown to effective in motion sickness. Interestingly, for people with migraine, a triptan may prevent motion sickness. For cruises or longer trips, transdermal scopolamine or clonazepam are preferable. The transdermal scopolamine patch can be applied behind one ear 4-8 hours before exposure to motion. Wash your hands thoroughly after touching the patch; if you don't, and inadvertently touch your eye, your pupil will be dilated for hours. Side effects include confusion, memory problems, dry mouth, dry eyes, and blurry vision. It should be avoided in people with prostate enlargement and glaucoma. To reinforce an important point: do NOT use transdermal scopolamine for more than 72 hours!

Noise Sensitivity & Tinnitus

Noise sensitivity and tinnitus usually improve when vestibular migraine is controlled. Chapter 12 discusses several measures to help hyperacusis. Here are some additional therapies if hyperacusis does not improve.

Hearing aids are a useful treatment option if a person also has hearing loss.

White noise machines produce simulated environmental noise like rain to help distract the brain from tinnitus. Pillow speakers could be a good option to help with sleep. If preferred, one can also have a fan, or humidifier on to distract from the ringing. Masking devices are worn in the ear and produce white noise to suppress the ringing.

Pink noise therapy: Pink noise closely matches the spectrum of everyday noises. Pink noise therapy can help improve tolerance for everyday noises over time.

Cognitive behavioral therapy (CBT): CBT targets overt emotional reactions to tinnitus and uncomfortable sounds through graded exposure, reduce the stress response, and provide people with the tools to manage situations and re-start normal activities.

Tinnitus retraining therapy: A device that delivers customized tonal music that matches the frequencies of the tinnitus can help acclimatize a person to the tinnitus. It can also help with noise sensitivity.

Supplements may also help tinnitus, including vitamin B12, melatonin, zinc, Ginkgo, and Pycnogenol.

Medications: In some, medications may be needed if noise sensitivity and tinnitus is severe enough. Antidepressants like duloxetine (Cymbalta) and sertraline (Zoloft) may help. Mirtazapine and bupropion can potentially aggravate tinnitus and should be avoided. Benzodiazepines are effective treatments but because of potential sedation and dependence, should not be used as a first-line therapy. Antipsychotic medications may be used in those with severe tinnitus and noise sensitivity that don't respond to other medications.

Headache

A detailed history and examination can help determine the cause of the headache. Is this headache due to chronic migraine? Medication overuse headache? Occipital neuralgia? Tension-type headache? Once the cause of the headache is determined, the appropriate treatment can be instituted. For example, if vertigo is well-controlled but a person continues to have headaches due to chronic migraine, Botox injections can be considered. If occipital neuralgia is the cause of pain, occipital nerve blocks can be very effective. Other headache disorders to consider in people with migraine are discussed in my book *The Migraine Manual*.

Neck, Back & Shoulder Pain

Because the vast majority of us work with computers, it is important to ensure that our workstations are set up ergonomically. Ergonomics is defined as the study of people's efficiency in their working environments. Basically, ergonomics is making sure that the position of your desk, chair, computer, and equipment does not place undue stress on your joints and body. There are volumes of books dedicated to ergonomics and a detailed discussion is beyond the scope of this chapter. Some tips for an ergonomic workstation include:

• Ensure that the weight of your arms is supported to prevent neck and shoulder pain.

• Keep your head's center of gravity aligned with your neck. Don't push or crane your head forward.

• Ensure that your computer monitor is at eye level.

• Keep the keyboard in front of the monitor to avoid turning your head repeatedly

• Your hands should be at, or below, elbow level.

- Ensure that your wrists are supported while working on your keyboard and mouse.

- Sit tall. Don't slouch and slump at your workstation.

- Use a chair that allows your knees to be level with your hips and your feet on the ground. Don't dangle your legs. If you are short, plant your feet on a stool.

For those with neck, shoulder, and back pain, physical therapy can often be very effective. Neck therapy is a specialized form of physical therapy aimed at helping those with neck pain. Dry needling is a method used by physical therapists to treat muscle pain. Acupuncture provides relief in some. Neck exercises, chiropractic manipulation and massage therapy (Chapter 10) are also potentially helpful.

Rest and apply ice to acutely injured muscles and joints. For chronic pain, applying heat to the affected areas is more effective. You can also apply magnesium oil, diclofenac sodium 1% gel (Voltaren), menthol-containing creams or patches (e.g., Bengay, Icy Hot, Salonpas), ethyl chloride 100% (e.g., Biofreeze), or lidocaine patches. Vibrating or percussion massagers can help relieve spasmed or right muscles. Transcutaneous electrical stimulation (TENS) can also treat musculoskeletal pain. I generally prefer to avoid muscle relaxants if possible because they cause drowsiness and sometimes weight gain.

Consulting a pain specialist or physiatrist (a doctor trained in physical medicine & rehabilitation) can be helpful. They can perform spine or trigger point injections, or nerve blocks. Surgical consultation is needed if you have degenerative disc disease, particularly if it is pressing on the spinal cord.

Sleep

By now, I hope that I have convinced you about the importance of regular sleep. Proper sleep hygiene was discussed in Chapter 12. These are other problems that can interfere with sleep quality and ways to manage them.

Obstructive Sleep Apnea (OSA)

OSA is a common condition that usually affects middle-aged men; overweight individuals have a higher incidence of OSA as well. Due to the collapse of the upper airway during sleep, the airflow is reduced or cut off, causing the person to awaken to breathe. As a result, a person with OSA typically does not get restful sleep, which leads to a persistent low-grade inflammatory state in the body.

This carries with it a whole host of other health problems, including cardiovascular disease, hypertension, and a worsening of migraine. If your partner tells you that you snore loudly, or observes periods where you stop breathing and suddenly gasp or snort for air, you may have OSA. See a sleep specialist to confirm the diagnosis and find the best treatment for you.

Sleeping on your side can help. Strapping a tennis ball to your back was an old technique to keep you from sleeping on your back but there are currently devices that monitor your sleep position and alert you if you happen to roll on your back during the night. Positive airway pressure treatments are the gold standard for OSA.

A CPAP device provides air pressure that keeps the airway open during sleep. Unfortunately, CPAP masks are not the most comfortable contraptions and can cause claustrophobia.

Oral appliances that prevent the lower jaw and tongue from falling backward during sleep are an option but could potentially aggravate TMJ problems.

Surgical procedures like tonsillectomy and uvulopalatopharyngeoplasty, which involve cutting away excess tissue from the back of the airway could be helpful but are not without risks. The pillar procedure involves placing three stiff plastic sticks in the soft palate to stiffen it but there is a high risk of extrusion.

In early 2021, the FDA approved a novel device called the eXciteOSA; it is used during the day for 20 minutes to strengthen the posterior tongue muscles.

Bruxism

Bruxism is teeth grinding and jaw clenching in sleep. It can cause jaw muscle pain, wearing down of teeth, and TMJ problems. Using a dental splint or mouth guard can help. A specialist can help you determine the best splint, as sometimes the jaw has to be repositioned to correct the misalignment.

Restless Leg Syndrome

RLS is an unpleasant sensation in the legs that is only relieved by moving them. It typically occurs in the late evening, and is most severe at night. It can also occur during long drives, and compel a person to take breaks to walk around for relief. It can interfere significantly with sleep quality and has been linked to migraine. If you have RLS it is important to see a neurologist to undergo an evaluation for potential causes. The most common cause of RLS is iron-deficiency and iron replacement often results in improvement. A neurologist will help discuss the best treatment options for RLS with you.

Periodic Limb Movement Disorder (PLMD)

PLMD is a movement disorder consisting of repetitive, rhythmic cramping or jerking of the legs during sleep. These movements range from slight movements of the knee, ankle, and feet, to wild kicking or thrashing. These last for a few seconds but recur every 20-40 seconds. A person with PLMD is often unaware of this problem, unlike RLS, unless informed of it by their bed partners. PLMD results in daytime drowsiness and trouble thinking. It is more common in people with migraine, and often coexists with RLS.

TMJ Dysfunction (TMD)

TMD is the term for disorders related to pain and problems affecting the jaw muscles and temporomandibular joint (the joint connecting the jaw to the skull). It typically results in jaw pain but also causes headaches, jaw noises when chewing (clicking, creaking, popping), clicking noises in the ear, ear pain, tinnitus, ear fullness, neck pain, and dizziness. TMD can worsen migraine and vestibular migraine.

Avoid hard, tough, and crunchy foods (e.g., nuts, jerky). Icing your jaw muscles and using dental guards at night to prevent bruxism may also be helpful. If the pain is severe, NSAIDs, muscle relaxants, and corticosteroids may be used. Trigger point injections or Botox may relieve the symptoms as well. Some physical therapists specialize in TMD. Some people may need surgical intervention to repair the joint or realign the teeth/jaw.

Vestibular Co-Morbidities

Persistent Postural Perceptual Dizziness (PPPD)

I often find that treating the vestibular migraine leads to improvement in PPPD symptoms in most. If it does not, I will try other treatments. Antidepressants like SSRIs or SNRIs are typically used to help treat PPPD. I generally prefer to use venlafaxine if a person also has vestibular migraine since it can help both conditions. If a person cannot tolerate it, or if it does not help, other antidepressants can be used. Benzodiazepines like clonazepam or lorazepam may be needed if antidepressants do not work adequately. Generally, benzodiazepines are not a first-line treatment due to the risk of sedation and dependence.

Vestibular rehabilitation therapy is one of the main treatments for PPPD, and can be very effective. Cognitive behavioral therapy may also be effective but requires a psychologist who is familiar with the condition. If anxiety and depression are severe, you should see a psychiatrist.

Mal De Debarquement Syndrome (MDDS)

I often find that treating the vestibular migraine leads to improvement in MDDS symptoms in most people. In those in whom it does not, other treatments may be considered, including antidepressants and benzodiazepines. Vestibulo-Ocular Reflex (VOR) readaptation therapy is a non-pharmacological treatment that "retrains" the vestibular system to cancel the maladaptive changes that caused MDDS in the first place. For more information about MDDS, please refer to my book *Disembark*.

Benign Paroxysmal Positional Vertigo (BPPV)

BPPV is caused by loose otoconial crystals that become dislodged from their usual place in the inner ear and wander into the canals where they trigger vertigo when the head is moved in the direction of the affected canal. The treatment for BPPV is aimed at dislodging the crystals so they no longer cause vertigo. There are several ways to treat BPPV. Here are two of the simplest ways you can treat BPPV at home:

Brandt-Daroff Exercises

1. Sit on the edge of the bed. Turn your head 45 degrees to the left.

2. Quickly lie down on your right side so that your right ear is touching the bed.

3. Hold this position for 30 seconds, or until vertigo stops.

4. Return to the seated position.

5. Now turn your head 45 degrees to the right.

6. Quickly lie on the left side, with your left ear touching the bed.

7. Hold this position for 30 seconds, or until vertigo stops.

8. Return to the seated position.

9. Repeat 6 times for each side. Do the exercises twice a day for 2 weeks.

Dix-Hallpike & Epley Maneuvers

1. Sit on the bed with enough distance from the edge of the bed to ensure that when you lie back, your head will be hanging comfortably off the edge of the bed.

2. Turn your head 45 degrees to the right. Lie back quickly and let your head hang off the edge of the bed (still turned to the right). Wait for 30 seconds, or until vertigo stops, then sit back up.

3. Turn your head 45 degrees to the left. Lie back quickly and let your head hang off the edge of the bed, turned to the left. Wait for 30 seconds, or until vertigo stops, then sit back up.

4. The side that caused vertigo is the side that the loose crystals are. Now perform the Epley maneuver for the affected side.

Epley maneuver for right-sided BPPV:

a. Start by sitting on the bed with enough space to allow your head to hang off the edge of the bed when you like back.

b. Turn your head 45 degrees to the right.

c. Lie down quickly with your head off the edge of the bed turned to the right. Wait for 30 seconds.

d. Turn your head 90 degrees to the left. Your head will now be looking 45 degrees to the left, and hanging off the edge of the bed. Wait for 30 seconds.

e. Roll onto your left shoulder to turn your head another 90 degrees to the left. In this position, you will be lying on your left shoulder, and you will be facing the floor. Wait 30 seconds.

f. Sit up on the left side of the bed.

Epley maneuver for left-sided BPPV:

a. Start by sitting on the bed with enough space to allow your head to hang off the edge of the bed when you like back.

b. Turn your head 45 degrees to the left.

c. Lie down quickly with your head off the edge of the bed turned to the left. Wait for 30 seconds.

d. Turn your head 90 degrees to the right. Your head will now be looking 45 degrees to the right, and hanging off the edge of the bed. Wait for 30 seconds

e. Roll onto your right shoulder to turn your head another 90 degrees to the right. In this position, you will be lying on your left shoulder, and you will be facing the floor. Wait 30 seconds.

f. Sit up on the right side of the bed.

One treatment is usually enough to treat BPPV. If not, you can repeat the Epley maneuver for the affected side a few times. Remember that experiencing vertigo during these maneuvers is a *good* thing. It confirms that you are performing the maneuvers correctly! If you are worried about nausea during the maneuvers, you can take your anti-nausea medication, or smell some peppermint oil, before you start.

For 24 hours after performing a successful Epley maneuver:

a. Do NOT bend over (head below horizontal).

b. Do NOT tilt your head too far backward.

c. Kneel or squat down if you have to tie your shoes or pick something off the floor.

d. Do not go to the dentist or hair stylist.

e. Do not swim free-style (or crawl style).

f. If you need to use eye drops, pull your lower eyelid down and place the eye drops on the inside of the lower eyelid.

g. To shave, protrude your chin forwards to access the area between your chin and neck.

h. Sleep in a recliner or use a few pillows at a 45-degree angle.

12. If your home maneuvers do not help, call your physician or vestibular therapist.

Chapter 18: Migraine & Hormones

Hormones are nature's three bottles of beer.
Mary Roach, Bonk: The Curious Coupling of Science and Sex

The relationship between migraine and hormones was alluded to many times in previous chapters, and in this, we shall tackle it head-on. The role of hormones in migraine cannot be underestimated. Migraines occur at almost similar rates in pre-pubertal boys and girls, but after menarche, the incidence in women increases, often triggered around the time of menstruation, fluctuates with pregnancy, and declines after menopause.

It appears that vertigo and dizziness are predominant migraine manifestations before puberty (benign recurrent vertigo, the childhood version of migraine, occurs in young children almost exclusively), and as menopause sets in. The material in this chapter is to educate you about treatment options, and any treatments should be discussed with your obstetrician/gynecologist and/or endocrinologist.

Migraine & Menstruation

Menstruation is a common migraine trigger, most likely due to the drop in estrogen levels. About half of women experience migraine attacks related to the menstrual cycle, the majority of attacks starting two days before the onset of menstruation. Pure menstrual migraine is defined as migraines that only occur 2 days before up to 3 days after the onset of menses. Menstrually-related migraine is defined as migraines that occur during this time, as well as attacks that occur at other times of the cycle. Menstrual migraines tend to be more severe, both in intensity and duration, and less responsive to rescue medication. Similarly, menses often trigger vestibular migraine attacks that are more severe than episodes that occur during other times of the cycle. Nausea is often more severe with menstrually-related migraine attacks.

Interestingly, women are more vulnerable to motion sickness during the menstrual cycle. Migraine attacks can also occur during ovulation, when estrogen levels spike during the middle of the cycle (about two weeks before menstruation).

One option for treating menstrually-related vestibular migraine is using treatments around the time of menstruation. The treatment should be started two days before the expected date of menses, and continued for 6 days. These treatment options include (1) eletriptan 20 mg three times a day, or; (2) frovatriptan 2.5 mg once a day, or; (3) zolmitriptan 2.5 mg once a day, or; (4) estradiol (a transdermal gel or patch), or; (5) rimegepant 75 mg every other day, or; (6) acetazolamide 125 mg once to twice a day, or; (7) vitamin E 400 IU daily.

Of course, your menstrual cycles will need to be fairly regular and predictable for this approach to work. Estrogen preparations (oral, gels, or patches) should be given two days before the anticipated start of menses to mitigate the drop in levels leading up to menses, It should not be used for more than a week; starting estrogen too early can cause a bump in migraine attacks when estrogen is stopped. A fixed, daily dose of estrogen can also be considered to prevent the hormonal fluctuations that drive menstrually-related migraine. Progestins can be combined with estrogens in women who also desire contraception.

Magnesium started on day 15 of the cycle in those who have less predictable menstruation. You can take 500 mg once daily. In those already on magnesium for migraine prevention, taking an additional 300 mg once daily may be helpful. Vitex is a supplement that could potentially relieve the flare-ups around menses (see Chapter 8), and can be taken daily. Another non-pharmacologic option for controlling menstrually-related migraine is to take soy isoflavones 60 mg (standardized to 40% isoflavones), dong quai or female ginseng (*Angelica sinensis*) 100 mg, and black cohosh (*Actaea racemosa*) 50 mg every day [Burke,

2002]. One study reported that laparoscopic uterosacral nerve ablation (LUNA) relieved menstrual migraine [Juang, 2007]. It is also reasonable to use an oral contraceptive with low or very low estrogen content (see later).

Using your rescue medications to treat acute attacks during the menstrual cycle can also be effective. Triptans and NSAIDs are efficacious. Mefenamic acid can be a good NSAID option during menstrual migraine, since it blocks the production of prostaglandins.

Migraine & Sex

Even though many people with migraine suffer from sexual dysfunction, this topic is rarely discussed aside from that famous "not tonight, I have a headache" line. Human sexuality is highly complex, and multi-dimensional. Sexual dysfunction can be categorized as problems of desire (lacking interest in sex), arousal (feeling in the mood, but the body does not respond as it should), orgasm (difficulty with climax), or pain (the act of sexual intercourse causing pain).

This problem is not solely related to headache frequency or severity. Vestibular symptoms can affect sexual activity as well; quick head movements or certain head positions can provoke vertigo or dizziness. Neck and shoulder muscle pain can interfere with sexual enjoyment. Depression and anxiety are major causes of sexual dysfunction. Serotonin and dopamine are important in sexual function; both neurotransmitter systems are dysfunctional in migraine. Some migraine preventive medications (e.g., antidepressants and beta-blockers) cause sexual dysfunction by affecting libido, orgasm, and erectile function Other comorbid disorders, like endometriosis and interstitial cystitis, can cause pelvic pain and painful sexual intercourse.

Because sex is still considered taboo, both physicians and patients are reluctant to discuss sexual dysfunction. Sexuality plays an important role in a person's sense of well-being and health. As such, sexual dysfunction should be discussed with your physician to find, and address its cause.

Migraine & Pregnancy

The first trimester is a somewhat mixed picture. About 25% of women (particularly those with menstrually-related migraine) have an increase in migraines, as well as morning sickness. About 10-15% of women develop migraine for the first time during the first trimester, and some women develop new aura symptoms during this time. However, others experience an improvement in migraines during the first trimester.

The high and stable estrogen state in the second and third trimesters brings about an improvement in migraines in the majority of women. Migraine increases the risk of some complications in pregnancy, including preterm delivery, gestational hypertension, and pre-eclampsia [Purdue-Smithe, 2023]. After delivery, the drop in estrogen levels usually exacerbates migraines (typically in the first week). Furthermore, post-partum depression and the stress of a new parental role (including sleep deprivation) result in a worsening of migraines, especially during the first month. In women with more than one child, migraines tend to worsen with subsequent pregnancies. Note that any worsening of headaches during pregnancy or the post-partum period, particularly if accompanied by new neurologic symptoms, must be brought to your neurologist's attention to rule out other potentially more serious causes (e.g., a blood clot in the veins around the brain, stroke).

The first trimester is when the fetus is most vulnerable to medications because the brain and many important organ systems are being formed. For women of childbearing age, planning for pregnancy is important to ensure the wellbeing of the baby. All women of child-bearing age should take folate daily. If possible, use medications that are safe for pregnancy even if you are not pregnant since most pregnancies are unplanned. If you need to use medications that may not be safe for pregnancy, use contraception, and discuss transitioning to a safer option with your neurologist before getting pregnant.

Rescue treatments during pregnancy:

Acetaminophen is safe to use for rescue; however, frequent daily use during pregnancy may be associated with a higher risk of ADHD in the child. Timolol eye drops are safe and can be effective. Neuromodulation appears to be safe as well. Nerve blocks and trigger point injections appear to be safe and effective [Govindappagari, 2014]. For headache and muscle pain, cyclobenzaprine (Flexeril) may be used.

Triptans are generally safe for pregnancy. In one study, mothers who used triptans prenatally had a slightly higher risk of having children with externalizing behavior problems (maladaptive behavioral problems directed at an individual's environment, e.g., ADHD) [Wood, 2016]. However, most studies indicate that triptans are not associated with major adverse pregnancy outcomes [Dudman, 2021; Marchenko, 2015].

NSAIDs carry a risk of low birth weight, vaginal bleeding, reduced amniotic fluid production, and asthma in the baby. Some recommend avoiding NSAIDs in the first and third trimesters of pregnancy. Butalbital-acetaminophen-caffeine medications (e.g., Fioricet) are often prescribed by obstetricians for headaches in pregnant women. As discussed before, such medications have a very high risk of medication-overuse headache. Furthermore, butalbital is a barbiturate, and readily crosses the placental barrier and enters the fetal circulation. It is a sedative and the effect on the developing baby's brain is unknown. Moderate to high caffeine exposure in pregnancy has been linked to miscarriage, low birth weight, and preterm delivery.

Dihydroergotamine (DHE) should not be used in pregnancy. Opioids should be avoided due to the risk of dependence and medication overuse headache. Furthermore, opioids can cross the placental barrier and affect the fetal brain; opioid withdrawal has been reported in babies exposed to it in utero. Some obstetricians allow its use in mothers with chronic pain and difficult-to-control migraine.

Benzodiazepines should be avoided as well as they can cross the placental barrier. However, some obstetricians allow the use of lorazepam from the second trimester onwards if the need arises.

For nausea, ginger, ondansetron (Zofran) and metoclopramide (Reglan) are safe. Promethazine appears reasonably safe, although withdrawal in babies has been reported when it is used in the third trimester. Doxylamine (Unisom) is safe, and can also help with insomnia and allergies; it is usually combined with vitamin B6. Diphenhydramine (Benadryl), meclizine and dimenhydrinate also appear safe for pregnancy.

Corticosteroids may carry a small risk of cleft lip with or without palate if used in the first trimester. However, the results of the studies are mixed. It may be prudent to avoid corticosteroids in the first and early second trimester. Corticosteroids are safe to use in the third trimester.

Gepants (ubrogepant, zavegepant, and rimegepant) should be avoided as there have been reports of fetal abnormalities in lab animals. There is no pregnancy data on lasmiditan at the time of this writing; as such, it would be best to avoid it when you are pregnant.

Preventive treatments during pregnancy:

Supplements that are generally safe for pregnancy include B2, B6, folate, B12, vitamin D, magnesium, CoQ10, ginger, L-tryptophan, and peppermint oil. There may be a theoretical possibility that melatonin could alter the baby's biological clock. Herbal supplements (e.g., feverfew) should be avoided.

Most migraine preventives have no proven safety or risks in pregnancy. Generally, propranolol, timolol, metoprolol, amitriptyline, nortriptyline, cyproheptadine, verapamil, lamotrigine, and memantine are reasonably safe. I find that timolol eye drops are very safe and effective. Atenolol should never be used due to the risk of intrauterine growth retardation. Neuromodulation devices are reasonably safe to use as well.

Caution should be exercised with gabapentin, SSRIs, and SNRIs. Venlafaxine used to be considered reasonably safe but there is some data to suggest it may carry a higher risk of preterm delivery and birth defects [Anderson, 2020]. Topiramate, valproate (divalproex), ACE inhibitors, and ARBs can cause fetal abnormalities and should be avoided.

CGRP may play a role in placental blood flow, fetal bone formation, and regulation of maternal blood pressure. Therefore, we currently recommend that pregnant women avoid CGRP monoclonal antibodies and gepants. Those on CGRP monoclonal antibodies should stop them for 6 months before trying to get pregnant. Those on rimegepant or atogepant should stop them for one week before trying to get pregnant. However, it is important to note that our knowledge continues to evolve. No fetal or pregnancy-related harm has been observed in pregnant lab animals exposed to CGRP monoclonal antibodies. An analysis of a safety database showed no maternal or fetal adverse effects in pregnant women exposed to CGRP monoclonal antibodies [Noseda, 2023]. Gepants in pregnant lab animals may cause fetal skeletal abnormalities.

Nerve blocks involving the administration of lidocaine or bupivacaine are reasonably safe for pregnant women. Botox acts on local nerve endings when injected into the head and neck muscles. It does not cross the placenta. Therefore, Botox is theoretically safe for pregnancy. There are case reports of women who are paralyzed from botulism (from food contamination) giving birth to normal babies with no evidence of Botox in their blood. More recently, an analysis of the Allergan (the manufacturer of Botox) Global Safety Database of 397 pregnancy exposures to Botox showed that the prevalence of major birth defects was no higher than that of the general population [Brin, 2023].

Migraine & Breastfeeding

Interestingly, breastfeeding seems to be protective against migraine in the post-partum period. One study showed that women who breastfed had half the risk of migraine recurrence compared to women who bottle-fed [Sances, 2003].

The medication restrictions while breastfeeding are less strict than those for pregnancy. Medications that are secreted in breast milk in large amounts should be generally avoided. However, if needed, rescue medications can be used with measures taken to minimize transfer to the baby. *Pre-pump and save*: Pump your breast milk beforehand, take the medication, and time the breastfeeding to avoid peak levels in breast milk. Use the saved breast milk your baby needs to feed during the peak levels. *Pump and dump*: Breast milk can be expressed and discarded for 24 hours after using the medication.

Rescue treatments during lactation:

Acetaminophen is safe to use while breastfeeding. NSAIDs also appear safe; the only exception is aspirin, which may cause Reye's syndrome in infants and should be avoided. Neuromodulation is safe while breastfeeding.

The data on triptan use during lactation is limited. However, there have been no reports of major adverse effects on breastfed infants exposed to triptans [Amundsen, 2021]. Eletriptan, sumatriptan, and rizatriptan are very minimally transferred to breast milk and appear safe. Naratriptan has the highest proportion of transference to breast milk and therefore, is not recommended as a first-line triptan in lactating mothers.

Rimegepant appears safe when breastfeeding due to very low levels in breast milk While low levels of ubrogepant are found in breast milk, there is insufficient data with regards to breastfeeding. There is no data on zavegepant use in lactating mothers.

For nausea, ginger and ondansetron (Zofran) is safe to use. Metoclopramide and promethazine (Phenergan) may affect prolactin (the hormone responsible for lactation) levels. Prochlorperazine (Compazine) appears to be reasonably safe during lactation.

Lorazepam (Ativan) is the best choice if a benzodiazepine is needed. Lorazepam has a shorter half-life, only very low levels make it into breast milk, and the metabolites are inactive. For vestibular migraine attacks, I typically recommend my patients take a bedtime dose. Pump some milk before taking lorazepam, and do not breastfeed until 8 hours later. If your baby needs to be fed during the night, use the milk you pumped before taking lorazepam. Avoid diazepam (valium) since the active metabolites can be passed into breast milk for many hours to days.

Corticosteroids appear safe during breastfeeding. Prednisone is safe and only minute amounts make it into breast milk. Some recommend not breastfeeding for 4 hours after taking a dose.

DHE, butalbital-containing drugs, and opioids should be avoided. The manufacturer of DHE nasal sprays recommends not breastfeeding for 3 days after treatment. Opioids and butalbital can sedate breastfed infants and lead to poor feeding. Lasmiditan is secreted into breast milk in animals and should be avoided until more data becomes available.

Preventive therapies during lactation:

Safe supplements while breastfeeding include B2, B6, folate, B12, vitamin D, magnesium, CoQ10, ginger, peppermint oil, L-tryptophan, and NAC. Breastmilk naturally contains melatonin; the levels in breast milk rise in the evening, mirroring the changes in the mother's circulating levels. Supplementing with melatonin in the evenings appears to be safe for infants. The amount of melatonin in breastmilk is safe; higher doses have been safely administered to infants in clinical studies [LactMed, 2006].

Generally, almost all migraine preventive medications are reasonably safe (with only a small amount making it into breast milk) with a few caveats. Higher levels of zonisamide, atenolol, and tizanidine are secreted into breast milk and as such, may cause adverse effects in infants. In mothers on high doses of lamotrigine, it may be important to monitor the levels in the infant. There is very limited data regarding ACE inhibitors and angiotensin II receptor blockers (ARBs) when breastfeeding. Small amounts make it into breast milk; they should be avoided in premature babies and the first 2 months as they may cause low blood pressure.

There is not much data on CGRP monoclonal antibodies in breastfeeding mothers. There have not been any reports of adverse effects in breastfed infants at the time of this writing. The likelihood of these antibodies being secreted into the breast milk is very low since these antibodies are very large molecules. Furthermore, when ingested by the infant, these antibodies are broken down in the gut (just like how any protein is digested). Rimegepant appears to be safe during lactation. There is no data about the safety of atogepant while breastfeeding.

Botox, nerve blocks, and neuromodulation appear safe during lactation.

Migraine & Polycystic Ovarian Syndrome

Polycystic ovarian syndrome (PCOS) refers to a condition where the ovaries produce excessive male hormones (androgens). Manifestations of PCOS include menstrual abnormalities, excessive body hair, acne, male-pattern hair loss, infertility, skin tags on the neck or armpits, and acanthosis nigricans (dark patches of skin around the nape of the neck, armpits, and under the breasts). Obesity, hypertension, and insulin resistance are commonly associated with PCOS. Ultrasonography often reveals multiple small cysts on the ovaries, hence the name.

While there are many anecdotal reports of women with migraine and PCOS, the research into PCOS and migraine is surprisingly scant. In my search of the medical literature, I came across only one small study that investigated the link between PCOS and migraine [Pourabolghasem, 2009]. Surprisingly, it did not elucidate a significant relationship between the two disorders. It is not unreasonable to draw connections between PCOS and migraine. Firstly, depression, obstructive sleep apnea and obesity are more common in PCOS; these conditions are linked to higher migraine incidence. Secondly, hormonal changes are inextricably linked with migraine. Thirdly, valproate, a migraine preventive medication, can induce PCOS in about 5-10% of women.

If you have migraine and PCOS, addressing insulin resistance, reducing weight, using the appropriate oral contraceptives, and/or using a male hormone-blocker may also improve migraine control. Consult a gynecologist or endocrinologist for the best treatment of PCOS.

Migraine & Endometriosis

The endometrium is the tissue that lines the uterus; during the menstrual cycle it thickens and develops a rich blood supply in preparation for the fertilized egg. If that does not occur, the lining breaks down and sheds. Endometriosis is a condition defined by the presence of abnormal endometrial tissue outside the uterus. The condition is characterized by chronic pelvic pain, painful menstruation, irregular or heavy periods, painful sexual intercourse, and infertility. Less common symptoms include painful urination, constipation, fatigue, nausea, or diarrhea.

The prevalence of migraine is two to five times higher among women with endometriosis. The risk of endometriosis among women with migraine is almost three times higher compared to women without migraine [Maitrot-Mantelet, 2020]. Furthermore, among women with migraine, those with endometriosis have a higher risk of chronic headache, anxiety, depression, chronic fatigue syndrome, fibromyalgia, interstitial cystitis, and irritable bowel syndrome [Tietjen, 2007]. Underscoring the relationship between the two disorders, there are shared genetic influences in migraine and endometriosis [Adewuyi, 2020; Nyholt, 2009]. Women with endometriosis and migraine may benefit from progestin-only or combined oral contraceptives. If medical treatments are ineffective, surgical intervention may be needed.

Migraine & Fertility

There is emerging evidence that migraine may affect fertility and family planning. The impact of the symptoms on relationships and the negative effect of some migraine preventive treatments on sexual function are partly to blame. Furthermore, vestibular migraine flares tend to occur around ovulation and leading up to menstruation, making intimacy difficult during these times. Migraine is also linked to hormonal abnormalities that negatively affect fertility. Some migraine medications may also potentially affect fertility. NSAIDs inhibit the production of prostaglandins, an important chemical involved in reproduction. Indomethacin, diclofenac, and naproxen are associated with lower rates of ovulation and fecundability (the likelihood of achieving pregnancy) [McInerney, 2017]. Ibuprofen does not seem to affect fecundability [McInerney, 2017]. Beta-blockers may lower testosterone levels and semen quality [Guo, 2017].

Ovarian hyperstimulation is sometimes used in IVF to induce the development of multiple follicles that will produce eggs. Gonadotropin-releasing hormone agonists or antagonists may be used depending on the protocol used. These medications alter the levels of estrogen and as such, can trigger migraine attacks. One-third of women undergoing IVF and embryo transfer suffered headaches, predominantly with the use of medications that induce very low estrogenic states [Ben-Yehuda, 2005]. Furthermore, the stress of the IVF process can aggravate migraine. This presents a tricky situation. On one hand, we want to keep migraine under control. On the other, we do not want to use any medications that could interfere with the IVF process or potentially harm the fetus. Working closely with your headache specialist and fertility expert is important in this process.

Migraine & Oral Contraceptives

Migraine with aura tends to worsen with combined oral contraceptives, while not affecting most people with migraine without aura. The World Health Organization and American College of Obstetricians and Gynecologists advise against the use of estrogen-based combined oral contraceptives in women over the age of 35 who have migraine with aura due to the increased risk of stroke and cardiovascular disease. According to these bodies, smokers under the age of 35 with migraine with aura also should not be on these contraceptives. However, the rationale for these recommendations was based on contraceptives that used high doses of estrogen, i.e., over 50 micrograms of estradiol.

New contraceptives use much lower estrogen doses (20-30 micrograms of estradiol). Most studies show that the risk of stroke is not substantially higher with estradiol doses below 20 micrograms. Very low-dose combined oral contraceptives (10-15 micrograms of estradiol) can inhibit ovulation and prevent estrogen from rising to levels that usually occur during a normal menstrual cycle. In women with migraine without aura, this may help decrease migraine attacks while minimizing stroke and cardiovascular risk. Generally, in migraine with aura, estrogen-free contraceptive measures are preferred. Progestogen-only contraceptives may be beneficial for migraine control. If estrogen-containing preparations are used to treat conditions like acne, pelvic pain, or menstrually-related migraine, very low-dose estradiol preparations can be considered, provided that there are no other stroke risk factors (e.g., smoking, hypertension).

Migraine & Menopause

The perimenopausal period is characterized by fluctuating ovarian hormone levels and can be associated with a worsening of migraine attacks. The post-menopausal period is characterized by a stable decline in hormone levels. It usually brings an improvement in headache frequency in the majority of women, while some experience no change, and 10-20% report a worsening of headache.

Interestingly, natural spontaneous menopause is usually characterized by improvement in headaches, but induced menopause (either through medications or surgery) causes a worsening of migraine headaches. Vestibular migraine typically begins in the years leading up to the perimenopausal period in most and in the post-menopausal period in some.

Women with migraine may be at higher risk of developing menopausal symptoms like poor sleep, hot flashes, and night sweats. Hormone replacement therapy can be considered in women who become menopausal before age 45, due to the risks that come with early menopause. Studies into the impact of hormone replacement therapy on migraine have produced mixed results, with most suggesting that hormone replacement therapy worsens migraine. An interesting observation is that a worsening of headaches in the peri-menopausal period predicts a worsening of migraine headache with hormone replacement. Hormone replacement can be considered if a woman's physician(s) feel that is indicated for other medical purposes, but hormone replacement for the sole goal of migraine control is not beneficial.

Gabapentin and venlafaxine are non-hormone medications that can treat both vestibular migraine and peri-menopausal symptoms like hot flashes. They may be useful for women suffering from both conditions, who prefer not to be on hormone replacement therapy.

Migraine & Testosterone

Yes, testosterone levels also play a role in migraine. Testosterone is not just needed for sexual function. Men with chronic migraine have lower testosterone levels [Shields, 2019]. Women also need adequate testosterone levels for optimal health. Testosterone replacement in pre- and post-menopausal women improves migraine severity [Glaser, 2012]. Low testosterone is linked to depression and cognitive impairment in both men and women.

I have seen men with vestibular migraine that began after they were put on testosterone blockers for prostate cancer. I have also seen men with vestibular migraine who were found to have low testosterone, and improved significantly once testosterone replacement therapy was instituted. In men and women with vestibular migraines and migraines that are difficult to control with preventive medications, it may be prudent to check testosterone levels. If these levels are low, working with a urologist, endocrinologist, or gynecologist on testosterone replacement may have life-changing results. I also prefer not to prescribe beta blockers to men without hypertension due to their potential to lower testosterone levels and semen quality [Guo, 2017].

ON

ONward!

Harnessing the power of your mind, building your social network, and preparing for the future

If you are distressed by anything external, the pain is not due to the thing itself, but to your estimate of it; and this you have the power to revoke at any moment. You have power over your mind, not outside events. Realize this, and you will find strength. Reject your sense of injury, and the injury itself disappears.
Marcus Aurelius, Meditations

The body and the mind are intimately connected. Vestibular migraine is more than a physical ailment; it affects the mind in profound ways. Vertigo and dizziness are extremely distressing, and there is no doubt about the connections between vertigo, dizziness, stress, vestibular migraine, PPPD, anxiety, depression, and insomnia. Chronic vestibular symptoms most definitely impact a person's emotional and mental state, causing substantial long-term harm.

Ignoring the emotional and mental dimensions of vestibular migraine while only treating it as a physical illness degrades treatment outcomes. Treating it holistically, by addressing all aspects of vestibular migraine helps guarantee the best possible outcome. As such. equipping yourself with the proper mindset and mental tools to deal with vestibular migraine will help you control it, mitigate its impact, and get your life back.

Neuroplasticity

The brain is made up of approximately 86 billion neurons. Each neuron is a cell that receives information from, and sends information to, other neurons. Information within a neuron is conveyed as electrical signals. Neurons "talk" to each other via connections called synapses. Information is conveyed across the synapses using compounds called neurotransmitters. Our brains are always altering these synapses, reconfiguring the connections between the billions of neurons, in response to our experiences. The ability of our brains to re-wire and re-organize, essentially by forming new synapses and disconnecting old ones, is called neuroplasticity. From the time we are formed in the womb until the day we die, our brains are constantly re-wiring the synapses.

With every new experience, new synapses form, and old ones are broken. While reading this book, your brain is forming new synapses to interpret and remember the information herein, while breaking the synapses formed while you browsed People magazine a week ago. Our individual experiences, personalities, skills, and knowledge, can be distilled into the distinct neuronal network in our brains. We are unique because our brain networks are unique. We evolve and adapt because our brains constantly evolve and adapt synaptic connections. In essence, we are the sum of our synapses.

Neuroplasticity is a very important characteristic of our brains, essential for us to survive and thrive. Allostasis, a concept coined by Peter Sterling and Joseph Eyer in 1988, refers to our brain's ability to predict, anticipate, and adapt to the constantly changing environment around us. Allostasis does not aim for rigid constancy, but a flexible variability that anticipates the needs of the organism, to meet them promptly. Sung Lee refined this concept and introduced the "paradigm of allostatic orchestration". According to Lee, the allostatic state represents the integrated totality of brain-body interactions in which health represents an allostatic state of optimal anticipatory oscillation, while diseases are allostatic states of impaired anticipatory oscillations demonstrated by the rigidification of set points.

The brain continuously monitors and integrates data from the body's internal milieu (interoceptive information) and the external environment (exteroceptive information). It must balance oft-conflicting needs and prioritize what is best for us. The interoceptive system conveys information about the internal state of the body to the insular cortex which integrates this with exteroceptive data, and communicates with the amygdala and hypothalamus. Notably, the insular cortex is also tasked with processing vestibular information, and plays a role in perpetuating states of anxiety. It is thus unsurprising that vestibular disorders often result in anxiety, panic, and hypersensitivity to interoceptive input.

Using both interoceptive and exteroceptive data, as well as its previous experiences, the brain predicts what is most likely to happen to chart the best course of action. The brain can respond more rapidly and efficiently if it knows what to expect. To refine its prediction models, the brain constantly compares incoming data with what it predicted. The better it can predict potential outcomes, the better it becomes at anticipating challenges and adapting. The brain aims to build the most accurate and complete model of the world to ensure the most adaptive (and thus, successful) behaviors. Sensory input is constantly compared with anticipated signals, and errors are fed back to improve the prediction models. If the brain finds that its predictions are incorrect, it attempts to make adjustments to minimize the differences between anticipated and actual input. In essence, allostasis is not about maintaining the status quo and rigidity, but fitness and growth in the face of uncertainty and challenges. Ideally, after an unexpected stress or challenge, we not only return to our previous state (resilience), but grow stronger and thrive (antifragility). In his book Antifragile, Nassim Nicholas Taleb emphasizes this difference: "Antifragility is beyond resilience or robustness. The resilient resists shocks and stays the same; the antifragile gets better".

However, at times neuroplasticity can go awry, resulting in disease states. Tinnitus is a prime example of maladaptive (i.e., bad) neuroplasticity. The auditory nerve's synapses that detect high frequencies are sensitive to noise damage and aging. As hearing begins to deteriorate, neuroplastic changes occur in the brain regions responsible for detecting these frequencies. Because sound input from the ear is lacking, the brain dedicates more neurons to "detect" these sound frequencies. Over time, these neurons fire more frequently and synchronously, causing the brain to "hear" a constant high-pitched ringing noise. With worsening tinnitus, maladaptive neuroplasticity affects other brain regions, for example, those that control mood and emotions, leading to depression and anxiety.

Neuroplasticity is extremely important in the vestibular system. Following vestibular neuritis, input from one inner ear is disrupted, resulting in vertigo. Within 2-3 days, the brain learns that the asymmetric vestibular signal is not normal and uses vision and proprioception to re-calibrate the balance networks. Within 3-7 days, the vertigo stops but a person will continue to feel unsteady and "off" for several weeks. During this phase, the brain adapts to the asymmetric vestibular signals (its "new normal"), and learns how to use visual and proprioceptive input to optimize balance and orientation. This process is called central compensation and can be disrupted by using meclizine, or benzodiazepines for too long after vestibular neuritis. On the other hand, central compensation is enhanced with vestibular rehabilitation therapy. If neuroplasticity goes wrong, chronic unsteadiness and dizziness may occur. In some, maladaptive neuroplasticity results in PPPD, characterized by constant dizziness, anxiety, and symptom hypervigilance.

The Power of Beliefs & Thinking Patterns

Vertigo and dizziness are powerful experiences with subconscious, emotional, and even spiritual dimensions. Out-of-body experiences usually are associated with spiritual events but vertigo is such a profound symptom that it can also produce out-of-body experiences. People who experience vertigo, even during vestibular testing, often describe feeling like they were hovering above their bodies, looking down at themselves.

How we interpret a symptom has a powerful impact on how it affects us. For example, we are much less affected by muscle soreness after an intense workout because we know that it is part of the process of getting stronger. However, we feel miserable when we are sore all over after the flu shot. Similarly, a person who believes his/her headache was because of a hangover perceives it very differently from one who believes the headache was because of a brain aneurysm. While most consider vertigo and dizziness extremely unpleasant, the whirling dervishes (*semazens*) of Turkey believe it is a vehicle to attain spiritual ecstasy. They spin in repetitive circles in rapturous meditation to connect with the Divine and embrace humanity. This shows how powerful our mental and emotional states can be – we can use our minds to redefine an extremely unpleasant experience into a positive and uplifting one.

Negative thoughts and emotions cause and are perpetuated by bad neuroplasticity. Neuroscientist, author, and executive coach Robert Cooper uses the term "upwiring" for neuroplasticity that betters ourselves, and "downwiring" for the default mode of the lower, instinctual animal brain. When we endeavor to change our lives, and use our mental powers to manifest positive outcomes and conquer vestibular migraine, we are "upwiring". Making the necessary changes needed to control migraine, and pro-actively managing your illness is "upwiring". When we allow negative thoughts and emotions to hijack our brains, we are "downwiring" and perpetuating the vicious cycle of dizziness. Refusing to believe that you will get better, being physically inactive all day, disbelieving that medications can help ("I'm too sensitive for any medication"), and accepting defeat ("I'm just going to be disabled") is "downwiring" and leads to chronification and worsening of vestibular migraine.

The Fear Circuit

Fear and anxiety are similar emotional responses that differ in terms of timescale. Fear is a transient response to a stimulus that may be a threat, stress, or danger. On the other hand, anxiety is a persistent and diffuse state of defensiveness and exaggerated sensitivity to threat detection. The same neural circuit controls both fear and anxiety; it can be called the fear circuit. The fear circuit plays a central role in downwiring and chronic symptoms of vestibular migraine.

There are many structures involved in the fear circuit; only three (amygdala, hippocampus, and frontal cortex) are pertinent to our discussion. The *amygdala* (plural: *amygdalae*) and *hippocampus* (plural: *hippocampi*) are part of the limbic system, an ancient brain network that controls emotions and memory. The amygdalae are two almond-shaped structures located deep in the brain's temporal lobes. They detect danger and threats, driving the emotional reaction to these situations, i.e., anxiety, fear, rage, and aggression. The amygdala's connections to the hypothalamus underpins how emotional states can influence the autonomic system.

The amygdalae are crucial for encoding, storing, and retrieving fear memories. They also drive changes in other brain regions that perpetuate states of anxiety. Fear is an essential evolutionary feature. Hence, the brain has evolved to quickly learn to fear potential threats and not easily forget them. Innate fears are primal, hardwired fears, and include a fear of spiders, snakes, heights, and pain. Many innate fears can be seen in infants and animals. Of interest, humans, monkeys, and rodents possess an innate fear of looming (i.e., rapidly approaching) objects, because such stimuli indicate an impending collision. Many people with vestibular migraine, PPPD, and MDDS have difficulty driving in traffic or navigating crowds, often describing it feels like cars or objects are "coming right at them", suggesting an amplification of this innate fear.

Most human fears are the result of learning, a process called fear conditioning. Fear conditioning is a behavioral model in which an organism learns that certain stimuli or experiences are unpleasant, threatening, or even traumatic. If you pair a certain sound with an electric shock, a lab rat learns to associate the sound with the unpleasantness of the shock; just playing that sound will be enough to activate the amygdala and a stress response. This is also called Pavlovian conditioning. Fear conditioning may arise from personal experiences or by observing another person's fearful experience. For example, a fear of large dogs may occur if you were attacked by one, or if you witnessed someone being mauled by a dog.

In fear conditioning, the amygdalae and hippocampus record stressful and threatening situations. The hippocampus stores information about the situation, deciding which details are important and activating the amygdalae every time it detects a similar situation. The hippocampus-amygdala complex can also remind the brain of potential threats or stressors. For example, if malls and crowds trigger your dizziness, the thought of going to the outlet mall for Black Friday is enough to make you tremble.

If the stimuli are unpredictable, uncontrollable, and ambiguous, the amygdala's response is stronger. This anticipatory dread can induce a state of sustained anxiety and fear where the amygdala remains in a state of hyperactivation. Over time, the brain is less able to distinguish threat from safety, resulting in a state of persistent anxiety, which in turn increases the chances of triggering fear responses. As a consequence, the brain is stuck in a vicious cycle of anxiety and fear to a constantly growing list of stimuli.

The frontal cortex is the most evolutionarily-advanced part of the brain and is connected to the limbic system, helping regulate its responses. The frontal cortex controls executive function, working memory, strategizing, organizing, planning and initiating actions, regulating emotions, delaying gratification (self-control), and controlling our impulses. The frontal cortex is the last part of the brain to fully mature, not achieving full development until our mid-20s. The frontal cortex is the mature parent that controls the emotional, impulsive, irrational teenager which is the limbic system.

The frontal cortices are connected to the amygdala and hippocampus. The prefrontal cortices, in particular, are responsible for regulating the amygdalae, preventing the limbic system from running riot. In this role, the prefrontal cortex can reverse fear conditioning. If the lab rat conditioned to associate a sound with an electrical shock is exposed to a different situation where a shock does not follow the sound, the rat begins to learn that the sound is not necessarily an unpleasant and stressful trigger. This is the role of the prefrontal cortex, which actively learns that a particular stimulus may no longer be a threat or danger, a process called extinction learning.

Central Sensitization Syndrome

Central sensitization is the result of maladaptive neuroplasticity of the fear circuit. It is a state where the brain amplifies and focuses excessively on a specific sensory input or symptom. This state is well described in pain disorders, including fibromyalgia, IBS, pelvic pain syndromes, interstitial cystitis, and TMJ syndrome. They are more common in people with depression, anxiety, PTSD, and migraine, and also share overlapping symptoms like fatigue, sleep disruptions, and brain fog.

The brain is overly vigilant and watches for any stimuli it perceives as threatening. This ever-increasing awareness feeds a vicious cycle of symptom hypervigilance, anxiety, and perceived threat. The brain loses the ability to distinguish threat from safety. For example, in chronic migraine, central sensitization amplifies the brain's sensitivity to pain to such a degree that non-painful stimuli (e.g., touching one's hair) are perceived as agonizing pain (a condition called allodynia). In vestibular migraine, frequent attacks of vertigo and dizziness cause the brain to fear anything that could provoke dizziness. It grows anxious and hypervigilant of any stimuli that could make it dizzy. If visual motion causes dizziness, central sensitization causes the brain to become extremely sensitive to movement in the visual field; the slightest unexpected movement in one's visual periphery sends the brain into a frenzy. This constant state of high alert is the brain's coping mechanism, an attempt to protect itself from what it considers threatening, but unfortunately, this only fuels a vicious cycle of exponentially increasing dizziness.

Personality also plays a role in aggravating central sensitization. Most people with migraine are type A personalities and perfectionists. They tend to be very self-critical when they don't attain the goals they set. When vestibular migraine disrupts the ability to accomplish job activities, and family and social engagements, frustration and anger simmer. Most people bottle up their frustrations, rather than express these emotions healthily, and this pent-up, self-directed anger aggravates central sensitization.

Transforming Thinking Patterns

To understand how to rewire one's brain to promote adaptive neuroplasticity and break away from maladaptive neuroplasticity, we will briefly review briefly. The brain should respond to threats and challenges rapidly and rationally. Context is essential; the brain must decide whether a quick response is essential to survival or if a careful analysis is better. The frontal cortex and amygdala work closely together to respond appropriately to threats and dangers. In Dr. Daniel Kahneman's bestselling book, *Thinking, Fast and Slow*, he outlines two systems our brains use to respond to the world.

System 1 is predominantly driven by the limbic system. It is automatic, quick, and uses very little cognitive resources; it is unfortunately inaccurate and prone to bias and errors. System 1 was extremely important to our cavemen ancestors, allowing them to quickly react to any danger. Sensory information can bypass the cortex and go straight to the amygdala. Thus, the amygdala can detect fleeting threat signals even if they are not consciously perceived. The amygdalae are activated in experiments where pictures of fearful or angry expressions are flashed so quickly that subjects are not even aware of them. This is important in many vestibular disorders; stimuli that provoke dizziness may be quick and imperceptible (e.g., flickering fluorescent lights, a small but sudden head turn, something moving in the periphery of one's vision) but can activate the amygdalae. Reinforced by strong emotions, these shortcut sensory connections to the amygdala become stronger than the cortical-amygdala connections that govern the conscious perception of sensory stimuli. These shortcuts are often inaccurate; we may mistake a cellphone for a gun or a dust ball for a spider. Furthermore, certain interoceptive signals may also be mistaken as potential danger signals. For example, dizziness can trigger anxiety which is accompanied by increased heart rate. Over time, the amygdala associates increased heart rate with dizziness; thus, any time one's heart rate goes up, a stress or fear response is triggered (e.g., exercise, caffeine, excitement).

The second is a slower, cognitive processing of the stimulus; Dr. Kahneman's slow or System 2 thinking. This involves a more deliberate process that demands more cognitive resources, but usually ensures a more intelligent outcome. System 2 is controlled by the frontal (particularly, the prefrontal) cortex, the most evolutionarily advanced part of the brain and what distinguishes us from apes. System 2, as you can expect, helps us navigate a social world. It works with or tempers System 1, to ensure we do the right thing by integrating multiple streams of information, including the context of the situation, knowledge from similar experiences, and personal values. From a neuroscientific standpoint, the "right" thing is not the morally correct response but the best adaptive response for the organism. The frontal cortex is tasked with regulating and monitoring the threat responses, and ensuring the amygdala's response is appropriate. It teaches us that it is fine to freak out if a rat scurries across our kitchen floor but not appropriate to scream if you see a rat in the subway.

Transforming thinking patterns, and rewiring the dysfunctional networks in vestibular migraine involves engaging System 2 thinking. Extinction learning is the process by which the brain re-learns that conditions and stimuli that it associated with severe vertigo and dizziness were not as debilitating as it once believed. Recall the fear-conditioned lab rat discussed earlier. The rat learned that a tone was followed by a painful shock. In a new experimental setting, if the tone is not followed by a shock, the rat learns a new reality, "the tone *was* associated with a shock, but not now" and will no longer react in terror every time it hears it. Extinction learning does not erase the original fear memory but rather, reconditions the brain to not immediately activate anxiety and fear responses when a person encounters the previously triggering event(s).

Exposure (or desensitization) therapy is a psychological treatment for anxiety disorders that involves gradually exposing a person to a feared object or situation to allow extinction learning, where the brain re-learns the associations between the fear trigger(s) and safety. Exposure to the stimuli can be in real life (walking in a supermarket), imagined (imagining you are walking in a supermarket), virtual reality (simulating supermarket aisles), or interoceptive (exposure to the internal sensations generated by the brain's reaction to supermarkets, e.g., higher heart rate, more rapid breathing). Extinction learning allows us to use conscious thoughts (i.e., System 2 thinking) to control and regulate emotional responses, particularly the fear circuit. There are two ways to regulate the emotional response to a particular trigger: expressive suppression and cognitive reappraisal.

Expressive suppression is an attempt to stifle the expression of emotion. This method is ineffective at best and amplifies the emotional response at worst. If I told you not to think about a monkey, you'll immediately think of one. The more you try not to think about a monkey, the more your brain will conjure up images of monkeys. Try harder and a whole troop of monkeys will dance through your mind. Similarly, suppressing emotions only worsens the situation; if you don't believe me, try telling an upset person to stop crying. In addition, expressive suppression is reactive, i.e., it takes place only after the emotional response is in full swing. Expressive suppression is chasing the runaway emotional horse once it has escaped the barn. This is a more exhausting and stressful process and creates a feeling of inauthenticity, poorer self-esteem, depression, and anxiety.

Moreover, expressive suppression is detrimental to social functioning; because stifling emotions takes up a lot of focus and energy, the person cannot pay as much attention to interacting with others.

The more effective method is cognitive reappraisal, which is a reinterpretation of an emotion-provoking situation to alter its meaning and thus, transform its impact. Cognitive reappraisal occurs at an earlier stage, before the emotional response is fully activated. Cognitive reappraisal closes the barn door before the emotional horse flees. For example, telling yourself "I know exercise will make me dizzy but this is to be expected and will help me heal" before exercising helps mitigate the perceived severity of the dizziness and its emotional response. Cognitive reappraisal increases prefrontal cortex activity and diminishes fear network activity, especially in the amygdala and hippocampus. Essentially, it helps prefrontal cortex to regulate the amygdala and hippocampus; in other words, it helps System 2 control System 1.

Vestibular therapy is, in a way, a form of exposure therapy that desensitizes the brain to stimuli that provoke dizziness, by teaching the brain that such stimuli (e.g., moving one's head, walking in unfamiliar environments, going into a supermarket, driving, or busy visual scenes are not threats or dangers) may be uncomfortable but are not overly-threatening, thus extinguishing the fear a person has developed with these stimuli. The brain gradually learns that stimuli associated with crippling vertigo and dizziness are no longer as potent triggers.

Cognitive reappraisal techniques can be used to mitigate the limbic system's reaction to stimuli that provoke dizziness by using System 2 to replace old ways of thinking ("Exercise makes me so dizzy") with new truths ("Exercise may briefly make me dizzier, but will help me heal"). Cognitive behavioral therapy (CBT) is a psychological treatment that identifies faulty thinking patterns and behaviors and replaces them with adaptive ways of thinking and behaving. In a way, CBT enables a person to be his/her own therapist, providing them with tools to identify problematic thoughts, emotions, and behaviors, then correcting and replacing them with more adaptive patterns.

Frontal cortex requires a lot of energy to function. Adulting *is* exhausting. Brain fog is partly due to frontal cortex dysfunction when excessive resources are dedicated to dealing with the ongoing vestibular symptoms. Unsurprisingly, it takes effort to use System 2, instead of just relying on the gut instincts of System 1. It can be exhausting and frustrating in the beginning as you actively monitor negative thinking patterns or behaviors to correct them. The good news is that this process gets easier with practice. As you diligently work to extinguish maladaptive thoughts and behaviors, the process gets easier and even becomes automatic. For example, when you start a new diet, it is insanely tough to replace bread, cookies, cakes, pastries, and sweets with fruits, but if you persevere, these urges become less powerful, and choosing healthier options eventually becomes second nature.

Conscious thoughts can alter how we perceive vestibular sensations. This is very important because how we think and what we believe can make our vestibular symptoms worse, or better. In a fascinating Dutch study [Reuten, 2022], blindfolded healthy volunteers sat on a swing. In one scenario, they were told that the swing would be moving the whole time they sat on it and were instructed to focus on the movements. In the second scenario, they were told the swing would only move in the beginning and would eventually stop; in this scenario, the researchers also distracted them by asking irrelevant questions about the pitch differences of a tune. In both scenarios, the swing was moved briefly at the beginning of the experiment but was quickly brought to a stop. The first group reported feeling that the swing was moving much more and for much longer. This study elegantly illustrated how cognition can alter our perceptions of vestibular signals; on one hand, maladaptive beliefs can intensify vestibular symptoms, but adaptive thoughts and beliefs can actually diminish these symptoms. We can harness the power of System 2 thinking and prefrontal cortices to mitigate and reduce the severity of dizziness and vertigo.

Mindfulness & Metacognition

We live in an utterly distracted world. The number of things vying for our attention is endless... texts, emails, phone calls, social media, television, errands, etc. We so often lose ourselves and our focus in this maelstrom of distractions. To manage these intrusive distractions, a technique called mindfulness can function as a gatekeeper that walls off our psyches and monitors any stimulus that tries to enter. Mindfulness refers to "conscientiously being in the moment" by being fully present and carefully paying attention to the experiences of the current moment.

The opposite of mindfulness is mindlessness, which is essentially being on autopilot and allowing your mind to wander in any direction it likes. It occurs on that familiar drive to work or home, where your mind no longer pays attention to road conditions and begins thinking of what to do at work or once you get home. It occurs during boring meetings, when you start planning what to cook while a co-worker babbles through his interminable presentation. Mindlessness occurs when you are watching a television program or browsing social media while having dinner, and end up finishing the meal without really tasting it.

A simple exercise in mindfulness is to eat a small meal alone. No phone, no TV, no distractions. As you eat it slowly, notice the colors, flavors, textures, and temperature of each bite. How does each bite make you feel? That meal would have been the most pleasurable experience for many people. It highlights the power of mindfulness, being in the moment, and fully immersing yourself in the present.

Mindfulness can help improve your awareness of your body and emotions. You will notice unpleasant sensations, heart rate, breathing, and muscle tone. You will learn how to recognize changes in your internal state of being. With roots in ancient

Buddhist teachings, mindfulness entered modern medicine through the work of Professor Jon Kabat-Zinn among people with chronic illnesses. Since his pioneering work, mindfulness has become a proven therapy for stress management, anxiety, depression, pain, eating disorders, and many other diseases. Multiple studies have confirmed the power of mindfulness on chronic illnesses, including migraine.

People with vestibular migraine can benefit immensely from mindfulness. It improves your resilience to stress, helps your cognitive abilities, breaks the dizziness-anxiety cycle, enhances your sense of well-being, and brings you into harmony with your body. It re-directs your attention from worrying about how the dizziness and vertigo are making you feel miserable, to why you feel that way and about how to manage it. Mindfulness can help you learn your body and brain's limits, work within those limits, and work on expanding those limits. It can help you identify negative thoughts and emotions, and neutralize them before they gain a foothold.

Misreading interoceptive and vestibular information is a common problem in people with vestibular migraine. For example, it is normal for everyone to feel slightly disoriented if they get up too fast, or if they stare too hard at the TV while someone is scrolling quickly on Netflix. Because of central sensitization, any hint of dizziness is associated with the anticipation of terrible vertigo. When a person with vestibular migraine experiences slight disorientation (even if normal), the brain goes bananas screaming about an impending vertigo attack. Similarly, in those with anxiety, racing thoughts and heart rate are instantly associated with panic attacks, even though they may occur in other situations (e.g., exercise, caffeine). Mindfulness can stop this spiral, allowing a person to step back and interpret the interoceptive signals correctly.

Mindfulness and metacognition also help you deal with negative thoughts and emotions that come with vestibular migraine. Our bodies "listen" to our internal monologues. If we constantly tell ourselves that we are ill and will not get better, we deteriorate. I am by no means promoting "positive thinking" – you don't have to go around with a forced smile on your face and pretend everything is honky-dory. I am also not endorsing the law of attraction (i.e., thinking about good things attracts them, and vice versa).

Negative thoughts and emotions are a normal and natural part of dealing with a chronic invisible illness like vestibular migraine. The key is not to let them take root and poison your mind. Recognize and analyze them and don't let them consume you. Metacognition refers to the process of analyzing your thoughts in a detached manner; you become your own therapist and "think about how you think". Metacognition can help you gain awareness of your strengths, and weaknesses while arming you to manage negative thoughts and emotions.

When a negative thought or emotion intrudes, pause, and address it. The first step is to recognize the negative thought. Be mindful when a negative thought or emotion enters your mind, and take a moment to identify it.

The second step is to classify that thought. These negative thoughts or emotions fit into several categories.

"If only" thoughts: Self-defeating thoughts that make you feel less than your pre-vestibular migraine self. "If only I was well", "If only I was not dizzy", "If I only I could attend my son's graduation party", or "If only I could attend that concert". These thoughts serve no good purpose and only depress you.

Filtering: The filter sieves out positive thoughts but allows negative ones in. For example, a person with vestibular migraine who has improved significantly might focus on how they are *still* slightly dizzy when they look at busy patterns and ignore how much progress they have made and how infrequent their vertigo attacks are. Such thoughts are discouraging; they demotivate you from working at changing your life for the better.

Disqualifying the positives: Similar to filtering, this pattern is characterized by a pessimistic *rejection* of anything positive. A person may think their improvement is just a fluke and everything is bound to worsen again. They reject any positive results and dwell solely on the negative.

Magnification & minimization: These thoughts magnify perceived negatives and minimize positives. A person who finds it difficult to work under fluorescent lighting at work may think they are a poor employee while completely discounting the fact that their performance remains above average. A more severe form of this pattern is *catastrophic thinking* where a person focuses excessively on the worst possible outcome, however unlikely ("I'm definitely going to get a bad rash from this medication"). Catastrophic thinking is common during vertigo attacks, and during periods of increased dizziness. Frequent thoughts that occur are "Oh my God, this is going to be horrible", "I am going to fall and the whole office will come running to stare", "I won't be able to drive home", "What if I collapse in the store?". Catastrophic thinking worsens anxiety and may trigger panic attacks.

"What if" questions: This type of thinking makes a person focus on the negative outcome. What if I get dizzy at the store and cannot leave? What if I embarrass myself? What if this medication causes a bad side effect? What if I never get better? What if I lose my job? These are thoughts that keep you beaten down, discouraging you from picking yourself up and getting better.

Polarized thinking: Also called "black-or-white" or "all-or-nothing", this pattern fails to appreciate the shades of gray. An example is a person who thinks "I still have a vertigo attack when the weather changes, therefore I'm not better" instead of paying attention to how the frequency of vertigo attacks has improved. It is closely related to psychological inflexibility, the mentality of "either I am completely well, or I cannot do anything to enjoy life".

Overgeneralization: This causes a person to make an unfounded generalization based on one or two pieces of evidence (i.e. jumping to conclusions). For instance, one may think "I had side effects with medications A and B, therefore I am too sensitive and will have side effects with every medication". An extreme form of it is called global labeling, where a person attaches an emotionally loaded and unhealthy label to themselves; for example, they may say "I'm a failure" because they have trouble coping at work because of their dizziness.

Fortune telling: This thought distortion causes people to think that the future is pre-ordained and there is nothing they can do about it. For example, they may think that their parent had horrible migraine, and that they are also destined to suffer from horrible migraine no matter what they do. This fatalistic attitude stops you from even trying to improve your life; these thoughts whisper "Why even bother?".

"I should" thoughts: These thoughts force a judgmental attitude on oneself and create guilt when one cannot live up to them. Examples include: I should finish the laundry, I should always cook dinner for my family, I should not have to take breaks at work, I should be able to do more around the house. Self-judgement produces and worsens depression, and must be rooted out.

Emotional Reasoning: the essence of this distortion is "If I feel this way, it must be true". Examples include, "If I feel my migraine won't get better, it will never get better" or "If I feel this medication will cause side effects, it will". This irrational, and closed-minded attitude robs you of being open to new experiences and treatments.

Personalization: This pattern makes you take everything personally and irrationally blame yourself. This pattern erodes relationships and friendships. For example, if the food at a dinner party is not good, you subconsciously blame yourself ("Maybe if I didn't ask them to exclude MSG, dinner wouldn't have been such a disaster") although you had nothing to do with the chef's lack of culinary skill.

The process of recognizing and categorizing a thought or emotion is called *affect labeling*. It is the act of verbalizing your internal emotional experience and is a subtle but highly effective way of disempowering that emotion or thought. The simple act of explicitly labeling a negative thought or emotion reduces its emotional load, physiological response, and behavior. This is why journaling or blogging is therapeutic and why one talks about feelings in psychotherapy. Studies prove that affect labeling changes the pattern of brain activity, by reducing activity in regions responsible for threat perception.

The third step is to analyze the thought rationally. Is it a really logical thought? For example, if you think that you are a failure because your dizziness makes it difficult to complete certain chores, think about how your family loves you, how you can care for them in other ways, and whether asking for some help in completing certain chores really makes you a failure. You will realize that most negative thoughts are irrational and don't deserve any mental space whatsoever.

The fourth step is to release it. Once you realize that negative thought or emotion has no basis in reality, release it and go on with life. Don't entertain it any longer. Move on.

The Mindful Metacognitive Approach to Negative Thoughts and Emotions
1. Recognize it 2. Label it 3. Analyze it 4. Release it

When you feel dizzy, don't just suppress it or panic. Use the mindful approach. First, recognize that you are dizzy. Second, label it; describe the sensation to yourself. Use the definitions of vestibular symptoms in Chapter 2. Third, analyze why you are dizzy; is it a vestibular migraine attack, motion sickness, or caused by visual stimuli. If it is a migraine attack, use your rescue medication. If it is not an attack, analyze how you can avoid it in the future; perhaps consider moving your head more carefully, taking a break from using the computer, or not scrolling too fast on your phone. Fourth, feel the dizziness dissipate. This will not only help you identify the cause of your dizziness and recognize your brain's limits but also prevent your mind from spiraling into negativity.

The first rule is to keep an untroubled spirit. The second is to look things in the face and know them for what they are.
Marcus Aurelius, Meditations

Perceived Control, Self-Efficacy & Learned Helplessness

Psychologist Julian Rotter introduced the concept of perceived control in 1966 in his publication entitled "Generalized Expectancies for Internal versus External Control of Reinforcement". Perceived control is the belief one has in one's ability to influence a particular outcome, behavior, or process. Put simply, it is the belief in one's control over one's destiny. A person takes positive actions to better the future if he/she believes in his/her ability to influence it. For example, one adopts a migraine-friendly diet if one believes this will reduce migraine attacks.

Self-efficacy, a concept introduced by psychologist Albert Bandura, is closely related to perceived control. It is defined as one's belief in one's ability to successfully accomplish a particular task. Self-efficacy is formed by your personal experiences and from interacting with others. Our previous experiences, observation of other's experiences, and feedback from others influence our self-efficacy. It affects all aspects of our life, but is not global –self-efficacy may be strong in some areas but weaker in others. For example, I feel quite capable of treating vestibular migraine but definitely cannot fly a plane or knit a sweater.

Learned helplessness, a concept introduced by psychologist Martin Seligman, is a condition where humans or animals learn to behave helplessly in particular situations after experiencing some failure to escape adversity. Learned helplessness is the moral of the elephant rope story. In this fable, a man at the circus sees full-grown adult elephants tethered by small ropes around one leg. He asks the trainer why the elephants just stood there when they could easily snap the ropes. The trainer informs him that a similar rope effectively restrained the elephants as small calves and even though they had grown into massive beasts, they were conditioned to believe that they could never break free. These elephants learned to be helpless.

Chronic unpredictable illnesses like vestibular migraine erode perceived control and self-efficacy. You must be aware of this psychological dynamic to avoid falling into learned helplessness. People with chronic illnesses who believe they can manage their symptoms do much better than those who believe that their symptoms are beyond their control. Unsurprisingly, higher self-efficacy translates to better treatment outcomes. This is the primary reason for this book —to equip you with the tools to manage your vestibular migraine and help you take control of this condition. *You* are the CEO of your health and *you* can control what happens. Vestibular migraine is incurable but it is very treatable; many get their lives back.

Meditation & Prayer

Some have valid concerns about merging religion and science, but for the treatment of a chronic invisible illness like vestibular migraine, we should embrace as many therapies as possible. If something is safe and potentially effective, let us embrace it. I am not, of course, endorsing any particular religion, or claiming that one specific religion holds the cure for vestibular migraine. If a particular belief or faith resonates with you, I encourage you to participate in it. Do something that holds meaning for you.

Prayer and meditation have such profound and fascinating effects on the brain that a field called neurotheology was created. Regardless of your faith, prayer is an effective therapy for improving the quality of life and well-being in chronic illnesses, including cancer and migraine [Matthews, 2000; Coleman, 2006; Olver, 2012; Tajadini, 2017].

A fascinating study found that praying actually changes brain activity in people with depression and breaks the link to the trauma that triggered their depression in the first place [Baldwin, 2016]. Like prayer, meditation is effective at improving a range of chronic disorders. Spiritual meditation reduces migraine frequency [Wachholtz, 2017]. Like prayer, meditation alters brain activity. Prayer and meditation appear to elevate activity in the dopamine and serotonin pathways (which is why they promote a sense of well-being), which are important in migraine.

Meditation enhances activity in the prefrontal cortex and insula, and regulate the limbic system. Regular mediation improves the practitioner's consciousness of their internal body states because of higher insula function. These changes occur during and persist after meditation. Recall that the insula processes interoceptive (internally generated) and exteroceptive (externally generated) information. In regular practitioners, meditation enlarges these parts of the brain.

Mindfulness meditation preferentially enhances the prefrontal cortex, essentially harnessing System 2 to calm the turbulent System 1. Mindfulness meditation improves attention, self-awareness, stress levels, and emotional regulation. It is effective in treating people with vestibular disorders, improving the severity of dizziness and limitations, and improving mood and functional abilities [Naber, 2011]. In mindfulness meditation, the person focuses on only one thing during the session (e.g., breathing) and pushes out all distracting thoughts. The following are some ideas for meditation that can help in certain situations.

Daily Mindful Meditation

Make this a habit. It would be great to do it three times a day but you start with once a day. Find a quiet spot and allocate 5 minutes to meditate as such:

1. Sit in a comfortable position with the back straight or lie down.

2. Begin performing controlled breathing. Inhale for 5 seconds, pause and hold the breath for 10 seconds, exhale over 5 seconds, then take 5 ordinary breaths. Repeat this over 5 minutes.

3. Be aware of each breath, and count the seconds. If you cannot hold the exhale for 10 seconds, hold it for as long as you can but work your way on building up to 10 seconds.

4. If your mind begins to stray, return it to your breathing.

5. If any unpleasant sensations or thoughts arise, spend a few moments analyzing and describing them and then feel them dissipate with every breath.

Mindful meditation when you are dizzy

If the mindful approach to dizziness does not work, you can try this technique:

1. Pay attention to the discomfort and analyze it as logically as you can, what does it feel like? How bad is it? What caused it?

2. Close your eyes, tilt your head down slightly, and put yourself in a "grounded position" (sit on a solid chair with a firm back and neck support if possible, or stand with your back against a pillar or wall with your feet apart)

3. Perform controlled breathing (see Daily Mindful Meditation).

4. Use your mind to perform a body scan to analyze for other unpleasant sensations like nausea, tremors, pain, weakness, or numbness. Start in the feet and move towards the head slowly.

5. Spend a few moments on each unpleasant sensation, and feel them dissipate with each exhaled breath

6. If negative thoughts or emotions enter your mind, label them as you feel each one dissipate with every exhalation.

Guided Imagery Meditation

This easy relaxation technique is highly effective for stress control. It produces physiological relaxation and is clinically proven to reduce anxiety, headaches, insomnia, and psychological stress. Guided imagery utilizes all the senses to build an experience in your mind that your body perceives as real. Apps like *Headspace* walk you through the entire experience, providing a narrative to help you build that mental experience. There are also many free videos of guided imagery meditation available online. Set aside 5-10 minutes once a day to perform guided imagery meditation. You can perform it at work to mitigate stress levels or at bedtime to unwind and sleep.

A quick guided imagery meditation when you are dizzy is to sit on a firm chair with back support, close your eyes, and lean your head back against the chair. Begin controlled breathing. Use your mind to focus on how stable you are in that grounded position, as you imagine yourself as a large tree firmly rooted in the earth. Visualize the deep roots extending into the earth and rocks for support, the thick stable trunk, and the branches that rise to the heavens firmly connected to the trunk. Smell the earth and grass around the tree. Feel the breeze around you, and hear the leaves rustle. Repeat the phrase "I am grounded, stable, and strong" as you perform this guided imagery meditation. After 5 minutes, your dizziness will improve.

A useful guided imagery meditation technique for insomnia is performing controlled breathing exercises, while visualizing gentle dark waters slowly enveloping you until you are completely submerged and drawn into a deep sleep. Imagine hearing the soft lapping sounds of the waves around you, and feeling the breeze against your skin. Do this until you fall asleep.

The Mind's Eye: The Power of Visualization

For anyone with dizziness and vertigo, the very thought of certain activities can be daunting and intimidating. The instinctual animal brain reminds you of the dizziness and vertigo associated with those activities and warns you away from them. Remember that you must "upwire" to build up your tolerance and ability for these activities. You must not "downwire" and avoid everything you fear may make you dizzy.

Visualization is a scientifically proven method of improving your performance and abilities. Visualizing how to play a music piece improves one's ability to do so. Visualizing golf swings enhances your golfing skills. The brain uses visualizations to simulate future experiences, priming the neurons and brain regions responsible for controlling a specific activity for optimal performance when the time comes. Visualization can improve your confidence, motivation, and ability to achieve a specific goal.

You can use visualization to your advantage when it comes to exercising or performing any activity you feel may make you dizzy. Before vestibular exercises, visualize yourself going through that entire exercise, executing it perfectly. For example, before you perform the tandem walking exercises, take a few seconds to picture yourself walking heel to toe forwards and backward in a perfectly straight line. This will improve your confidence and ability to do so. You can combine visualization with mindfulness; as you imagine tandem walking, doubts, anxiety and negative thoughts may creep in. Take a moment and perform the Mindful Metacognitive Approach to deal with those negative thoughts and emotions.

Similarly, if you have to a grocery store, take a few minutes to perform a visualization exercise before even getting into your car. Use your mind's eye to see yourself driving to the store, the traffic conditions, entering the store, going to specific aisles to pick out the items you need, getting to the checkout lane, going back to your car, and heading home. Be as specific as possible and add as many details as possible. Imagine the parking lot, familiar cashiers, the aisles, and even your cart. The more detailed your visualization, the more impactful this exercise will be. As you visualize the trip, be aware of negative thoughts and emotions that intrude and use the Mindful Metacognitive Approach to deal with them. Visualize yourself navigating the store with perfect balance, without any dizziness whatsoever. You will find that this improves your experience and builds your confidence.

Biofeedback

Biofeedback is a mind-body technique that helps a person alter their physiological responses to improve physical, mental, and spiritual health. Biofeedback is the process of gaining awareness and insight into physiological functions by utilizing instruments to measure specific functions and generate actionable feedback, enabling the person to consciously influence these functions.

A biofeedback therapist uses specific instruments to help bring unconscious physiologic processes to conscious awareness, allowing the person to alter these processes. In a sense, we perform biofeedback whenever we learn a new task. When learning how to write, a child scribbles and scrawls, and learns from his/her own observations and critique from adults, until writing becomes effortless. When learning a new dance, a person watches his or her reflection in a mirror and corrects mistakes until the dance routine is perfected.

Biofeedback reduces the frequency, duration, and severity of migraine attacks. It is also effective for a variety of vestibular disorders, including PPPD. Effective biofeedback therapy requires a certified and experienced therapist to identify the most appropriate physiologic marker. For example, a temperature probe can be attached to the index finger so the person can practice how to increase blood flow to the finger. An electromyographic (EMG) skin probe on the neck muscles can help a person learn relaxation techniques to reduce neck muscle spasms and tightness. Neurofeedback (or neurotherapy) refers to a specific form of biofeedback that uses electroencephalography (EEG) to measure real-time changes in brain waves and help a person alter them.

Be sure that the biofeedback therapist is qualified. The Biofeedback Certification International Alliance (formerly the Biofeedback Certification Institute of America) is a non-profit organization that certifies those who possess the education, training, and experience for biofeedback and neurofeedback.

Never let the future disturb you. You will meet it, if you have to, with the same weapons of reason which today arm you against the present.
Marcus Aurelius, Meditations

Chapter 20: Build Your Support Network

We do not heal in insolation, but in community.
S. Kelley Harrell

In Chapter 19, we discussed how the brain responds to challenges and stressors via System 1 (the quick, but imprecise, emotional response), and System 2 (the slower, but more accurate, intelligent response). As social creatures, humans have evolved another adaptation to help with challenges and stress: seeking help from others.

Ironically, the increased connectivity afforded by the internet and social media apps has led to a breakdown in social bonds and a rise in isolation. Loneliness is a growing problem in developed societies and sharply worsened by the COVID-19 pandemic.

Loneliness is associated with pro-inflammatory states, degenerative diseases, cardiovascular disease, and premature death. Loneliness is an insidious epidemic slowly eroding the health of many. Social ties and the assurance that one is cared for by those in one's social network positively affect health.

Since many migraine symptoms (e.g., light sensitivity, noise sensitivity, dizziness, motion sickness) make it difficult to engage in many social settings, loneliness and social isolation are major problems among people with migraine. A vicious cycle can ensure – social isolation worsens migraine symptoms, which leads to greater social isolation.

Decreased intimate relationships are associated with a higher migraine headache prevalence [Cohen, 2011]. People with migraine who are lonely also tend to have poorer self-management capabilities [Lui, 2020], which refer to abilities to regulate one's actions, emotions, and thoughts. The importance of a support network is often forgotten when discussing migraine treatment.

For people with chronic invisible illnesses like vestibular migraine, building a support network helps equip them to face the challenges of their journeys, learn from the experiences of others, make new friends who share similar challenges, and help others heal. There are many allies to help you on your journey, each providing crucial forms of support for you to heal.

Medical Allies

You will need a physician who is familiar with vestibular migraine to serve as your quarterback and guide your treatment plans. This is a life-long journey and you will need a physician who can help you through it, step by step. As such, you need to ensure that you build a good working relationship with your treating physician. A specialist in vestibular disorders and/or migraine is usually best since they are more aware of the condition and the latest treatments, and can diagnose and treat other conditions that cause vertigo and dizziness.

Another critical ally to your overall health is a good primary care physician, who can help coordinate care across various specialties. Your vestibular migraine expert will usually be a neurologist (typically a headache specialist), or an otolaryngologist (usually a neuro-otologist) and therefore, may not be as well-versed in other medical problems, like diabetes, high blood pressure, or thyroid disorders that can affect migraine control and aggravate dizziness. For this, you will need a primary care physician who can oversee your care and treat other medical conditions or refer you to the appropriate specialists if needed.

If you plan to get pregnant or get on hormone replacement, you will need an obstetrician and gynecologist to guide you along the way. Your OBGYN will provide you with the most up-to-date information on medications that are safe for pregnancy and breastfeeding, as well as the risks of hormone replacement.

If you have significant anxiety, depression, PTSD, or a psychiatric disorder, a psychiatrist would be important to your care. Most neurologists and primary care physicians are comfortable managing antidepressant medications to an extent but if these first-line treatments are ineffective, consulting with a psychiatrist is important. Psychiatrists also work closely with psychologists to help provide medication(s), psychotherapy, or cognitive-behavioral therapy.

If the physician managing your vestibular migraine is a neurologist, you may need to have an ENT specialist if you experience ear-related symptoms, like tinnitus, hearing impairment, or ear pressure. While some of these symptoms may be migraine-related, it is always important to monitor for otolaryngologic disorders.

A well-trained, experienced vestibular therapist is invaluable to your team. A vestibular therapist can help reduce your visually-induced and head motion-induced dizziness, help improve your gait and balance, and help treat conditions like BPPV and PPPD. It is important to look for a vestibular therapist, not just a physical therapist who performs basic vestibular exercises. A vestibular therapist will customize a specific exercise plan for your *individual* needs. I have seen many patients who report no benefit from vestibular therapy but were actually treated by physical therapists who were not experienced in treating vestibular disorders and only gave these patients the simplest of vestibular exercises rather than tailoring specific exercises according to their needs.

Family & Friends

Your partner, children, family members and close friends are your most important allies in this journey. These are the people who are with you the most, and your relationship with them is crucial in your healing.

Your partner will be your closest ally, helping you through this journey. Research shows that partners of people with chronic illnesses experience positive emotional and personal growth during their journeys. In fact, facing a chronic illness together strengthens the bond between partners. Bring your partner along with you to your doctor visits if possible. Talk to your partner about migraine and help them understand how it affects you. Discuss your triggers and the lifestyle changes you need to control your migraine. For example, discuss food triggers and what you have to avoid, then discuss options that both of you would enjoy. There are many things you can do to help your spouse help you. Tell your partner what you need and what you can do. Be specific; do not expect your partner to read your mind. Your partner also needs personal time; let them know that this is ok with you, so that they do not feel guilty. It is ok for your partner to go to the gym or attend social or family functions alone; you do not want them to feel isolated and lonely. Spend quality time with your partner on your good days. This is important to help keep the relationship thriving. Gifts are also a great way of showing your appreciation to your spouse.

Your children will be great allies as well. You will be surprised at how understanding, mature and dependable your children can be when you explain your limitations to them. Offer different activities, like reading together or an art project to replace more rambunctious play. Try to make everything a game to keep them engaged. There are many game ideas online, including those that involve being as quiet as possible. For example, the *graveyard* is a game where everyone has to be as still and quiet as possible; the first person to move or speak loses. In the statue game, children have to pose as particular statues (e.g., cat, dog) for as long as possible. Let other adults in the family help take care of them. Allow them more time to play with their friends. Take the time to explain what vestibular migraine is and how it affects you. To allay their fears, emphasize that vestibular migraine is not contagious or fatal. Get them to help you with house chores; make a game out of it so that it is fun for them, and you can bond with them over the activities. Reward your children for helping you around the house and if they are well-behaved.

Adult family members and friends can also be a great source of support. Just having them check on you and knowing they are there for you through the highs and lows can do wonders for your sense of well-being. They can help watch your kids if you feel unwell or if you need some alone time with your spouse. They can also help with tasks or errands. When you are feeling better, reciprocate by offering to help them, cook them a meal, or give them a gift.

Many mistakenly isolate themselves from family and friends because they are afraid of being a burden and an inconvenience. Realize that your loved ones are not judging you. They want to help and feel powerless when they see your suffering but cannot make it better. They feel trapped between the helplessness of not knowing how to help, and the fear of making your condition worse. If you sublimate self-judgment as judgment by others, you alienate others and isolate yourself. Reach out, let them know you need them, and let them know how they can help. Be specific. For example, ask for help unloading the dishwasher if that makes you really dizzy. Or ask for help cleaning the top shelves if looking upwards for too long makes you dizzy. Ask someone to help you with grocery shopping if the store is too overwhelming. Help them understand how to help you.

When they do offer help, don't take it as a personal insult or an attempt to coddle you; they are genuinely concerned. Tell them politely if you don't need help this time but may need it in the future, and thank them. Learn to say no sometimes; if you have a migraine attack, it is ok to decline social or family functions. If you get an invitation, it's ok to say "I'm sorry, but this may be a bit too much for me". They need you to be truthful about your boundaries and limitations.

Unless your friends and family members accompany you to your doctors' appointments, they will most likely not be very familiar with vestibular migraine. You will need to explain what vestibular migraine is, how it impacts you, what treatments you are on, and what to expect. However, avoid the TMI (too much information) trap. Don't overwhelm people with information. Let them learn at their own pace. Answer the questions they have, keep it sweet and short, and spare them the details unless they are genuinely curious and want to learn.

Community Support

Far from being simple, our inner life has something like a double center of gravity. On the one hand is our individuality... on the other is everything in us that expresses something other than ourselves.
Émile Durkheim

The great French sociologist Émile Durkheim promulgated the concept of *homo duplex*, the two-level human. On one level is the biological creature, driven by base instincts for survival and pleasure, and on the other level is the elevated moral and social being. Professor of social psychology, Jonathan Haidt, speaks of a "staircase" experience, the warm uplifting feeling of moral elevation, as we transcend ourselves, rising from selfish biological organisms to ascendant moral beings focused on the welfare of others and the community.

This staircase experience elevates us to become part of something much larger than ourselves, a community with a greater purpose. Finding and plugging into a community of people who are going through similar experiences as yourself will transform you. You will focus less on your own symptoms and sufferings and dedicate more energy to the betterment of your fellow community members, and this will improve your physical, emotional, and spiritual well-being.

Find an online community. There are many online groups and patient support associations. Ensure that the group you join is non-hostile and supportive. Check to ensure that it is not infiltrated by crooks trying to peddle quack cures.

These online groups can be very helpful. You will be able to tap into the experiences of people from all around the country and even the world. Such communities can often help you discover new treatments or new ways of doing things to improve your quality of life. They can also put you in touch with specialists who can guide your treatment.

Blogging, vlogging, or producing art about your experiences with vestibular migraine can be a therapeutic outlet, allowing you to vent your frustrations and emotions, and connect with others.

Find in-person support groups. It is one thing to read comments on a computer screen but nothing beats being in the same room with people who understand and empathize with your symptoms. There is just something about gathering in a group to share experiences and ideas.

In-person support groups can also be platforms for organizing events like outings, easy-to-watch movies, and migraine-friendly dinners. If no such in-person support group exists in your area, take the initiative and form your very own group. You can start by looking for people with vestibular migraine online who happen to live in the same town or city, plan a meeting, and *voila*, you have just had your inaugural meeting. Another option is forming a support group as a branch of an existing support group; for example, if you are part of a large support group for vestibular disorders, you can form a support group with other members who have vestibular migraine. You could also ask your vestibular migraine specialist to forward your contact information to other patients with vestibular migraine, so you can connect with them and form a support group.

Join an organization. Many organizations help people with chronic diseases like migraine. These organizations provide information about the health conditions they were formed to address, put people in touch with the right specialists and organize educational lectures or other events.

The *Vestibular Disorders Association* (VEDA) is a non-profit organization that aims to inform and support people who suffer from vestibular disorders, including vestibular migraine. *Miles for Migraine* is an organization that raises awareness for migraine, and organizes walks to raise funds to sponsor training for future headache specialists; it has local chapters that also organize in-person group meetings. Other organizations include the *Mal de Debarquement Syndrome Foundation, Migraine Strong*, and the *Association of Migraine Disorders*.

Find spiritual support. Regardless of your religious beliefs, there is a subconscious or spiritual impact from chronic illnesses like vestibular migraine. Religious organizations can often provide volunteers who will check in on you and help you with errands and chores. They may even help you build your own in-person support group by providing logistical support (venue, food, publicity, etc.).

Dealing with Doubters

Unfortunately, you will encounter people who may doubt your symptoms and illness. Such is the fate of those afflicted with chronic invisible illnesses. It will be frustrating, but you will need to prepare yourself for this.

The Doubting Physician. If you have a physician who does not believe you or your symptoms, you may need to find a new one if the doubting physician's continued care may negatively impact your health. I have a few patients whose family physicians did not believe they had migraine and discontinued their migraine medications due to an irrational fear of side effects, causing their migraines to flare up again, after many months of superb control.

One particular physician (fresh out of residency training) wrote in a clinic note that my patient's treatment consisted of "exotic and unproven combinations of antidepressants" without realizing that the combination was the result of two years of tweaking doses and formulations to find just the right balance between efficacy and side effects.

I encourage my patients to advocate for themselves and not allow other physicians to discontinue their migraine meds without first consulting with me. Another physician can (and should) recommend stopping a particular migraine treatment if there is a more pressing or urgent health problem (e.g., stopping topiramate if you have kidney disease); we can always transition to a different migraine medication. However, if you have a physician who insists on stopping your vestibular migraine medications without clear reasons to do so, you may need to find another physician.

The Doubting Spouse/Partner. A spouse who does not believe your diagnosis or symptoms is a more challenging problem. Fortunately, most of the people with migraine I know have amazingly supportive partners. What if your spouse accuses you of making things up? What if they don't believe that you are as sick as you say you are? The first step is to avoid getting into an argument and fighting back. This will only worsen the situation.

Inquire about their family members or friends who have had chronic illnesses to look for clues about their current attitudes. Is there some resentment stemming from their parents devoting their time to a sickly sibling at the expense of their healthier children? Did they have a sick parent who missed family, school, and important life events? Did they have a relative with a chronic illness whom everyone called a hypochondriac behind her back? Often, our childhood experiences shape our views and attitudes of the world.

Help your spouse learn about migraine by bringing them to support group meetings and doctor's appointments, so that they can also ask questions about the disease. Share material about migraine with them. If they are not interested in learning about your illness, or focusing on how to help you, they are probably not with you for the right reasons. Couple therapy or counseling may be needed in cases where friction and suspicion become more pervasive.

Doubting Family & Friends. Family members and friends who don't believe you can be very negative influences. Similarly, look into their history to see if there is a source of this disbelief or perhaps resentment. You can also explain your symptoms, what vestibular migraine is, and what to expect. Share informational resources with them. If they take no interest in learning and continue to undermine your credibility and cast doubt on your symptoms, you may need to disengage from them. Some people are just not sympathetic and will never understand. A crisis often brings out people's true character. When you have a chronic invisible illness, you will see which family members and friends truly care about you.

Well-meaning but misinformed friends and family members are trickier. They are genuinely concerned and feel strongly that their misinformed ideas are the best for you. Their doubts and fallacious information are more insidious and can be harder to manage.

A situation I often encounter is when a patient is told by a friend, "Oh, I know someone who had horrible side effects with antidepressants. You should never take antidepressants!" or "You shouldn't take these pills. You'll get addicted to them!". Remember, medications affect everyone differently, and the choice to use a particular one for your migraine depends on the benefit-to-risk ratio of your unique situation.

You may need to take friendly advice with a grain of salt. Gently try to educate them about migraine, but don't argue. Though well-meaning, not every bit of advice is sound or suitable for you.

Beware toxic negative personalities

While support groups are usually wonderful places that inform and support, look for groups that motivate and avoid those filled with toxic, negative people. Everyone has some negative experiences, of course, and it is perfectly healthy to share those and discuss them. However, when someone complains of bad experiences almost all the time, they are most likely a toxic negative personality.

These chronically unhappy souls never have anything good to say about anyone or anything. They find fault in every little thing and perpetually feel that the world has wronged them. Toxic negative people find perverse fulfillment in publicizing their suffering and complaining. A deep, subconscious, insidious psychopathology drives them to *embrace* the role of victim and the perpetual martyr. They spout negativity about everything, even offering their unwanted opinions about matters of which they really know nothing. Even if the vast majority report amazing positive experiences, toxic negative people *always* find something to gripe about. These bitter souls try to discourage everyone else from getting better. They *want* to be miserable and they want you to be miserable with them.

Often, they sabotage their own treatment plans with irrational prejudice, refusing treatments because they believe nothing will work or that everything will cause side effects. Many destroy their relationship with their doctors by being unreasonable, rude, and overly demanding. Perversely proud, they then declare, "No doctor can help me! Nothing works for me! The medical field has failed me!" Toxic negative personalities will see the best specialists in their field but still gripe and complain that they could not help them at all. Subconsciously, they really don't want to get better because their warped sense of identity is bound to their perpetual suffering. They are the ones who will always find some way to criticize what you are doing to heal. They will instill doubt and fear in your mind ("Better don't take that medication. I hear bad things about it" or "Why go see that doctor? All doctors are the same!") to keep you in the same poisonous misery they stew in.

Learn how to recognize these toxic negative individuals. Avoid them at all costs. Don't be seduced by their "straight talk" or "honesty". Don't give them the attention they crave. Ignore them and cut them off. Isolate and ostracize them. They will sap your strength and infect you with their venom. They are not worth your time and energy. When you see their comments (they *love* to express their wretched cynicism online – it's like a full-time job for them), skip past and don't even bother to read them. Quickly label these personalities "toxic negative" in your mind and ignore their bitter grumblings. Block them if possible.

Conclusion

Remember, you are not alone. You are not alone in your journey with vestibular migraine. Find medical allies and help your loved ones help you. Find a community of support that uplifts, motivates, and encourages each other. This network of support will be invaluable to your healing and journey.

You won't understand the unabashed power of a community until you're a part of one
Anonymous

Chapter 21: Planning for the Future

The most reliable way to predict the future is to create it.
Abraham Lincoln (1809-1865)

Throughout this book, we understand that vestibular migraine is a chronic invisible illness that is incurable *but* can be very effectively controlled in the vast majority of people. In a very small number, the symptoms can be very difficult to control despite our best efforts. In most, even though we can control it well, there may be periods where it flares up and causes significant debility. Vestibular migraine can affect many aspects of life, including relationships, finances, school, and work. It can help tremendously to be prepared to face these scenarios.

First, I prepare. Then I have faith.
Joe Namath

Advocating for Yourself

Advocating for yourself as a patient means assuming an active role in your care and taking the necessary steps. Self-advocacy enables your physicians to care for you more effectively and ensure that your needs are being addressed.

Information is power. Earlier in this book, we discussed the characteristics of vestibular symptoms. Diagnosing vestibular disorders requires a detailed history. You must be cognizant of your symptoms (including the characteristics, triggers, and temporal profile) and previous treatments (those that worked and those that failed) to provide all the data your physician needs to accurately diagnose your illness. Keeping a journal of symptoms is an objective way of tracking them. I have created a Vestibular Journal to help you log your symptoms more effectively.

Documentation. Keep copies of your tests and medical notes to ensure continuity of care. Although the physician referring you to a specialist often provides their medical records, this is sometimes incomplete because they may not have access to tests and notes from other physicians' offices. If you have seen multiple physicians for vertigo and dizziness, ensuring that all these records are faxed to a specialist you are consulting can be as difficult as herding cats. Keeping a copy of your records will greatly facilitate this process. Time and resources will not be wasted searching for information or repeating tests.

Maximize your time with your physician. The constraints imposed by rising costs and diminishing insurance reimbursements mean that physicians are being forced to see more patients. This means shorter and rushed visits. The average medical appointment is now 17 minutes. Having a copy of your medical records, being aware of your symptoms, and preparing a list of questions to ask can help make full use of your visit.

Get to your appointment early. I know it's frustrating to wait at the doctor's office for your appointment, but physicians often run late as unexpected issues often arise during patient visits. You need to get there early so as not to miss your appointment. Most physicians will still see you if you are late but the visit will be shorter so that other patients are not kept waiting too long. If you are seeing a physician for the first time, be sure to complete all necessary paperwork (e.g., insurance details, contact information, review of systems) beforehand. Don't waste time in the waiting area filling out paperwork when you could be speaking with the physician.

Don't expect your physician to review every single record and note you send to them. This takes away valuable time that could be spent talking with you. Most of the information may be irrelevant to the diagnosis and your care. For example, I don't need to see your cholesterol test from 3 years ago or childhood tonsillectomy report when you consult me for vestibular migraine. Your physician will take a history from you first then pick out the relevant and important information from your records.

Be informed. I wrote this book to inform and educate people with vestibular migraine. Knowledge empowers you. The more you understand about your illness and available treatments, the better choices you will be able to make. Now, don't confuse being informed with obsessing over every single detail. It is essential to be aware of the common and serious side effects of medications, but being overly worried about every single side effect listed on Google or WebMD will cause paralysis by analysis. Remember, if you believe that you will suffer a particular side effect, guess what... you will.

Be inquisitive, not an Inquisitor. Ask questions but remember you are not the Spanish Inquisition. Ask questions to find out more about your condition and treatments. Clarify issues that you don't understand. I love it when my patients ask questions about vestibular migraine, vertigo, dizziness, and treatments because I have the chance to empower them and enrich my own understanding. I learn a lot from my patients. They often ask about different treatments or ideas, which inspire me to think outside the box and sometimes leads to completely new treatments. For example, after some patients told me that the Cefaly device helped improve visually-induced dizziness, I began using it more for this condition and found that it really does seem to work. Being inquisitive about your condition and treatment(s) empowers you to be in control of your health.

It is imperative to avoid being adversarial and argumentative. It is a dialog, not a debate. Remember that your physician, his/her staff, and you must all work together for your health. If you are oppositional and confrontational in your approach, you bring out a defensive response, and this will lead to an unproductive relationship that will ultimately harm your health. You can be assertive and questioning, yet polite and cordial at the same time. There is a difference between inquisitive questions and rude, interrogative behavior. Building a respectful working relationship with your medical allies will benefit you. If you feel that you are not getting what you need from your physician, you should look for another one.

Dating

You deserve to be loved and to love. For single people, a chronic invisible illness like migraine can make dating challenging. Traditional dating activities like movies, bars, and dinner may be more difficult while dealing with light sensitivity, dizziness, motion sickness, food triggers, and maintaining a healthy sleep routine. Dating for people without migraine is complicated enough. Navigating the dating minefield is ten times more difficult for people with migraine. The following are some helpful tips.

Use dating apps to meet, chat, and decide if you would like to take it further and go on an actual date. Meeting online is a more comfortable way to screen potential partners, before expending the time and energy to meet in person.

Be honest and open. Be upfront about some aspects of your illness and limitations, for example, avoiding crowds, 3D movies, or certain food triggers. Mention that you have migraine but keep it short and sweet. Don't overwhelm with information right off the bat. Some dates may have more questions. Allow room for curious questions. It may be a good sign if your date truly wants to learn about your condition.

Don't be a victim. Play up your best assets. Remember that people mirror your mood; if you are sad and miserable, your date will also feel the same. Learn to laugh at yourself – not only will it help break the ice, but it also projects confidence which in itself is highly attractive.

Be creative. Find new ways to date that don't aggravate your symptoms. You don't have to go to the movies, restaurants, or bars. A walk in the park, picnic, board games, watching programs on TV, reading together, or cooking together can be very romantic.

Keep your rescue medication handy on dates. If you don't use your rescue treatments frequently, you can consider using them before a date (provided it doesn't cause unwanted side effects).

Beware of the codependent personality. Codependent individuals are drawn to people with chronic illnesses, drug addiction, or personality disorders. Codependent persons "nurture" their partners when they are in the sick role or engaged in bad behavior, creating a dynamic that reinforces this role or behavior. Basically, codependents feel a deep need to be caretakers or enablers and enjoy having partners who are ill and dependent on them. The attention can be very flattering initially but remember that they subconsciously prefer that you remain ill and completely reliant on them. Codependents have a deep need to be martyrs and make visible sacrifices for a partner in need. Red flags of codependency to look out for include a history of intense but unstable relationships, a fear of being alone, chronic feelings of emptiness, low self-esteem, a victim mentality, blaming others for their own faults, and clinginess.

Recognize when to break it off. Some people are not looking to commit, much less be with a person who has a chronic invisible illness. Some people are not mature or empathetic enough to have a partner with a chronic invisible illness. That's ok. Don't waste your energy and time trying to make them into something they are not. Move on. In the book *Think Like a Freak*, the authors of Freakonomics discuss the concept of the self-weeding garden where you let problems sort themselves out. The people who are unsuitable for you will reveal their true intentions when they criticize you as being "difficult" or "neurotic" and attempt to guilt you into focusing solely on their needs. Some may break off a relationship with you if they cannot accommodate your needs. Let these weeds remove themselves from your garden and move on.

Finances

Healthcare is expensive. Almost two-thirds of all bankruptcies in 2007 were medical-related; 92% of these arose from medical debt, and the remainder had lost substantial income due to illness, or had mortgaged a home to pay for medical bills [Himmelstein, 2009].

Unless you suffer from severe dizziness, the chances of vestibular migraine causing financial ruin are quite small. Nevertheless, migraine attacks may result in days where you have to call in sick, or may be unable to work effectively. Particularly severe attacks may necessitate a visit to the emergency department or urgent care clinic, which can be expensive. It is prudent to prepare a financial cushion and plan for any potential financial impact from migraine.

Budget and live within your means. Keep a record of your finances to ensure that you are not spending more than you earn. Live within your means. Don't spend money you don't have. Don't take on unnecessary debt, like car payments or high mortgages if you can help it. Don't splurge on stuff you don't need. Many apps can help you keep track of your expenses.

Create an emergency fund. The 2018 Federal Reserve's Survey of Household Economics and Decision Making showed that 40% of American households would struggle to come up with even $400 to pay for an unexpected bill. Try saving a portion of your income every month. This will help create a financial buffer to help cushion any unexpected medical bills.

Keep good records. Track your medical expenses, and insurance claims. Try to simplify your financial records and consolidate accounts so that you can easily access them quickly when needed.

Use credit cards responsibly. A credit card is not free money. Credit cards can provide some perks like cashback, points, or airline miles, but be sure to pay off the credit card balance every month. Do not let credit card balances accumulate. Unpaid credit card balances are high-interest loans that can destroy you financially. Keep a credit card to use for emergency or urgent bills in case you do not have enough cash to pay for them.

Learn about insurance. Insurance companies like to confuse people with all their jargon, and gotcha fine-print. They're very clear on how much you have to pay them, but try to make the process of obtaining payment from them as opaque and mysterious as they can. Learn as much as you can about insurance plans before your annual open enrollment. Understand your health insurance policy coverage, co-payments, deductibles, and maximum out-of-pocket costs.

Use a flexible medical spending or health savings account. This will help you use pre-tax dollars for out-of-pocket medical expenses. Remember to use it up before the end of the financial year.

Tax deductions. If your medical costs are high, you can deduct expenses that exceed 10% of your adjusted gross income. For example, if your adjusted gross income is $50,000, and your medical expenses are $7000, you will be able to deduct $2000 from your taxable income. This amount may change and it is best to consult your accountant to keep up with the current rules. You will need to keep your bills and premiums to submit these deductions; keep these bills organized in a folder.

Ask for assistance. If your doctor is part of a large health network, ask the billing department about special discounts or assistance programs for patients who are financially constrained.

Cut drug costs. Some tips to help you save on drug expenses:

• Choose generic drugs where possible. There is no evidence that branded medications work better for migraine.

• 90-day prescriptions may be cheaper compared to 30-day supplies. However, when starting a new medication, 30-day supplies are usually best because the dosage may need to be adjusted, or the drug causes side effects.

• Ask for higher-dose pills that you can split. These are often cheaper than lower-dose pills. For example, if you take lamotrigine 50 mg twice a day, ask for 100 mg tablets that you can then split.

• Use free programs like GoodRx, Script Relief, SingleCare, WellRx, RxSaver, US Pharmacy Card, and Blink Health that provide free coupons for you to purchase generic medications and bypass insurance companies. In my experience, GoodRx is the best program; it is very user-friendly and provides excellent savings by providing the prices for all pharmacies in your geographic area, allowing you to compare prices. Many times, the cash price is lower than the co-pay amount. Mark Cuban's Costplus Drugs online pharmacy is also a great option; they offer cheap prices on generic medications.

- If you are on Medicare, review your Part D prescription drug or Advantage plans.
- Programs like Partnership for Prescription Assistance (www.pparx.org) and RxAssist (www.rxassist.org) can help you find patient assistance programs offered by drug manufacturers.

Above all, remember that your health is priceless.

Insurance Denials

One of the most frustrating experiences you will encounter is insurance denial of treatments or tests that your physician orders. Insurance companies are driven by profit. They don't care for patients or physicians. The sole purpose of their existence is profit and shareholder enrichment. Insurance company executives are only interested in fattening their wallets. Understanding this and you will understand why they behave the way they do.

Prescriptions are sometimes denied by insurance companies. For people who pay substantial premiums every month (almost all of us!), it comes as a surprise that insurance companies do not always approve the tests, procedures, or prescriptions ordered by their doctors. They greedily devour your premiums but when it comes time to pay for your health, they behave as if you have no right to expect anything from them. They think they know better than the patients and doctors, and assume it is their right to dictate how you should manage your health.

Most of the time, insurance companies deny prescriptions for medications that are more costly (typically branded drugs) or tests that they do not feel are appropriate. However, at times, there is no logical reason for denial; they even deny cheap generic drugs. I have seen insurance companies deny prescriptions for nortriptyline, which costs $4 a month (cash price) at Walmart. Now, insurance companies will claim that they are not denying a prescription or test, but are only "reviewing" prescriptions or tests that have been ordered. Don't be fooled – these restrictions are intended to obstruct, delay, and hopefully dissuade patients and physicians from ordering treatments or tests that they don't approve of.

The first hurdle an insurance company throws out is called prior authorization or pre-authorization. This process basically requires that the ordering physician fill out more forms for the insurance company. The website Cover My Meds (www.covermymeds.com) has helped streamline this process.

Usually, the prior authorization is just a hurdle to overcome and once the physician performs the ritual demanded, the prescription or order is approved. However, in some cases, it is denied and the legion of bureaucrats hired by insurance companies produce more forms that "need" to be completed.

Insurance companies claim that prior authorization is only meant to review a prescription or test. This excuse is as real as hen's teeth – prior authorization requirements cause almost half of the prescriptions to be abandoned [Rubin, 2017]. Prior authorizations cost practices 20 hours per week and almost $70,000 per year. This translates to over $30 billion annually [Casalino, 2009]. The next hurdle insurance companies throw at patients and physicians is misleadingly called "peer-to-peer". When a prior authorization is denied, the next obstacle is a telephone call between your physician and some physician who works for the insurance company. Your physician has to take time out of the busy day for this call. To top it off, it's almost never a "peer" – I've had to speak to pediatricians and gynecologists to get treatments approved for my adult neurology patients. Furthermore, many of the doctors who work for the insurance companies are very early in their careers, not very successful, or are close to retirement. These bureaucratic obstacles may save the insurance company money but it costs our health system more. In essence, insurance companies are taking this money away from physicians and patients. They know what they are doing – they know that adding layers of bureaucracy will discourage most patients and physicians.

Many insurance companies try to deceive patients by telling them that they are "working with" the physicians to get the ordered test or prescription approved. This is nothing more than a shameless attempt to blame the physician's practice for the delays they cause by creating ridiculous red tape.

As a patient, you can try to pressure your insurance company to approve your treatment or test. Call them daily, write complaint letters, and demand to speak to supervisors or managers. You can also consider complaining to your state's insurance commissioner.

If your insurance company denies a generic medication, check out programs like GoodRx, US Pharmacy Card, or WellRx for coupons for cash purchases of generic medications. Using these coupons, the cash price for your prescriptions will very likely be quite affordable. If you are prescribed a branded medication, look up the manufacturer's website for patient savings cards or patient assistance programs. Often, the manufacturers will provide you with a supply of the medication while the insurance company processes your prescription.

Emergencies

Make sure your emergency contacts are up to date. Keep an updated list of your current medications, physicians (with their contact information), and medical problems handy, either on your phone or in your purse. Have a list of family members and friends who would be willing to help you to the emergency department (ED), and help take care of matters at home (e.g., feeding your pets, bringing you a change of clothes).

Be aware that some medical emergencies like strokes can also present with vertigo/dizziness. These are rare, but not impossible. These are some red flags to look out for:

• Dizziness or vertigo that feels different or worse from your usual vestibular migraine symptoms

• Any new neurological signs, including double vision, loss of vision, slurred speech, drowsiness, loss of consciousness, muscle weakness (e.g., one side of the body not moving as strongly), loss of sensation, facial weakness (drooping of one side of the face), or language changes (inability to speak or comprehend).

• Sudden loss of hearing in one ear

• Inability to walk without assistance

• New-onset neck pain or stiffness

• Preceding neck manipulation or trauma

For headaches, look out for these headaches:

• New-onset headache

• Headache that feels different or worse from your usual headaches

• Thunderclap headache: the worst headache of your life that reaches its peak within a minute

• Any new neurological signs (as detailed above)

• New-onset neck stiffness or pain

• Visual loss

• Preceding head or neck trauma

If any red flags for vertigo/dizziness or headache are present, you need to be evaluated emergently i.e., in the emergency department. Do not waste time calling your primary care physician or neurologist. Go straight to the closest emergency department.

Keeping a sphygmomanometer (blood pressure monitor) at home is important to measure your blood pressure and heart rate. If you experiencing vertigo/dizziness and your blood pressure is consistently too high (systolic blood pressure above 140 mmHg, or diastolic blood pressure above 90 mmHg), or too low (systolic blood pressure below 90 mmHg, or diastolic blood pressure below 60 mmHg), or if your pulse is consistently too high (above 100 beats per minute) or too low (below 60 beats per minute), you need to be evaluated urgently.

If you have been unable to keep any fluids down and have been vomiting a lot, you may be dehydrated and need to go to the ED. If you develop severe side effects from a migraine medication, go to the ED. EDs are loud, bright, chaotic places in general. Bring your blue light-blocking glasses, earplugs, water, and snacks along just in case the wait is long.

School

While most college students struggle with coursework, those with chronic invisible illnesses face additional burdens. It may be difficult to meet the attendance policy due to doctors' appointments, or vestibular migraine attacks. It may be challenging to be in class for the whole day, or use electronic screens for a prolonged period. The US Department of Education enforces Section 504 of the Rehabilitation Act of 1973 and the Office for Civil Rights enforces Title II of the Americans with Disabilities Act of 1990. These laws prohibit discrimination based on of disability in schools and colleges. All colleges have dedicated services to address the needs of students with disabilities; familiarize yourself with these services and work with them.

Notify your school of your diagnosis and needs where appropriate, and as early as possible. If you feel that your symptoms may interfere with school, be sure to specify what your limitations are. You must be as specific as possible. Does being in a class for too long aggravate your vestibular migraine? Do you have difficulty walking down long hallways? Are you light-sensitive? Do you have to limit the amount of screen time?

Authorize the exchange of information between your healthcare provider and your school. Get documentation from your doctor, preferably a specialist in vestibular migraine. It is best to document your diagnosis, symptoms, and impact on your school performance.

Speak to counselors or advisors to see if it is possible to adjust class schedules, make accommodations for testing requirements, or take fewer credits per semester. Speak to your vestibular migraine specialist and list all the accommodations you need so that they can be documented in your medical records. These records will help support your requests.

As a general rule, your approach should be: don't ask, don't tell. This depends on your job requirements, of course. If your job requires you to fly planes, drive commercial trucks, or wash the windows of a skyscraper, vestibular migraine may need to be disclosed because of safety and legal implications. If you don't anticipate a significant impact on your job performance (for example, in an office-based environment), you don't have to tell your employers about your diagnosis. It is none of their business. Legally, employers are not entitled to any disclosures about your health, and are prohibited from discriminating against people with physical limitations according to the Americans with Disabilities Act.

If you do not want your employer to learn about your diagnosis, beware of what you post on social media. If you share a lot of details of your vestibular migraine, you may not want to add anyone from your place of employment and make sure that your posts are only visible to friends so that your employer cannot spy on them. While an employer cannot legally fire you for having an illness, they may try to look for other reasons to get rid of you if they have some concerns about your health. Why even give them that opportunity?

If you find that your symptoms interfere with your job (for example, if working on multiple computer screens simultaneously makes you dizzy or if fluorescent lighting at the office triggers migraine attacks) and you would like to request accommodations, consult with a neurologist, preferably a specialist in vestibular migraine, to clearly document your diagnosis, symptoms, and job impact. You must be as specific as possible. The impact of migraine in an office environment is often unclear to the uninitiated. Outsiders like HR employees and disability-claims paper-pushers won't see a problem working in your job unless you specify what the problems are. Do screens aggravate your headache? Do long hallways or warehouse aisles make you feel off-balance and dizzy? Do screeching school children or loud machines trigger migraine attacks? Does the cloying smell of perfume make it difficult to work in the cosmetic section of your department store? Does your desk by the window aggravate your visual height intolerance? You need to precisely document the sort of limitations you face at work.

Once you have identified the problem areas in your work environment, be specific about the accommodations you need. Specify if you would like a change in lighting, the need to work from home, how many hours you can work per day, a need for breaks every so often, or a need to take certain medications or wear blue light-filtering glasses. If you have two vestibular migraine attacks per month, do you need two sick days per month? How about flexible hours? Can you miss a few hours but make up for it later in the day or the weekend? Do you need to move your office to a quieter, less bright area with no blinds? Don't be afraid to ask for accommodations. Speak to your vestibular migraine specialist, and list all the accommodations you need so that they can be documented in your medical records. These records will help support your requests. When my patients ask me to fill out documents for workplace accommodations, I always ask them what exactly they need. You know your work environment and what you need far better than your physicians, and it is your responsibility to convey this information to them.

Consider drawing up backup plans if you feel that you may have to leave your job. Avoid the last-minute scramble for a new job. Look out for signs that you may have to leave your job, and start planning your exit in advance.

Disability

The process of applying for disability is beyond the scope of this book. It may be necessary to apply for short-term disability to allow time for migraine treatment to work. This is a decision that should be discussed with your employer, family, and physician. Long-term or permanent disability for vestibular migraine is rare since the disease can usually be controlled with the appropriate treatment.

Be sure that you have documented the impact of your vestibular migraine with your physician. Note that it is important that you have seen a physician for some time before asking for him or her to complete disability paperwork. It is difficult to honestly and accurately complete these forms without a clear clinical picture of a person's symptoms over time. Assessing a person's clinical picture over a reasonable duration gives me the information needed to accurately complete these documents.

It is in your best interest to consult a disability attorney to help you with the process. Disability insurance companies try their hardest to deny coverage because it will cost them money. The questions on disability forms are antiquated and (maybe intentionally) focused on physical jobs and not on office jobs, which the majority of adults have. They also are biased towards musculoskeletal diseases and not migraine, vertigo, or dizziness. For example, they ask if you can sit, stoop, walk, climb, balance, twist, and reach. They ask how much weight you can push or carry for how many hours a day. When it comes to computer work, they only ask if you can use a keyboard and mouse – they don't even consider if you have difficulty with computer screens. The disability forms fail to capture many disabling symptoms of vestibular migraine and disability insurance companies use this lack of information to deny disability applications. It's like saying an armless person is not disabled because their leg X-rays look perfectly fine.

Changing Directions

Our past is not our future and our fates are not set in stone. We create our own destinies. There are moments in life when we are compelled to look deeply at ourselves and our circumstances and think – is this really what we want? Is this the life we envisioned for ourselves? What is our purpose? What is our passion? These are questions only you can answer for yourself.

If your job is too stressful and is causing your vestibular migraine to deteriorate, you may need to ask yourself whether it is worth it to continue working in that job. There may come a time when you have to choose between your job and your health. What are your priorities – your professional career or health? If no interventions help your vestibular migraine and your job stress is clearly exacerbating your vestibular migraine, it may be time to consider a career change. Many of us identify with our jobs but in reality, that is not who we truly are.

If office jobs aggravate your vestibular migraine, consider jobs that enable you to work more from home, like creative writing, graphic design, marketing, and information technology. You may also consider pursuing something that has always interested you. If the river leads you away from your current job, flow with it and discover what lies ahead.

Changing career directions is scary but can open whole new worlds for you. Vestibular migraine could help you discover your purpose, and share your passion. My two patients, Kayla McCain and Alicia Wolfe are great examples of this. Instead of being defeated by vestibular migraine, both of them have found a way to channel their experiences dealing with the disease into careers and helping others who suffer from it. Kayla has used her experience with vestibular migraine to start a marketing business and blog, while Alicia has written a cookbook specifically for people with vestibular migraine. Both of them are active social media influencers who use their platforms to raise awareness of vestibular migraine and help educate people about the condition.

Alicia writes of her journey:

Managing vestibular migraine in the workplace is incredibly difficult. My journey with it was a 9-month battle before I finally gave in and decided to leave my career in watch design. It began with symptoms that were too debilitating for me to drive myself into work. The constant dizziness and vertigo episodes made it difficult for me to stare at a computer screen without vomiting.

Normally this type of illness would easily be approved through FMLA and short-term disability, but because none of the seven doctors I saw in Dallas could give me an accurate or official diagnosis, I struggled with my workplace believing that I couldn't do my job because I was "stressed" or had anxiety - which was basically how these doctors were diagnosing me.

With my job in jeopardy, I begged an ENT specialist to sign off on my forms without him being confident in my diagnosis.

It wasn't until I saw Dr. Beh that my life got a little bit easier. At this point, I was suffering from daily, debilitating symptoms and could still not drive, but I was able to easily get all the forms I needed for short-term disability signed and approved. Still, I felt the pressure of losing a promotion I was overdue for. On Dr. Beh's protocol, I was making slow progress, but I pushed myself to go back too early before I was really ready.

When I returned to my old job, I found out that I had a completely new manager and team and my desk had been moved to a high-traffic walkway under bright fluorescent lights - a nightmare for anyone with vestibular migraine. My workplace was less than accommodating, not understanding that migraine can be much more debilitating than a bad headache. Doctors' appointments, vestibular therapy, and attack days cut so far into my pay that I was only making about half my salary and getting overwhelmed with work. I asked HR for help multiple times, but things only seemed to get worse. I felt as though I was being forced out of my job, and the progress I had made towards feeling better was falling apart rapidly. I eventually decided this job, and half my salary, wasn't worth my health and I made the very difficult decision to leave. Later I found out half the things that happened weren't actually legal, but when you're so focused on your health it's tough to fight these situations.

I struggled for a while with my identity outside of my career, and who I was as a person with chronic illness. With my extra time at home, I began to research alternative treatments and also everything vestibular migraine. It was then I realized there weren't many helpful resources on vestibular migraine from a patients' perspective. I also realized there were literally zero good options for those wanting to try a migraine diet. I knew there was a need for a resource that presented information on vestibular migraine in layman's terms, as well as a fun food blog with genuinely good migraine diet recipes. This allowed me to combine my love for research with my joy of cooking and creating recipes. Little did I know my future publisher would have vestibular migraine and be searching for resources when she stumbled on my blog and offered me a book deal. "The Dizzy Cook: Managing Migraine with More Than 90 Comforting Recipes and Lifestyle Tips", debuted in February 2020 and became an Amazon best-seller. The Dizzy Cook now receives more than 100,000 page views a month and I can finally make my own schedule, adapting for any dizzy days.

As humans we instinctively fear change, preferring the comforting familiarity of our current bland circumstances to the unpredictability of a potentially brighter future. It behooves us to sometimes ask ourselves, what is our purpose in life? What is our passion? What do we really want from life? As Socrates said, the unexamined life is not worth living. Such introspection often comes during times of crisis, when we question ourselves, our purpose, and our raison d'etre. Rather than wait for crises to force such introspection, we should reflect on these questions, and prepare for the future.

It is good to have an end to journey towards; but it is the journey that matters, in the end.

Ursula K. Le Guin

CONCLUSION

The first and greatest victory is to conquer yourself.
Plato

The famous psychiatrist and psychoanalyst Carl Gustav Jung (1875-1961) referred to the unconscious portion of the personality as the "shadow". According to him, "Everyone carries a shadow, and the less it is embodied in the individual's conscious life, the blacker and denser it is". This shadow grows more powerful if it is ignored or denied. To conquer one's dark side, Jung believed that one must work to integrate the shadow into the consciousness, a process that adds depth and dimension to one's character. Vestibular migraine is like a shadow. It is a part of you, an unwelcome companion that is always there. To be victorious over vestibular migraine, you cannot ignore, deny, or fight against this reality, but must accept it. To be truly victorious over vestibular migraine, be conscious of it, and proactively take the measures needed to control it.

There is no shortcut or magic cure for vestibular migraine. Your journey to victory and healing will take time and effort. You are in control of your life and reality. As the CEO of your health, you are the only one who can take the necessary steps to control vestibular migraine, and improve your life. The power to heal lies within you. You *can* be victorious. You must persevere, and consistently work towards this goal. As Napoleon Bonaparte said, "Victory belongs to the most persevering." Your victory over vestibular migraine will not be won in a single war, but a series of battles as you journey along your river. Every battle won will take you closer to healing. Setbacks do not mean defeat; they mean education, an opportunity to learn and face the next battle.

In conclusion, I hope this book equips you with the tools and knowledge needed to be victorious over vestibular migraine. May it empower and encourage you to take the steps that will help you regain control over your life.

Victory at all costs, victory in spite of all terror, victory however long and hard the road may be; for without victory, there is no survival.
Winston Churchill (1874-1965)

387

INDEX

Dehydration, *70, 151, 180, 198, 199, 201*

Delivery, 317, 318

Depression, *12, 14, 16, 26, 28, 31, 32, 34, 35, 36, 40, 45, 55, 62, 65, 67, 69, 71, 72, 73, 74, 76, 81, 83, 84, 85, 86, 87, 88, 91, 92, 98, 105, 114, 119, 120, 137, 140, 149, 153, 154, 156, 158, 165, 169, 170, 171, 189, 203, 218, 219, 221, 222, 231,* 239, 254, 256, 262, 263, *274,* 277, *289, 301, 302, 310,* 317, 323, 324, 327, 330, 333, *337, 340, 344, 347, 351,* 359

Desipramine, 255

Desvenlafaxine, 264

DHE, *92, 281, 285, 286, 295, 318, 322*

Diamine Oxidase, *144, 227*

Diphenhydramine, *294, 319*

Divalproex, 261, 320

Dix-Hallpike, *95, 312*

Dopamine, *40, 117, 293, 316*

Doxylamine, *294,* 319

Dry eyes, 206

Duloxetine, 264

Ear pain, *52, 123*

Ear pressure, *51, 123*

Eating disorders, *88,* 344

Endometriosis, 316, 324

Epley, *95, 312, 313*

Eptinezumab, 268, 269

Erenumab, 268

Escitalopram, 265

Essential Oils, *155*

Estrogen, *31, 40, 92, 93, 137, 160, 196, 229,* 314, *315,* 316, 317, 325, 326

Fatigue, *10, 14, 27, 36, 40, 44, 49, 50, 54, 55, 71, 74, 75, 83, 85, 87, 106, 114, 115, 117, 120, 121, 122, 125, 126, 128, 148, 159, 191, 197, 238,* 256, 263, *299, 300,* 324, *337*

Fear circuit, *334, 335, 337, 340*

Fertility, *154, 161, 325*

Feverfew, *144, 145*

Fibromyalgia, *14, 69, 71, 72, 76, 126, 151, 153, 221, 255, 258,* 261, 264, 324, *337*

Flunarizine, 257

Fluoxetine, 265

Fluvoxamine, 265

Folate, *135, 136, 137, 166, 219, 238,* 240, 317, 319, 322

Fremanezumab, 268

GABA, *39, 85, 138, 162, 203, 219, 222*

Gabapentin, 260, 261

Galcanezumab, 268

Gammacore, *274, 275, 277, 280, 304*

Gastroparesis, *75*

Gepants, *270, 290, 319, 320*

Ginger, *145, 146, 240, 244, 303,* 319, 322

Ginkgo Biloba, *146*

Glutamate, *35, 39, 117, 141, 162, 219, 232, 233, 237, 241, 244*

Gluten, *74, 230, 242*

Glycine, *39*

Gut-brain axis, *6, 31, 73, 215, 222*

Hangover, 227

Helicobacter pylori, 75

Histamine, *82, 194,* 226, 227, *229, 255*

HPA axis, *37, 88, 128, 171, 188, 216, 217, 218, 221*

hyperacusis, *65, 206, 305,* 399

Hyperacusis, *65, 192*

Hypertension, 249, 256, 257, 262, 323, 326

Hypothalamus, *36, 37, 44, 63, 68, 152, 198, 199, 221, 231, 331, 335*

Infantile Colic, *25*

Interstitial cystitis, *72,* 316, 324

Irritable bowel syndrome, *40, 72, 144, 153, 221,* 264, 324

IVF, 325

Ketogenic Diet, *237*

Lacosamide, *262*

Lamotrigine, *259, 260, 262, 263*

Lasmiditan, *253, 285, 319*

Lavender, *156*

L-Carnitine, *148*

Levetiracetam, *261*

Light sensitivity, *47, 62, 153*

Lipoic Acid, *148*

Long COVID, *14, 112, 114, 115, 116, 117, 118, 120, 121, 122, 123, 125, 219*

L-tryptophan, 319, 322

Magnesium, 140, 149, 150, 151, 152, 315, 319, 322

Marijuana, *161, 162*

Mast cell activation, *101*

MDDS, *99, 100, 117, 118, 119, 122, 124, 125,* 264, *299, 311, 335*

Sertraline, 265

Sleep, *27, 36, 40, 44, 63, 67, 68, 69, 70, 72, 83, 84, 98, 114, 117, 120, 140, 141, 151, 152, 153, 159, 166, 187, 189, 197, 201, 202, 203, 212, 219, 264, 294, 297, 299, 300, 302, 303, 305, 307, 308, 309, 317, 323, 327, 337, 353, 372*

Smoking, *91, 92, 207, 326*

SNRIs, 255, 263, 264, 265, 266

Soy, 223, 229, 315

Spontaneous Intracranial Hypotension, *107*

SSRIs, 263, 265, 266

Stress, *30, 31, 37, 87, 150, 188, 189, 201, 208, 210, 217*

Stroke, *7, 11, 16, 30, 69, 92, 118, 128, 189, 207,* 269, 283, 285, 288, 290, 317, 326

Sugar, *231*

Sulfites, 227, *234, 237*

Superior Canal Dehiscence Syndrome, *108*

Sympathetic, *36, 37, 215, 366*

Temporomandibular joint disorder, *72*

Tension-type headache, *69, 122, 306*

Testosterone, *137, 163, 299, 325,* 327, *328*

Timolol, 257, *279, 296,* 319

Tinnitus, *22, 52, 65, 66, 97, 98, 101, 102, 104, 107, 108, 110, 114, 123, 147, 149, 158, 166,* 263, *277, 287, 304, 305, 310, 332, 359, 399*

Tolerance, *254*

Topiramate, 258, 263, 320

Transcranial magnetic stimulation, 277

Traveling, 211

Tricyclic Antidepressants, *254*

Trigeminal, *34, 35, 36, 39, 40, 52, 72, 73, 82, 112, 145, 149, 162, 190, 193, 197, 198, 262, 273, 274, 275, 276,* 297

Triptans, *50, 70, 71, 92, 122,* 253, 265, *279,* 282, 283, 284, 285, 290, *318, 321*

Tryptophan, *158*

Turmeric, *159, 160*

Tyramine, 227, 228

Ubrogepant, *290,* 319

Vaccination, *112, 123, 124, 125*

Vagus nerve, 35, 117, 182, 215, 216, 219, 222, 274, 275, 297

Valproate, 254, 260, 261, 320

Venlafaxine, 263, 264

Verapamil, 257

Vestibular Neuritis, *109*

Vestibular Schwannoma, *110*

Visual height intolerance, *80*

Visual snow, *54, 63*

Visualization, *354*

vitamin B2, *135, 136, 166, 300*

Vitamin C, *138*

Vitamin D, 139, 140, 319, 322

Vitamin E, 138, 139, 315

Vitex, *160, 161, 315*

Vomiting, *22, 25, 26, 27, 28, 41, 43, 46, 48, 56, 70, 74, 75, 82, 88, 94, 146, 163, 170, 216, 280, 286, 288, 289, 294, 295, 297, 379, 384*

Weather, *32, 187, 189, 190, 193, 201, 206, 346*

Yentl syndrome, *14*

Zavegepant, *291*

Zonisamide, 259

Appendix: Tests

Imaging Tests

Computed Tomography (CT)

CT scans use X-ray beams from different angles to build an image of the internal structures of the body. CT scans are quick to perform and as such, are preferable in emergency situations. The CT gantry is large and does not cause claustrophobia. Because of radiation, CT scans are usually avoided in pregnant women and limited in children. CT scans allows rapid visualization of the skull and its contents. It is useful for detecting acute bleeding and bone abnormalities (e.g., fractures, canal dehiscence) but does not provide good visualization of the soft tissue and brain.

Iodinated contrast is used to visualize the anatomy of arteries or veins (called CT angiogram or venogram, respectively). It is not uncommon to feel a warm sensation in the neck or throat as the contrast is injected. CT contrast may be toxic to the kidneys and should be used cautiously in people with renal disease. Sometimes, iodinated contrast may cause thyroid dysfunction. Allergic reactions to iodinated contrast are uncommon but may occur. It is usually mild and consists of a rash or itching but may be life-threatening in rare cases. A widely believed myth in medicine is that shellfish allergy increases the risk of an allergic reaction to iodinated contrast. Shellfish allergy is due to proteins in these animals (most commonly tropomyosins) and not iodine.

Magnetic Resonance Imaging (MRI)

MRI utilizes powerful magnetic fields to visualize the internal organs and structures of the body. Unlike CT scans, no radiation is involved. MRIs take longer to perform than CT scans. The MRI scanner is a small tube into which the patient must be inserted. As such, claustrophobia can be a problem. Because of the powerful magnet, MRI cannot be used in patients with metallic pieces (e.g., bullet fragments) or certain devices (e.g., older pacemakers, nerve stimulators) in their bodies. MRI is the best way to visualize soft tissue structures, i.e., the brain, vestibular nerves and inner ear structures. It is also the best way to visualize the spine, surrounding tissue, and the spinal cord.

MRI contrast agents are injected intravenously to look for any breach in the blood-brain barrier, where it leaks into the surrounding tissue. Such breaches may occur with infections, tumors, or inflammatory lesions in the brain. Gadolinium is the typical contrast used for MRIs. True allergy to gadolinium contrast is very rare. It is not toxic to the kidneys; however, it should be avoided in people on dialysis because it may cause a rare condition called nephrogenic systemic fibrosis if it accumulates in the body. Allergy to CT contrast does not mean you are allergic to MRI contrast.

MR Angiography is an MRI method to visualize the arteries. MR Venography evaluates the anatomy of the veins. They do not require the use of contrast but if abnormalities are detected, contrast can be used for a more accurate evaluation.

Audiometry

Hearing tests are important in people with vestibular disorders and those with hearing symptoms like tinnitus, hyperacusis, and difficulty hearing. Hearing tests help identify the type and degree of hearing impairment.

Pure Tone Audiometry

Pure tone audiometry is a standardized hearing test that measures the hearing thresholds for a set of sound frequencies. It tests two hearing pathways: air and bone conduction. It is usually performed in a sound booth to minimize external noise. A set of headphones are placed over the ears to test air conduction. For bone conduction, a small oscillating device is placed on the mastoid process, the bone behind the ear. The subject responds by pressing a button or raising their hand when they hear a sound.

Speech Testing

Speech testing measures the subject's ability to hear and understand spoken words. The audiologist says specific words through the headphones and the subject repeats them. The audiologist aims to detect the softest speech you can detect (speech detection threshold) and correctly repeat (speech recognition threshold).

Tympanometry

Tympanometry is a test of middle ear function. A probe is inserted into the ear canal and a tone is generated which causes the eardrum to vibrate. Some of the sound is deflected back and is detected by the probe. The device measures the difference between how much sound is transmitted through the middle ear and how much is reflected back to the probe. Tympanometry can help determine if there is fluid in the middle ear, a perforated eardrum, a tumor in the middle ear, or a problem with the Eustachian tube.

Auditory Brainstem Response (ABR)

In ABR, electrodes are placed on the forehead, top of the head, and earlobes. Clicks are played through the headphones and brain activity is measured at several locations. This tests the hearing pathway all the way from the inner ear to the cortex. Unlike pure tone audiometry, ABR does not require feedback or responses from the test subject and thus, can be performed in babies and children, or those who have difficulty cooperating with the pure tone audiometry.

Vestibular Tests

Video Nystagmography (VNG)

The VNG is the standard vestibular test for people with vertigo and dizziness. The VNG involves placing a pair of infrared goggles that detect the subject's eye movements. Electronystagmography (ENG) uses electrodes to measure electrical changes from eye movements. Nowadays, the VNG is preferred method of testing. The VNG tests several eye categories of eye movements: gaze stability (the ability to keep the eyes steady in a particular position), saccades (the ability of the eyes to "jump" to a target), smooth pursuit (the ability to track a moving target), optokinetic tracking (the ability to track a moving visual field), and nystagmus in several testing conditions.

Do not wear eye makeup as this can interfere with the infrared camera's ability to detect the eyes. Most audiologists advise stopping any medications that may suppress vestibular function, including meclizine and benzodiazepines, to ensure abnormalities can be detected.

Caloric Testing

Caloric testing is usually done as part of the VNG. It involves instilling warm and cold air/water into the external ear canals. This induces movement of the fluid in the semicircular canals and triggers vertigo and nystagmus. Yes, this is an unpleasant test. The degree of nystagmus is measured and these responses provide information about the function of the vestibular apparatus on each side.

Video Head Impulse Test (VHIT)

The VHIT is a convenient way to measure the function of the semicircular canals. A pair of goggles are strapped to the subject's head. The subject is then instructed to keep looking at a target on the wall while the examiner quickly thrusts the head in specific planes. Unlike caloric testing, it does not trigger vertigo. It measures the integrity of the vestibulo-ocular reflex pathway. The VHIT can be difficult to perform in people with droopy eyelids and those with very stiff necks.

Rotary Chair Testing

In rotational testing, the subject is strapped to a motorized seat inside a large drum. The seat is rotated and the subject's eye movements are recorded with a pair of infrared goggles. The chair can be moved at different speeds and the vestibulo-ocular reflex measured at these speeds. Because these chairs are expensive and take up a lot of space, not many centers have them. Rotational testing can provide some information if the VNG is ambiguous but in most cases, the combination of the VNG and VHIT provides sufficient information for diagnosis.

Vestibular Evoked Myogenic Potentials (VEMPs)

VEMPs are a vestibular test that involves recording a muscle response to a sound stimulation (click or pulse). Cervical VEMPs record the response over the sternomastoid muscle in the neck while ocular VEMPS measure the response of the muscles that move the eyes. The main use of VEMPs is to diagnose superior canal dehiscence syndrome. Some abnormalities may be seen in vestibular migraine but there are no specific diagnostic findings.

Computerized Dynamic Posturography (CDP)

CDP is a test that helps measure neural mechanisms used to control posture and balance. The subject stands on a forceplate that detects small changes in the posture. The forceplate is moved to generate a series of standardized conditions to test how the subject uses vestibular, visual and proprioceptive information to maintain balance.

Other Neurologic Tests

Electroencephalography (EEG)

The EEG is a test that measures electrical activity from the cortex. A series of electrodes are attached to several locations on the scalp. These are connected to a computerized device that amplifies these tiny electrical changes and records them. A video camera records the subject to capture any movements that may correlate with abnormal brain electrical activity. The EEG is performed in several different scenarios: awake with eyes open and closed, asleep, hyperventilation, and with a flashing light. An EEG is performed when there is a suspicion of seizures or epilepsy and is not a typical test for people with vertigo or dizziness.

Nerve Conduction Studies (NCS)

Nerves conduct electrical signals like wires. NCS involves delivering a small electrical shock at one part of the nerve and measuring it at another location to assess its speed and amplitude. This provides information about the integrity of the myelin covering (the insulation) and the axon (the internal conductor). NCS can be helpful in determining if a peripheral nerve disorder is responsible for causing numbness, tingling, pain, imbalance, or weakness.

Electromyography (EMG)

Although the EMG is a distinct test, it is often performed together with the NCS. The EMG involves placing a tiny needle in a muscle to measure its activity. It is performed at rest and with activation (i.e., when flexing the muscle). The information can help diagnose muscle disorders.

Cardiovascular Tests

Electrocardiogram (ECG/EKG)

The EKG is a standard test for measuring the heart's electrical activity. Several electrodes are placed on the chest wall to detect the electrical activity from different locations. An EKG measures the heart rhythm and can be used to diagnose conditions like arrhythmia, heart attacks, and electrolyte abnormalities. An EKG is also used during cardiac stress testing.

Holter & Event Monitors

The EKG provides a snapshot of the heart's rhythm but may miss arrhythmias that happen intermittently. The Holter monitor is a portable heart monitor that records the heart's electrical activity continuously for 24-48 hours.

An event monitor is a heart monitor that records over a much longer duration. It does not record continuously but instead, has to be activated by the patient. When a person feels something, they hit a button that activates the event monitor. A symptom event monitor records heart activity over the next few minutes. A memory looping monitor captures the information a few minutes before, during, and after it is activated.

Tilt table test

A tilt table test measures changes in blood pressure and heart rate caused by changes in one's posture from lying to standing. The subject is strapped to a bed with a footrest and safety belts. From a flat, lying position, the bed can be brought to an almost standing position. In certain circumstances, medications like nitroglycerin may be administered. A tilt table test is useful for evaluating patients who faint or report faintness when getting up from a seated or lying position.

The future, good or ill, was not forgotten, but ceased to have any power over the present. Health and hope grew strong in them, and they were content with each good day as it came, taking pleasure in every meal, and in every word and song.
J.R.R. Tolkien, The Fellowship of the Ring

About the Author

Shin C. Beh, MD, FAAN, FAHS

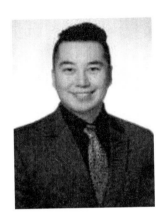

Dr. Beh is one of the few neurologists in the U.S. who specializes in vestibular disorders. He completed his neurology residency training at the University of Texas Southwestern Medical Center in Dallas. His fellowship training was a one-of-a-kind, triple fellowship in multiple sclerosis, neuro-otology, and neuro-ophthalmology that was completed at the University of Texas Southwestern, Johns Hopkins University Hospital, and New York University Medical Center. During his training, he had the privilege to be mentored by experts and luminaries like Dr. David Zee, Dr. Laura Balcer, and Dr. Steven Galetta. Dr. Beh has helped numerous patients with migraine, and vestibular migraine, including best-selling author Alicia Wolf. Dr. Beh has published and presented extensively about vestibular migraine, including ground-breaking studies on non-invasive vagus nerve stimulation and external trigeminal nerve stimulation as rescue treatments for vestibular migraine attacks. He founded and directs the Beh Center for Vestibular & Migraine Disorders located in North Texas, a practice dedicated to providing comprehensive care to people with vertigo, dizziness, and migraine. Follow Dr. Beh on Twitter (@thedizzydoc).